Pediatrics Essence

AUTHORS

Dr. Sunil Natha Mhaske
M.B.B.S., M.D. Pediatrics
Vice Principal (P.G.) and Professor-Head
Department of Pediatrics
PDVVPF's Medical College and Hospital
Ahmednagar - 414 111 (M.S.)

Dr. Nishad Yashawant Patil
M.B.B.S., M.D. Pediatrics
Department of Pediatrics
PDVVPF's Medical College and Hospital
Ahmednagar - 414 111 (M.S.)

PEEPEE

PUBLISHERS AND DISTRIBUTORS (P) LTD.

Pediatrics Essence

Published by
Pawaninder P. Vij and Anupam Vij
Peepee Publishers and Distributors (P) Ltd.
Head Office: 160, Shakti Vihar, Pitam Pura
Delhi-110034 (India)

***Correspondence Address:* 7/31, First Floor, Ansari Road**
Daryaganj, New Delhi-110002 (India)
Ph: 65195868, 23246245, 9811156083
e-mail: peepee160@yahoo.co.in
e-mail: peepee160@rediffmail.com
e-mail: peepee160@gmail.com
www.peepeepub.com

First Edition : 2015

ISBN: 978-81-8445-172-6

DEDICATED TO

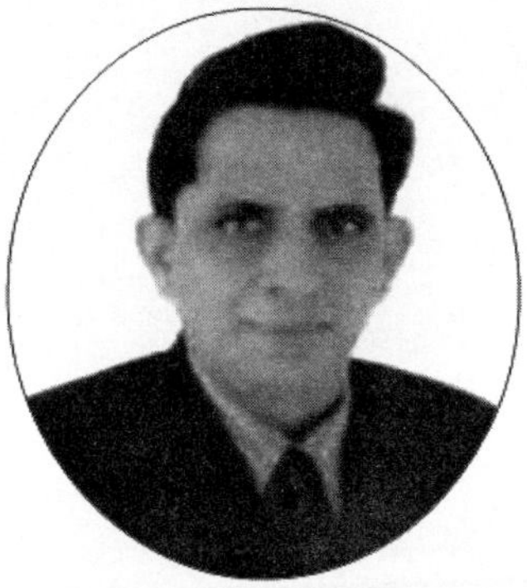

Lt. Gen. Dr. B. Sadananda

AVSM, VSM

MBBS, MD (Med), MD (CH), DHA NDC

Secretary General

Padmashree Dr. Vithalrao Vikhe Patil Foundation

Ahmednagar

PREFACE

This is our pleasure that we are contributing to medical fraternity in the form of **"Pediatrics Essence"** which is a multiple choice questions collection for approach of pediatric diseases. This book is useful for all who are in contact with children, basically MBBS students, Postgraduates, Nursing students, Private Practitioners and those who are in pediatric practice as general practitioners.

In this book, we have included multiple questions on all important topics based on various state and national entrance examinations along with special mention on pediatric pharmacology, pediatric pathology, pediatric microbiology, and pediatric radiology. In addition we have added multiple choice questions on history of pediatrics and nursing along with physiotherapy syllabus also.

In this journey, there are so many people who have helped us to achieve the target of completion of the book. We are very thankful to Dr. Sujay Vikhe Patil (C.E.O. Padmashree Dr. Vithalrao Vikhe Patil Foundation), Lt. Gen. (Retd) Dr. B Sadananda (Secretary General, Padmashree Dr. Vithalrao Vikhe Patil Foundation), Dr A. K. Pandey (Medical Superintendent) and Dr Ashok Raul (Principal).

Our departmental colleagues who blessed and helped us are: Dr. Ramesh Kothari and Postgraduate students Dr. Sandeep Deokate, Dr. Rahul Maski, Dr. Rajesh Gurjar, Dr. Vaibhav Nandgaonkar, Dr. Liza Bulsara, Dr. Kanchan Sakharkar and Dr. Aditya Sawla and interns Dr. Suraj Vyawahare, Dr. Khushal Sanghavi, Dr. Lucky Doshi, Dr. Madhurima S Nair, Dr. Mrunal Patil, Dr. Neena Phade, Dr. Padmin Patil, Dr. Krupa Sankhe, Dr. Pradip Phad, Dr. Resma Ranade.

Lastly, we are thankful to Peepee Publishers and Distributors (P) Pvt. Ltd., because of whom this book is born.

Suggestions and criticisms to further improve the book are welcome and can be mailed to sunilmhaske1970@gmail.com.

Dr. Sunil N Mhaske **Dr. Nishad Y Patil**

CONTENTS

Chapter 1

General Pediatrics

1. **What are components of definition of pediatrics?**
   (a) Child (b) His family
   (c) His environment (d) All of the above

2. **What is word meaning of pediatrics?**
   (a) Healer of children
   (b) Pharmacist of children
   (c) Counselor of children
   (d) Vaccinator of children

3. **What is age limit of pediatrics?**
   (a) Birth up to 10 years (b) Birth up to 1 month
   (c) Birth up to 15 years (d) Birth up to 18 years

4. **Which is the first printed book on pediatrics?**
   (a) Ebers Papyrus
   (b) Bagallarder's Little Book on Disease in Children
   (c) Soranus of Ephesu
   (d) None

5. **Who is father of pediatrics?**
   (a) Dr Waldo Nelson (b) Dr George Coehlo
   (c) Professor ST Achar (d) Dr Abraham Jacobi

6. **When was the Indian Academy of Pediatrics established?**
   (a) 1967 (b) 1982
   (c) 1962 (d) 2002

7. **Which is official publication of Indian Academy of Pediatrics?**
   (a) Elsevier journal
   (b) Indian Pediatrics
   (c) Journal of IMA (JIMA)
   (d) Current Pediatric Research

8. **Where is the head office of I.A.P.?**
   (a) New Delhi (b) Bangalore
   (c) Mumbai (d) Chennai

9. **Who founded Association of Pediatrics of India?**
   (a) Dr George Coehlo
   (b) Dr K. C. Chaudhuri
   (c) Professor ST Achar
   (d) Dr Abraham Jacobi

10. **Who was first pediatrician of India?**
    (a) Dr George Coelho (b) Dr K. C. Chaudhuri
    (c) Professor ST Achar (d) Dr Abraham Jacobi

11. **When pediatrics was started in India?**
    (a) 1918 (b) 1982
    (c) 1928 (d) 1996

12. **Who is "Father of Indian Pediatrics?"**
    (a) Dr George Coelho (b) Dr K. C. Chaudhuri
    (c) Professor ST Achar (d) Dr Abraham Jacobi

13. **Which is the first pediatric hospital in India?**
    (a) Niloufer Hospitals
    (b) St Stephen's Hospital
    (c) Bai Jerbai Wadia Hospital for Children, Mumbai
    (d) Necker Hospital

14. **Who was first professor of pediatrics in India?**
    (a) Professor ST Achar (b) Dr K. C. Chaudhuri
    (c) Dr George Coelho (d) Dr Stephen

15. **Who founded first Indian pediatric independent journal?**
    (a) Shri C. Chandramouli (b) Dr K. C. Chaudhuri
    (c) Professor ST Achar (d) Dr Abraham Jacobi

16. **Which organization of pediatricians was founded by Dr George Coelho?**
    (a) IAP
    (b) Association of Pediatrics of India
    (c) IMA
    (d) Indian Science Institute

17. **Which is the first pediatric hospital in the world?**
(a) Boston's children hospital
(b) Wadia Hospital
(c) Niloufer Hospitals
(d) Necker Hospital in France

18. **Which is the first pediatric hospital in English-speaking world?**
(a) Children's Hospital of Philadelphia
(b) Negi child world
(c) Great Ormond Street Hospital for Children
(d) Boston's children hospital

19. **Which is the largest and oldest children's hospital in the world?**
(a) Great Ormond Street Hospital for Children
(b) Boston's children hospital
(c) Children's Hospital of Philadelphia
(d) None

20. **Who were Registrar General and Commissioner of 2011 Indian census?**
(a) Dr K. C. Chaudhuri (b) Professor ST Achar
(c) Dr Abraham Jacobi (d) Shri C. Chandramouli

21. **What is 0-6 years sex ratio in 2011?**
(a) 814 females per 1000 males
(b) 914 females per 1000 males
(c) 983 females per 1000 males
(d) 1000 females per 1000 males

22. **What is literacy rate of India as per 2011 census?**
(a) 74.04% (b) 82.14
(c) 65.46 (d) None

23. **What is infant mortality rate in India?**
(a) 58 per 1000 births (b) 49 per 1000 births
(c) 74 per 1000 births (d) 111 per 1000 births

24. **What was population in the age group of 0-6 of India as per 2011 census?**
(a) 10,822,262 (b) 11,026,113
(c) 12,848,375 (d) 14,848,375

25. **What is population of India above the age of 7 years as per 2011 census?**
(a) 1,051,404,135 (b) 2,010,632,022
(c) 2,510,632,022 (d) 3,010,632,022

26. **What was annual birth rate of India during 2005-2010?**
(a) 17,271,000 (b) 20,271,000
(c) 27,271,000 (d) 37,271,000

27. **What was crude birth rate of India during 2005-2010 per 1000?**
(a) 3.1 (b) 23.1
(c) 13.7 (d) 17.9

28. **What was crude death rate of India during 2005-2010 per 1000?**
(a) 2.1 (b) 7.3
(c) 8.3 (d) 9.2

29. **What was total fertility rate (number of children per woman) of India during 2005-2010?**
(a) 1.73 (b) 2.00
(c) 2.73 (d) 4.21

30. **What was infant mortality rate of India during 2005-2010?**
(a) 23.1 (b) 87.5
(c) 68.4 (d) 52.9 per 1000

31. **What was 2011 census regarding India's live births?**
(a) 7092000 (b) 10092999
(c) 17221000 (d) 27092000

32. **What was crude birth rate of India during 2011?**
(a) 11.2 (b) 21.8
(c) 18.7 (d) 8.0

33. **What was crude death rate of India during 2011?**
(a) 1.7 (b) 2.0
(c) 7.1 (d) 9.7

34. **What was total fertility rate (number of children per woman) of India during 2005-2010?**
(a) 1.5 (b) 3.5
(c) 2.44 (d) 8.44

35. **What is birth rate of Maharashtra as per 2011 census?**
(a) 17.1 (b) 7.1
(c) 14.7 (d) 2.41

36. **What is infant mortality rate as per 2011 census?**
(a) 28 (b) 8
(c) 18 (d) 21

37. **As per 2001 census what is percent wise population of 0-14 years' age group in India?**
(a) 30.8% (b) 27.5%
(c) 42.3% (d) 2.0%

38. **As per 2001 census what is percent wise sex ratio at birth in India (males/female)?**
(a) 0.70 (b) 1.12
(c) 2.12 (d) 5.67

39. **What is life expectancy at birth in India as per 2011 census (years)?**
(a) 58.5 (b) 62.8
(c) 65.8 (d) 72.1

40. **What is total fertility rate in 2009 of India? (children born/woman)**
(a) 1.74 (b) 2.72
(c) 8.11 (d) 3.71

41. **What is average world's child population involved in prostitution?**
(a) 1 million (b) Around 10 million
(c) 5 million (d) 20 million

42. **What is India's average child population involved in prostitution?**
(a) 80 thousand (b) 1 million
(c) 1.1 million (d) 1.2 million

43. **Which is apex governmental body regarding to women and child development in India?**
(a) Ministry of Health and Family Welfare
(b) AIIMS, New Delhi
(c) Ministry of Women and Child Development
(d) None

44. **Under terminology of maternal death what is the duration after termination of pregnancy?**
(a) 42 days (b) 28 days
(c) 60 days (d) 3 months

45. **In India, when Children's Day is celebrated?**
(a) 1st July (b) 14th November
(c) 5th November (d) 1st December

46. **On what date Universal Children's Day is celebrated?**
(a) 14th November (b) 8th August
(c) November 20 (d) November 30

47. **Which is the International Day for Protection of Children?**
(a) 1st March (b) 23rd December
(c) 31st July (d) 1st June

48. **What is worldwide figure of child labour?**
(a) 27 million (b) 217 million
(c) 1 billion (d) None

49. **As per Factories Act of 1948 what is age limit of child which prohibits the employment?**
(a) 7 years (b) 12 years
(c) 18 years (d) 14 years

50. **As per Mines Act of 1952, what is age limit of child which prohibits the employment?**
(a) 7 years (b) 12 years
(c) 16 years (d) 18 years

51. **As per Child Labour (Prohibition and Regulation) Act of 1986, what is age limit of child which prohibits the employment?**
(a) 12 years (b) 18 years
(c) 21 years (d) 14 years

52. **As per "The Right of Children to Free and Compulsory Education Act of 2009" at what age group children free and compulsory education is given?**
(a) 6 to 14 years (b) 0 to 5 years
(c) 12 to 18 years (d) Not at all free

53. **Who is Father of Medicine?**
(a) Hippocrates (b) Kashyap and Jeevaka
(c) Bindusara (d) Rhazes

54. **Who is world's first pediatrician?**
(a) Charak (b) Kashyap and Jeevaka
(c) Shushrutu (d) Waldo Nelson

55. **As per Hindu mythology who is the first child born by caesarean section?**
(a) Bindusara (b) Kashyap and Jeevaka
(c) Shushrutu (d) Charak

56. **Who is referred as the Father of Anatomy?**
(a) Bindusara (b) Shushrutu
(c) Charak (d) None

57. **Who is Persian physician remembered as the 'father of pediatrics'?**
(a) Soranus of Ephesus (b) Avenzoar
(c) Rhazes or Rasis (d) Paolo Bagellardo

58. **Who has written the first known manuscript dedicated to pediatrics?**
(a) Rhazes or Rasis (b) Avenzoar
(c) Paolo Bagellardo (d) Soranus of Ephesus

59. **Who was first physician to do the postmortem dissections?**
(a) Paolo Bagellardo (b) Rhazes or Rasis
(c) Avenzoar (d) Jakob Nufer

60. **Who has written the first medical book in printed format?**
(a) Thomas Phaer (b) Jakob Nufer
(c) Avenzoar (d) Paolo Bagellardo

61. In medical history who had performed the first successful caesarean section where both baby and mother survived?
(a) Thomas Phaer (b) Jakob Nufer
(c) Avenzoar (d) Rhazes or Rasis

62. Who wrote the first English language book on pediatrics?
(a) Jakob Nufer (b) Thomas Phaer
(c) Rhazes or Rasis (d) Hieronymus

63. Who had written the first important printed book on children, entitled, 'De Morbus Pusiorum'?
(a) Hieronymus (b) Thomas Phaer
(c) Paul Gottlieb Werlhof (d) Edward Harrison

64. Who described rheumatic chorea?
(a) Paul Gottlieb Werlhof
(b) Antonie Philips van Leeuwenhoek
(c) Thomas Sydenham
(d) Friedrich Wilhelm August

65. Who is Father of Microbiology?
(a) Antonie Philips van Leeuwenhoek
(b) Sir Thomas Watson
(c) Paul Gottlieb Werlhof
(d) None

66. First description of idiopathic thrombocytopenic purpura was mentioned by:
(a) George Armstrong
(b) Antonie Philips van Leeuwenhoek
(c) Paul Gottlieb Werlhof
(d) None

67. Who is regarded as the founder of pediatrics and child health in Great Britain?
(a) Anthony Jenner (b) Wilhelm August
(c) Both (d) George Armstrong

68. Who is known as "the father of immunology"?
(a) Edward Anthony Jenner
(b) Edward Harrison
(c) George Armstrong
(d) Friedrich Wilhelm August

69. Who described Harrison's groove?
(a) George Armstrong (b) Edward Harrison
(c) Sir Thomas Watson (d) None

70. What was invented by Rene Theophile Hyacinthe Laennec?
(a) Tunning fork (b) Stethoscope
(c) B.P. Apparatus (d) None

71. Who was pioneer in the field of the kindergarten and foundation for modern education?
(a) Edward Jenner
(b) Thomas Watson
(c) Friedrich Wilhelm August Frobel
(d) Sir Dominic John

72. Who described water hammer pulse which is found in aortic regurgitation?
(a) Edward Jenner (b) Sir Thomas Watson
(c) Both (d) Sir Dominic John

73. Who was first to develop smallpox vaccine ?
(a) Thomas Hodgkin
(b) Dominic John Corrigan
(c) Edward Jenner
(d) Sir Dominic John

74. Who was first to describe Hodgkin's lymphoma?
(a) Edward Hodgkins (b) Thomas Hodgkin
(c) Duminac Mc Evan (d) Francis Captain

75. Who described Corrigan's pulse?
(a) Willium Henle
(b) Dorland Serk
(c) Adolf Henle
(d) Sir Dominic John Corrigan

76. Guillaume-Benjamin-Amand Duchenne described which disease?
(a) SLE
(b) DLE
(c) 'Wilson's disease
(d) Duchenne Muscular Dystrophy

77. Who is referred to as "the father of modern pathology"?
(a) Donald Gamble
(b) Dr Charles Littman
(c) Rudolf Ludwig Karl Virchow
(d) Dr Joan H. Admirand

78. Who described Kussmaul's breathing?
(a) Adolph Kussmaul
(b) Donald Gamble
(c) Theodor Bilharz
(d) John Langdon Haydon Down

79. Who was pioneer in the field of parasitology?
(a) Theodor Bilharz (b) Adley Brian
(c) Leonard Girnita (d) None

80. **Down syndrome was firstly described by:**
(a) John Langdon Haydon Down
(b) Dr Wei Yang
(c) Dr Charles Littman
(d) Willium Henle

81. **Who is father of incubator?**
(a) Stephane Etienne Tarnier
(b) Hermann Robert Koch
(c) Dr Charles Littman
(d) None

82. **Kernig's sign is named because of:**
(a) Waldemar Kernig (b) Adolphe Pinard
(c) Bernard Sachs (d) Etienne Tarnier

83. **Who introduced the lumbar puncture for diagnostic and therapeutic purposes?**
(a) Hermann Robert Koch
(b) Bernard Sachs
(c) Heinrich Irenaeus Quincke
(d) Etienne Tarnier

84. **Who isolated tuberculosis bacillus?**
(a) Hermann Robert Koch
(b) Bernard-Jean
(c) Bernard Sachs
(d) None

85. **Who invented fetal stethoscope or fetoscope?**
(a) Bernard (b) Adolphe Pinard
(c) Bernard Sachs (d) Conrad

86. **Who discovered the X-rays?**
(a) Jules Francois
(b) Wilhelm Conrad Rontgen
(c) Finse
(d) None

87. **Who described the anatomical defects of cyanotic congenital heart disease, which later named as "Tetralogy of Fallot"?**
(a) Joseph Jules
(b) Etienne-Louis Arthur Fallot
(c) Fhon Little
(d) None

88. **Who is known for the pathological plantar reflex indicative of corticospinal tract damage?**
(a) Joseph Jules Francois Felix Babinski
(b) Albert Calmette
(c) Fhon Little
(d) None

89. **Who described a hereditary disorder of connective tissue, known as Marfan syndrome?**
(a) Willium Turner
(b) Antoine Bernard-Jean Marfan
(c) Leonardo d Dagen
(d) Hunsele

90. **Who is known as father of pediatric neurology?**
(a) Bernard Sachs (b) Willkins
(c) Milton Rechards (d) Murphy Kapore

91. **Who invented the use of light-phototherapy in the treatment of neonatal jaundice?**
(a) Niels Ryberg Finsen (b) Milton Rechards
(c) Willkins (d) Leon Charles

92. **Who was first to describe the spastic diplegia in children?**
(a) William John Little
(b) Dumpen Gughoti
(c) Harshley Davenson
(d) Dodden Hagen

93. **Who discovered the Bacillus Chalmette-Guerin (BCG) vaccine against tuberculosis?**
(a) Anton Ghon
(b) Leonel Revald
(c) Leon Charles Albert Calmette
(d) None

94. **Who named primary complex of tuberculosis?**
(a) Anton Ghon
(b) Dodden Hagen
(c) Mandid Bogger
(d) Kutrics Gandre

95. **Maria Montessori is related to:**
(a) Montessori hospital (b) Montessori disease
(c) Montessori norped (d) Montessori schools

96. **Which neonatal reflex was discovered by Ernst Moro?**
(a) Moro reflex (b) Rooting
(c) Tonic neck reflex (d) None

97. **Who was first to describe 'Twin-to-twin transfusion syndrome'?**
(a) Beatle Bewen (b) Benjamin Harley
(c) Friedrich Schatz (d) Fousi chelate

98. **Johannes Orth was first to describe:**
(a) Jonas Edward Salk (b) Johannes Orth
(c) Dr Abraham Jacobi (d) Cicely Williams

99. Who was the first to describe Wilson's disease?
(a) Willium Jhon
(b) Edward Samuel
(c) Samuel Alexander Kinnier Wilson
(d) None

100. In India, National Doctor's Day is celebrated in memory of:
(a) Dr George Coehlo (b) Professor ST Achar
(c) Dr Abraham Jacobi (d) Bidhan Chandra Roy

101. Who invented a vaccine against pertussis (whooping cough)?
(a) Helena Kagan (b) Cisley Henrey
(c) Louis Wendlin Sauer (d) Alexender Fleming

102. Who was the first pediatrician of Israel?
(a) Helena Kagan (b) Cisley Henrey
(c) Henry H. Turner (d) None

103. Who made the description of Turner syndrome?
(a) Almroth Edward Wright (b) Mary Mallon
(c) Henry H. Turner (d) None

104. Whose work was pionear in kwashiorkor—A protein energy malnutrition in Africa?
(a) Almroth Edward Wright
(b) Mary Mallon
(c) Dr Cicely Williams
(d) Johann Sussmann Galant

105. Who invented inactivated whole-cell typhoid vaccine?
(a) Johann Sussmann Galant
(b) Mary Mallon
(c) Almroth Edward Wright
(d) None

106. Who invented the diagnostic tool for tuberculosis and is named after him as Mantoux test?
(a) Dorland Reverb (b) Gangman jerck
(c) Wilium Nelwager (d) Charles Mantoux

107. Who is father of modern chemotherapy?
(a) Sidney Farber (b) Frank
(c) Mary Mallon (d) Lawson Wilkins

108. Who was the world's first pediatric ophthalmologist?
(a) Albert Bruce Sabin
(b) Lawson Wilkins
(c) Professor Wong Hock
(d) Frank D. Costenbader

109. Who was inventer of an oral polio vaccine?
(a) Baruch Samuel
(b) Dilip Mahalanabis
(c) Albert Bruce Sabin
(d) Jonas Edward Salk

110. Who was known as Typhoid Mary?
(a) Edwin Carlyle Carl Wood
(b) Mary Mallon
(c) de Silva
(d) Harry Fitch

111. Who developed the Apgar scoring system for neonatal assessment?
(a) Lawson Wilkins
(b) Virginia Apgar
(c) Thomas Chalmers Peebles
(d) Professor Wong Hock

112. Who studied Klinefelter's syndrome?
(a) Harry Fitch Klinefelter Jr.
(b) William Thomson
(c) Charles-Augustin de Coulomb
(d) Ernst Werner von Siemens

113. Who discovered the first safe and effective polio vaccine?
(a) Jonas Edward Salk
(b) Lawson Red Wilkins
(c) William Thomson
(d) Heinrich Rudolf Hertz

114. Who described the deep abdominal reflex in newborn?
(a) Johann Sussmann Galant
(b) Antoine Henri Becquere
(c) Nikola Tesla
(d) Heinrich Rudolf Hertz

115. Who was founder of the first pediatric endocrine clinic in the world?
(a) Lawson Wilkins (b) John Napier
(c) Alexander Graham Bell (d) None

116. Who developed Brazelton Neonatal Behavioral Assessment Scale?
(a) Robert Bakewell
(b) Thomas Berry Brazelton
(c) Patrick Bateson
(d) Julian Huxley

117. Who was first to give blood transfusion through the umbilical vein in the newborn?
(a) Christopher John Lamb
(b) Sidbury
(c) John Maynard Smith
(d) Herbert Spencer

118. Who developed a scale for measurement of sexual development during puberty?
(a) Rosalind Franklin
(b) James Mourilyan Tanner
(c) St. George Jackson Mivart
(d) Alfred Russel Wallace

119. Who was first to isolate the measles virus?
(a) John Jenner Weir
(b) Thomas Chalmers Peebles
(c) Mary Osborn
(d) Ernest William Lyons Holt

120. Who was first to propose Ponderal Index for calculation of relationship between mass and height?
(a) John Kendrew (b) Miriam Rothschild
(c) Tim Hunt (d) Rohrer

121. Who designed first growth charts useful for children's progress of growth?
(a) John Kendrew
(b) Thomas Chalmers
(c) Osborn Ernest
(d) David Cornelius Morley

122. Who was the first professor of pediatrics in the National University of Singapore?
(a) Professor Wong Hock
(b) Sir Robert Geoffrey
(c) Heinrich Rudolf Hertz
(d) None

123. When International Children's Day is celebrated?
(a) 21st March (b) 30th June
(c) 7th August (d) 1st June

124. Who was pioneer in the successful conception through IVF which led to the birth of the first test-tube baby?
(a) Sir Robert Geoffrey Edwards
(b) Heinrich Rudolf Hertz
(c) Thomas Chalmers
(d) St. George Jackson Mivart

125. Who identified the hepatitis B virus and later also developed vaccine?
(a) Baruch Samuel
(b) Dharmendra Kumar Tyagi
(c) St. George Jackson Mivart
(d) Dilip Mahalanabis

126. Who invented the "Red Triangle" symbol as a branding effort to familiarize and popularize the idea of family planning?
(a) Dilip Mahalanabis
(b) Dharmendra Kumar Tyagi
(c) Subhash Mukhopadhyay
(d) None

127. Who is known as father of in-vitro fertilization?
(a) Louis Costaz
(b) Edwin Carlyle Carl Wood
(c) Louis K. Diamond
(d) Prof. Priyani Soysa

128. Who created the world's second and India's first in-vitro fertilization?
(a) Jean-Baptiste Dumas
(b) Subhash Mukhopadhyay
(c) Louis Costaz
(d) Pierre Louis Maupertuis

129. Who discovered the inexpensive method–oral rehydration therapy for the treatment of diarrhea and cholera?
(a) Prof. Priyani Soysa
(b) Dilip Mahalanabis
(c) Subhash Mukhopadhyay
(d) Louis Costaz

130. Who reported the first case of beta thalassemia in India?
(a) Dr Mukherjee
(b) Dilip Mahalanabis
(c) Subhash Mukhopadhyay
(d) S.T. Achar

131. Who was the pioneer for doing exchange transfusion via umbilical vein as treatment for erythroblastosis fetalis?
(a) Prof. C. C. de Silva
(b) Prof. Priyani Soysa
(c) Louis K. Diamond
(d) Louis Costaz

132. When World Health Day is celebrated annually?
(a) 1st November (b) 21st July
(c) 14th November (d) 7th April

133. Who was the first professor of pediatrics in Shri Lanka?
(a) Prof. C. C. de Silva
(b) Jean-Baptiste Dumas
(c) Subhash Mukhopadhyay
(d) Pierre Louis Maupertuis

134. When Children's Day is celebrated in India
(a) 1st November (b) 21st July
(c) 14th November (d) 18th February

135. Who was first to establish the pediatric intensive care unit?
(a) Goran Haglund
(b) Louis Costaz
(c) Jean-Baptiste Dumas
(d) Pierre Louis Maupertuis

136. Who is remembered as mother of phototherapy?
(a) Jean-Pierre Vernant
(b) Prof. Priyani Soysa
(c) Miss Sister Jean Ward
(d) Pierre Louis Maupertuis

137. When Universal Children's Day is celebrated?
(a) 20th January (b) 20th September
(c) 20th October (d) 20th November

138. Who was the first pediatric woman professor in the Shri Lanka?
(a) Jean-Picrre Vernant (b) Louis K. Diamond
(c) Prof. Priyani Soysa (d) None

139. When International Children's Literature Day is celebrated?
(a) 1st April (b) 2nd April
(c) 21st April (d) 1st May

140. Who developed an orchidometer—an instrument used to measure the volume of the testicles?
(a) Prof. Dr. Andrea Prader
(b) Subhash Mukhopadhyay
(c) Pierre Louis Maupertuis
(d) Jean-Pierre Vernant

141. Who is regarded as father of pediatric gastroenterology?
(a) Louis Costaz
(b) Professor John Walker Smith
(c) Jean-Baptiste Dumas
(d) Jean-Pierre Vernant

142. Who was the world's last indigenous patient with smallpox on the earth.?
(a) Louis K. Diamond
(b) Pierre Louis Maupertuis
(c) Jean-Pierre Vernant
(d) Louis K. Diamond

143. Who was the world's first human test tube baby?
(a) Pierre Louis Maupertuis (b) Louise Joy Brown
(c) Louis K. Diamond (d) Louis K. Diamond

144. Who was the pioneer in establishing Kangaroo Mother Care?
(a) Dr. Edgar Rey Sanabria (b) Louis K. Diamond
(c) Louis Costaz (d) Jean-Baptiste Dumas

145. When global eradication of smallpox was certified?
(a) December 1984 (b) December 1978
(c) 9 December 1979

146. What is mean by CRY?
(a) Child Rights and You
(b) Crème Rou Yasnane
(c) Child Rehabilitation and Yardsticks
(d) Child Resolution in Year 2000

147. Parental alienation syndrome was coined by:
(a) Pierre Louis Maupertuis (b) Richard A. Gardner
(c) Baptiste Dumas (d) Louis Costaz

148. As per World Health Organization when complete smallpox eradication was declared?
(a) 1979 (b) 1980
(c) 1984 (d) 1987

149. When National Youth Day is celebrated in India?
(a) 31st July (b) 12th January
(c) 1st March (d) 23rd December

150. Who was the first human test tube baby of the India, credited to T.C. Anand Kumar?
(a) Mukta (b) Sunidhi
(c) Ambalika (d) Harsha

151. Which is an international awareness day for hemophilia and other bleeding disorders?
(a) 17th April (b) 17th May
(c) 26th June (d) 8th September

152. When International Thalassemia Day is celebrated?
(a) 8th January (b) 27th November
(c) 8th May (d) 5th May

153. When International Youth Day is celebrated?
(a) 12th June (b) 5th May
(c) 23rd November (d) 12th August

154. Who created the International Breastfeeding Symbol in response to a contest hosted by Mothering magazine?
(a) Pambansang Alagad (b) Juan S. Salcedo
(c) Alfredo C. Santos (d) Matt Daigle

155. When is World Down Syndrome Day?
(a) 21st March (b) 21st April
(c) 21st May (d) 21st June

156. When is International Day for Street Children?
(a) 1st February (b) 12th April
(c) 12th March (d) 21st April

157. When is International Missing Children's Day?
(a) 25th May (b) 1st May
(c) 25th September (d) 11th January

158. Satyamev Jayate—a TV programme based on female foeticide in India was anchored by:
(a) Abhishek Bachchan (b) Aamir Khan
(c) Shah Rukh Khan (d) Karina Kapoor

159. In India, when Children's Day is celebrated?
(a) 1st November (b) 14th November
(c) 1st December (d) 27th July

160. On what date Universal Children's Day is celebrated?
(a) 1st November (b) 1st December
(c) 20th November (d) None

161. Which is the International Day for Protection of Children?
(a) 1st May (b) 8th August
(c) 30th December (d) 1st June

162. What is worldwide figure of child labour?
(a) 127 million (b) 217 million
(c) 250 million (d) 1 billion

163. As per Factories Act of 1948 what is age limit of child which prohibits the employment?
(a) 6 years (b) 10 years
(c) 12 years (d) 14 years

164. As per Mines Act of 1952 what is age limit of child which prohibits the employment?
(a) 7 years (b) 12 years
(c) 14 years (d) 18 years

165. As per Child Labour (Prohibition and Regulation) Act of 1986 what is age limit of child which prohibits the employment?
(a) 7 years (b) 18 years
(c) 21 years (d) 14 years

166. As per "The Right of Children to Free and Compulsory Education Act of 2009" at what age group children free and compulsory education is given?
(a) 6 to 14 years (b) 12 to 16 years
(c) 14 to 18 years (d) Less than 6 years

167. Pratham is concerned with:
(a) Education (b) Nutrition
(c) Marriage (d) Sexual assault

168. What is minimum age limit of marriage as per Child Marriage Restraint Act, 1929?
(a) 18 years
(b) 21 years
(c) A male 21 or a female 18
(d) A male 18 or a female 21 years

169. Sarda Act is related to:
(a) Child marriage (b) Child abuse
(c) Child education (d) None

170. As per definition of UNICEF what is minimum age for marriage?
(a) 12 years (b) 18 years
(c) 21 years (d) 24 years

171. When the Prohibition of Child Marriage Act was established?
(a) 2006 (b) 1984
(c) 1996 (d) 2014

172. Apni Beti, Apna Dhan programme is related to what?
(a) Child marriage
(b) Child abuse
(c) Child education
(d) Heigher education abroad

173. Physical, sexual or emotional maltreatment or neglect of a child is called as:
(a) Child abuse (b) Child retreat
(c) Child embodiment (d) Podigree

174. Pediatrics is concerned with the health of:
(a) Infants (b) Children
(c) Adolescents (d) All of above

175. Runaway is a youth younger than 18 years who is gone for at least __________ from his or her home without parental permission:
(a) One night (b) 12 hours
(c) 3 days (d) 1 month

Answers

1. **(d)** All of the above

Pediatrics is defined as the science which deals with continuous and comprehensive care of a child, his family and his environment. (Pediatrics–from Wikipedia, the free encyclopedia)

2. **(a)** Healer of children

Pediatrics is a Greek word composed of–pedio-pais means child and iatros means doctor or healer. (Pediatrics–from Wikipedia, the free encyclopedia)

3. **(d)** Birth up to 18 years

As per Convention on the Rights of the Child adopted by the United Nations General Assembly on 20 November, 1989–a child means every human being below the age of 18 years unless, under the law applicable to the child, majority is attained earlier. In India, the right to vote in political elections is attained at the age of 18. In the United States of America, Pediatrics covers up to 21 years of age.

4. **(b)** Bagallarder's Little Book on Disease in Children

The first printed book on pediatrics was in Italian (1472) – Bagallarder's Little Book on Disease in Children. (Pediatrics – from Wikipedia, the free encyclopedia)

5. **(d)** Dr. Abraham Jacobi

Abraham Jacobi (1830–1919) is known as the father of pediatrics because of his many contributions to the field. He was born in Germany, where he received his medical training, but later practiced in New York City. (Pediatrics – from Wikipedia, the free encyclopedia)

6. **(c)** 1962

Indian Academy of Pediatrics was established in 1962, in Patna, Bihar which is the unique association of pediatricians in India. (Pediatrics – from Wikipedia, the free encyclopedia)

7. **(b)** Indian Pediatrics

IAP's official publication is Indian Pediatrics, an indexed journal. (Pediatrics – from Wikipedia, the free encyclopedia)

8. **(c)** Mumbai

Head office of IAP is in Mumbai. (Pediatrics – from Wikipedia, the free encyclopedia)

9. **(a)** Dr George Coehlo

The Association of Pediatrics of India started in 1950 in Bombay by Dr George Coehlo. (Pediatrics – from Wikipedia, the free encyclopedia)

10. **(a)** Dr George Coelho

11. **(c)** 1928

Pediatrics made a beginning in Mumbai in 1928 by Dr George Coelho. (Pediatrics – from Wikipedia, the free encyclopedia)

12. **(a)** Dr George Coelho

In 1928, Pediatrics was started by Dr George Coelho first time in India at Bai Jerbai Wadia Hospital for Children, Mumbai. Later on he became superintendent in same hospital and also remained the head of the department of Pediatrics till 1953. Because of all his contributions he is rightly remembered as "Father of Indian Pediatrics". (Pediatrics – from Wikipedia, the free encyclopedia)

13. **(c)** Bai Jerbai Wadia Hospital for Children, Mumbai

In 1928, Pediatrics was started by Dr George Coelho first time in India at Bai Jerbai Wadia Hospital for Children, Mumbai – The first children's hospital in India. (Pediatrics – from Wikipedia, the free encyclopedia)

14. **(a)** Professor ST Achar

In 1946, Professor ST Achar has created a separate department of pediatrics in Government General Hospital, Chennai. Later on it became a separate Institute of Pediatrics and Children's Hospital in Egmore, Chennai. Dr. S.T.Achar was the first professor of pediatrics in this department and all over India. (Textbook of Pediatrics by Professor S.T. Achar)

15. **(b)** Dr K. C. Chaudhuri

In 1933, Dr K. C. Chaudhuri founded the first independent pediatric journal namely, the Indian Journal of Pediatrics, in Calcutta also started the Indian Pediatric Society in 1948. (Pediatrics – from Wikipedia, the free encyclopedia)

16. **(b)** Association of Pediatrics of India

The Association of Pediatrics of India started in 1950 in Bombay by Dr George Cohelo. (Pediatrics – from Wikipedia, the free encyclopedia)

17. **(d)** Necker Hospital in France

The Hopital Necker - Enfants Malades (Necker Hospital - Hospital for sick children) is a French teaching hospital, located in Paris, France. It is a hospital of the Assistance publique–Hopitaux de Paris group, and is affiliated to the University of Paris Descartes. It is historically the first pediatrics hospital in the world. (Pediatrics–from Wikipedia, the free encyclopedia)

18. **(c)** Great Ormond Street Hospital for Children

Great Ormond Street Hospital for Children (GOSH) is a medical institution specializing in the care of children. It was founded in London in 1852 as the Hospital for Sick Children, making it the first hospital providing in-patient beds specifically for children in the English-speaking world. (Patrick S. Pasquariello; Tessa Hilton, 1999–The Children's Hospital of Philadelphia Book of Pregnancy and Child Care. John Wiley.p. xvii.ISBN 0471320129, 9780471320128. Retrieved 5 January 2012)

19. **(d)** Children's Hospital of Philadelphia

The Children's Hospital of Philadelphia (CHOP) is one of the largest and oldest children's hospitals in the world. In 1855, Philadelphia physician Dr. Francis West Lewis, inspired by a visit to the new Great Ormond Street Hospital for Sick Children in London (which was founded in 1852). He along with Dr. T. Hewson Bache and Dr. R.A.F. Penrose founded this first children's hospital in North America. ("Best Children's Hospitals: General Pediatrics" U.S. News and World Report, Accessed October 5, 2008)

20. **(d)** Shri C. Chandramouli

Shri C. Chandramouli is the Registrar General and Commissioner of 2011 Indian census.

21. **(b)** 914 females per 1000 males

Child Sex ratio (0–6 age group) per 1000 males–914 females.

22. **(a)** 74.04%

Census year	Total (%)	Male (%)	Female (%)
2011	74.04	82.14	65.46

23. **(b)** 49 per 1000 births

Year	Infant (0-1 year) Male	Infant (0-1 year) Female
1998	70	74
2005	56	58
2009	49	52

24. **(c)**12,848,375

	Person	Males	Females
Maharashtra	12,848,375	6,822,262	6,026,113
India	158,789,287	82,952,135	75,837,152

25. **(a)** 1,051,404,135

India/State/UT	Persons	Males	Females
Maharashtra	99,524,597	51,539,135	47,985,462
India	1,051,404,135	540,772,113	510,632,022

26. **(c)** 27,271,000

27. **(b)** 23.1 per 1000

28. **(c)** 8.3 per 1000

29. **(c)** 2.73

30. **(d)** 52.9 per 1000

Period	Births per year	Deaths per year	Natural change per year	CBR[1]	CDR[1]	NC[1]	TFR[1]	IMR[1]
2005-10	27,271,000	9,757,000	17,514,000	23.1	8.3	14.8	2.73	52.9

[1]CBR = crude birth rate (per 1000); CDR = crude death rate (per 1000); NC = natural change (per 1000); TFR = total fertility rate (number of children per woman); IMR = infant mortality rate per 1000 births.

31. **(d)** 27, 092, 000

32. **(b)** 21.8 per 1000

33. **(c)** 7.1 per 1000

34. **(c)** 2.44

2011 Average population (x 1000)	Live births[1]	Deaths[1]	Natural change	Crude birth rate (per 1000)	Crude death rate (per 1000)	Natural change (per 1000)	Total fertility rate
1,242,738	27,092,000	8,823,000	18,268,000	21.8	7.1	14.7	2.44

35. **(a)** 17.1

36. **(a)** 28

37. **(a)** 30.8%

2001 Census – Age structure
0–14 years: 30.8%
Male: 188,208,196, Female: 171,356,024

38. **(b)** 1.12 males/female

2001 Census – Sex ratio
At birth: 1.12 male(s)/female under 10 years: 1.14 male(s)/female 15-24 years: 1.09 male(s)/female

39. **(c)** 65.8 years

Life expectancy at birth–total population: 65.8 years (Source: UN Human Development Report 2013)

40. **(b)** 2.72 children born/woman

Total fertility rate — 2.72 children born/woman (2009 est.) although more up to date statistics indicate that India's TFR was 2.6 in 2008. The TFR (Total number of children born per woman) according to Religion in 2001 was: Hindus — 2.0, Muslims — 3.4, Sikhs — 2.1 Christians — 2.1, Buddhists — 2.1, Jains — 1.4, Animists and Others — 2.99, Tribals — 3.16, Scheduled Castes — 2.89

41. **(b)** Around 10 million

Country	Number of children involved in prostitution	
Worldwide	10,000,000	
India	1,200,000	Children account for 40% of prostitutes in India

42. **(d)** 1.2 million

Child prostitution is a major problem in India involving around 1.2 million children.

43. **(c)** Ministry of Women and Child Development

The Ministry of Women and Child Development, a branch of the Government of India, is the apex body for formulation and administration of the rules and regulations and laws relating to women and child development in India.

44. **(a)** 42 days

According to the World Health Organization (WHO), maternal death is defined as the death of a woman while pregnant or within 42 days of termination of pregnancy, irrespective of the duration and site of the pregnancy, from any cause related to or aggravated by the pregnancy or its management but not from accidental or incidental causes.

45. **(b)** 14th November

In India, Children's Day is celebrated on 14 November, the birthday of the country's first Prime Minister Jawaharlal Nehru. Jawaharlal Nehru, who was fondly called Chacha Nehru (Uncle Nehru) or Chachaji (Uncle) by the kids, emphasized the importance of giving love and affection to children, whom he saw as the bright future of India.

46. **(c)** November 20

Universal Children's Day takes place annually on November 20. First proclaimed by the United Nations General Assembly in 1954. This day is observed to promote the objectives outlined in the Charter and for the welfare of children. On November 20, 1959 the United Nations adopted the Declaration of the Rights of the Child. The United Nations adopted the Convention on the Rights of the Child on November 20, 1989.

47. **(d)** 1st June

International Day for Protection of Children, observed in many countries as Children's Day on June 1 since 1950, was established by the Women's International Democratic Federation on its congress in Moscow (22 November 1949).

48. **(b)** 217 million

UNICEF defines child labour differently. A child, suggests UNICEF, is involved in child labour activities if between 5 and 11 years of age, he or she did at least one hour of economic activity or at least 28 hours of domestic work in a week, and in case of children between 12 and 14 years of age, he or she did at least 14 hours of economic activity or at least 42 hours of economic activity and domestic work per week.

The 2001 national census of India estimated the total number of child labour, aged 5–14, to be at 12.6 million. Worldwide, about 217 million children work, many full-time. In 2001, out of a 12.6 million, about 12 million children in India were in a hazardous job.

49. **(d)**14 years

The Factories Act of 1948: The Act prohibits the employment of children below the age of 14 years in any factory.

50. **(d)** 18 years

51. **(d)** 14 years

The Child Labour (Prohibition and Regulation) Act of 1986: The Act prohibits the employment of children below the age of 14 years in hazardous occupations identified in a list by the law.

52. **(a)** 6 to 14 years

The Right of Children to Free and Compulsory Education Act of 2009: The law mandates free and compulsory education to all children aged 6 to 14 years. This legislation also mandated that 25 percent of seats in every private school must be allocated for children from disadvantaged groups and physically challenged children.

53. **(a)** Hippocrates

460-370 BC: HIPPOCRATES OF COS—An ancient Greek physician who is often called as the "father of medicine". Hippocrates and his followers were first to describe many childhood diseases and medical conditions. He is given credit for the first description of clubbing of the fingers and description of

Hippocratic face. (Adams, Francis 1891 Works by Hippocrates, 1994–2000)

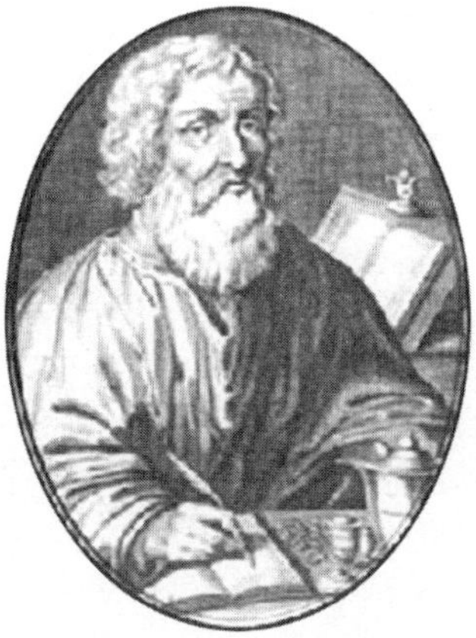

54. **(b)** Kashyap and Jeevaka

400 BC: World's first pediatrician—KASHYAP AND JEEVAKA (guru-shishya) were Indians, whose pioneering work on the child care and diseases are relevant today. The first manuscript on the management of children was included in Kashyap samhita and Vridha jeevka. (Viswanathan J, Desai AB, Editors, Achar's Textbook of Pediatrics. 3rd edition. Madras, Orient Longman 1991: pp1-16)

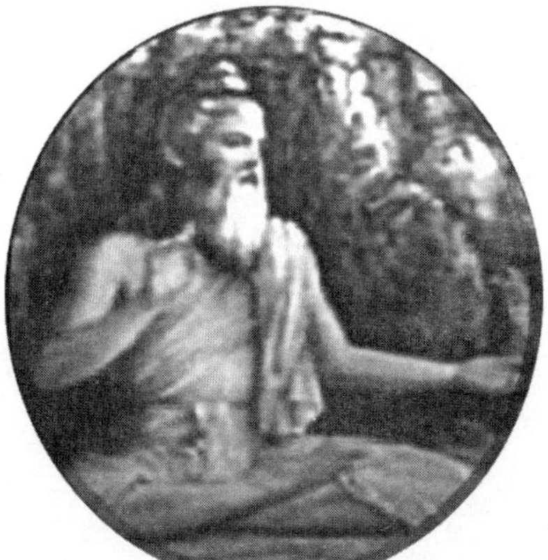

55. **(a)** Bindusara

320 BC: BINDUSARA (Second Maryann Samrat of India)–He was the first child born by Caesarean section. His mother (wife of Chandragupta Maurya) accidentally consumed poison and died; when she was close to give birth. Chanakya, the Chandragupta's advisor, opened the abdomen of the queen and took out the baby, thus saving the baby's life.(M. Srinivasacharitar -1989- History of Classical Sanskrit Literature, 3 edn. Motilal Banarsi Dass, p. 550.)

56. **(c)** Charak

300 BC: CHARAK—He was the first physician to state the concept of digestion, metabolism and immunity also was first to mention about the genetics and relevant disorders. He was first to suggest that prevention of disease is important than to cure. He is also referred as the "Father of Anatomy". (Pal MN. The Ayurvedic tradition of child care: Pediatric wisdom of ancient India Clinical Pediatr. Phila 1973; 12: 122-123)

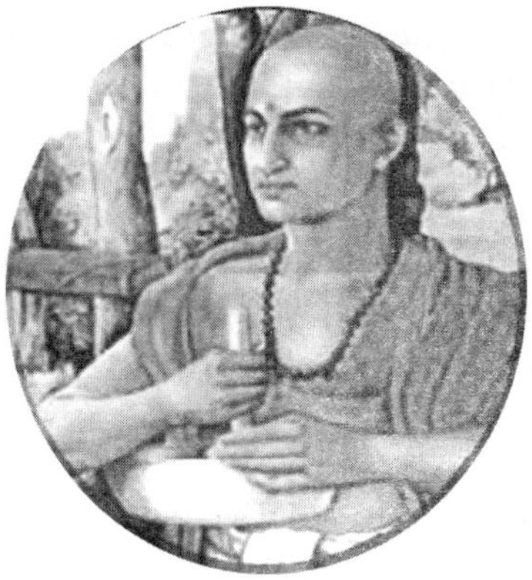

57. **(c)** Rhazes or Rasis

Rhazes or Rasis—He was a Persian physician, who made inventions in medical field including first to differentiate smallpox from measles and the discovery of alcohol and kerosene. He was also a pioneer of neurosurgery and ophthalmology. Because of this he is known as the 'father of pediatrics. (Kraus, P & Pines, s: 1913-1938—"Al-Razi". Encyclopedia of Islam pp. 1136)

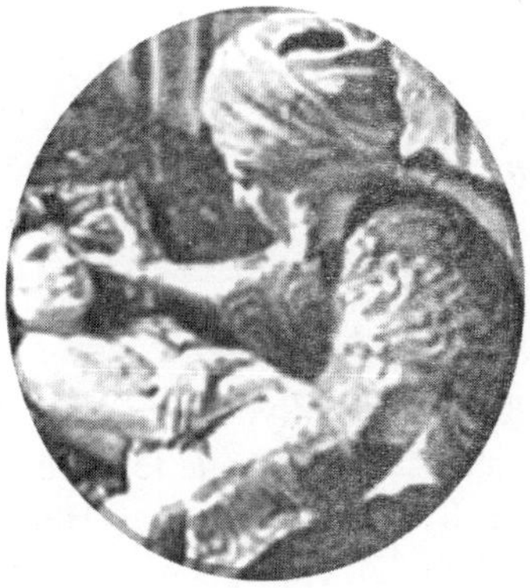

58. **(d)** Soranus of Ephesus

2nd century AD: Soranus of Ephesus (Greece)–He had written the first known manuscript dedicated to pediatrics. (Todman, "Soranus of Ephesus and the Methodist sect", Journal of Medical Biography 16 - 1: 51)

59. **(c)** Avenzoar

1091–1161: Avenzoar—He was the first physician to do the postmortem dissections. (Islamic medicine, Hutchinson Encyclopedia)

60. **(d)** Paolo Bagellardo

Paolo Bagellardo (1425–1495, Italy)—He has written the first medical book in printed format. It was based on Greek and Arab works, though it included some of his own experience such as medicines that could be used to soothe a crying baby. (Hook and Norman ***the Haskell F. Norman Library of Science and Medicine*** 1991 no. 102)

61. **(b)** Jakob Nufer

1500: Jakob Nufer—He was a Swiss pig-gelder who performed the first successful Caesarean section in history. In this surgery both baby and mother survived. (Henry, John 1991—Doctors and Healers: Popular Culture and the Medical Profession. New York: p197)

62. **(b)** Thomas Phaer

1545- 12 August 1560: Thomas Phaer—He was an English lawyer, pediatrician, and author who wrote the first English language book on pediatrics. This book of children included a long section on dentition especially teething, crying, fever, cramps, palsies, etc. He advocated washing the child in chamomile and applying oil of roses, fresh butter with barley flour or honey, or frank incense and licorice mixed in a fine powder. (Chisholm, Hugh, ed. 1911. Encyclopedia Britannica–11th ed. Cambridge University Press)

63. **(a)** Hieronymus

1583: Hieronymus—He had written the first important printed book on children, entitled, '***De Morbus Pusiorum***.' ("Achar's Textbook of Pediatrics, Third Edition. Desai, A.B. ed.1989, p.1. ISBN 81-250-0440-8)

64. **(c)** Thomas Sydenham

1624–1689: Thomas Sydenham—He described the clinical features of rheumatic fever and one of them is known as Sydenham's chorea. (Bloch, H, January 1994—the father of clinical observation. The Journal of family practice 38 -1: 80–1)

65. **(a)** Antonie Philips van Leeuwenhoek

1632 October 24-1723 August 26: Antonie Philips van Leeuwenhoek (Netherlands)—He was the first to observe and describe single celled organisms, muscle fibers, bacteria, spermatozoa, and blood flow in capillaries. He is known as "The Father of Microbiology" and considered to be the first microbiologist. (Frank N. Egerton 2006—A History of the Ecological Sciences, Part 19: Leeuwenhoek's Microscopic Natural History. Bulletin of the Ecological Society of America: Vol. 87, No. 1, pp. 47-58)

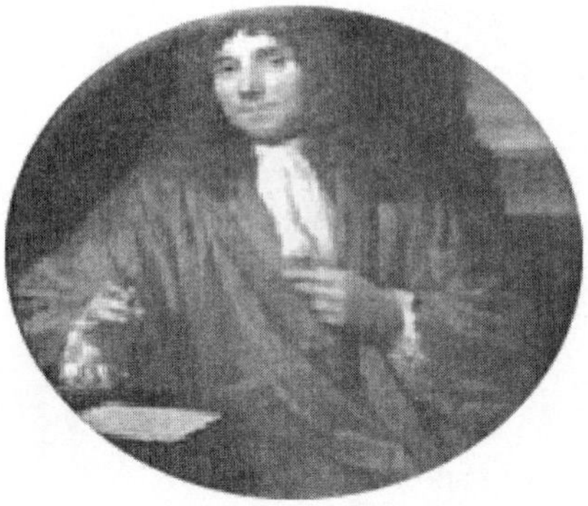

66. **(c)** Paul Gottlieb Werlhof

1699 March 24–1767 July 26: Paul Gottlieb Werlhof—A German physician, who mentioned the first description of idiopathic thrombocytopenic purpura. (Stasi R, Newland AC–May 2011–"ITP: A historical perspective". Br. J. Haematol 153-4-437–50)

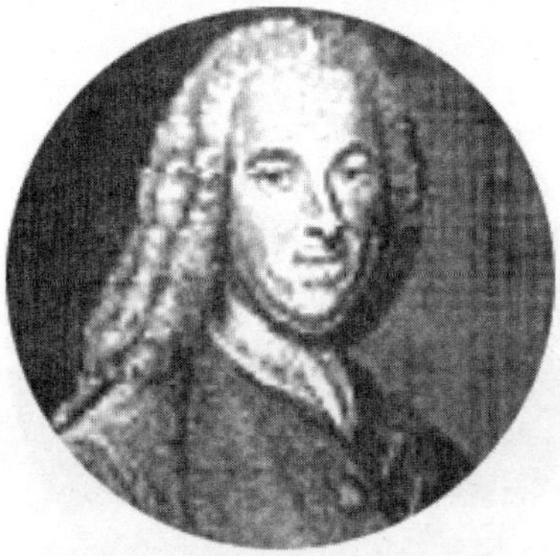

67. **(d)** George Armstrong

1719–1789: George Armstrong (United Kingdom)—He introduced clinical teaching and may be regarded as the founder of pediatrics and child health in Great Britain. He published one of the first textbooks on children's diseases in 1767. He was the founder of the world's first dispensary/hospital for sick children, for pioneering in children's diseases and child health, for his teaching of clinical pediatrics, and for his regard for the social welfare of children. (Web)

68. **(a)** Edward Anthony Jenner

1749 May 17–1823 January 26: Edward Anthony Jenner—An English physician and scientist from Berkeley, who was the pioneer in the development of smallpox vaccine. He is known as "the father of immunology" and his work is said to have saved more lives than the work of any other man. ("Dr. Edward Jenner and the smallpox vaccination". Essortment.com. Retrieved 28 July 2009)

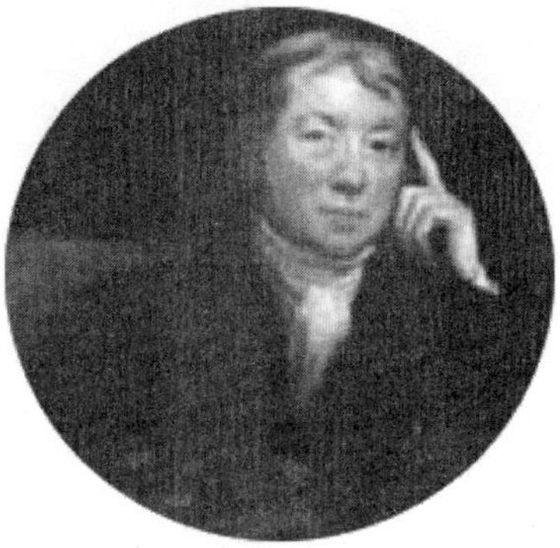

69. **(b)** Edward Harrison

1766-1838 May 06: Edward Harrison—A British physician who described Harrison's groove, which is a mark on the back, breast and ribs in children affected with spinal diseases. (London Medical and Physical Journal, 1820)

70. **(b)** Stethoscope

1781 February 17-1826 August 13: Rene Theophile Hyacinthe Laennec—A French physician, who invented the stethoscope in 1816 while working at the Hospital Neckerand. (Bloch, Harry 1993. "The inventor of the stethoscope: Rene Laennec Journal of Family Practice – Find Articles". Journal of Family Practice. Retrieved-2007-10-11)

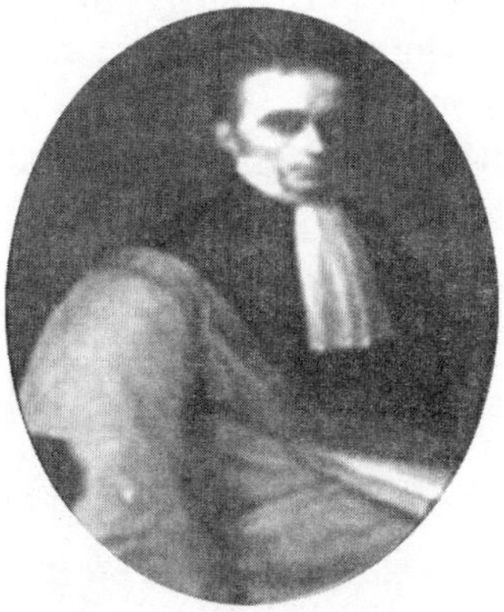

71. **(c)** Friedrich Wilhelm August Frobel

1782 April 21-1852 June 21: Friedrich Wilhelm August Frobel (German)—He was a pioneer in the field of the kindergarten and foundation for modern education based unique needs and capabilities of children. Also he developed the Frobel Gifts educational toys.

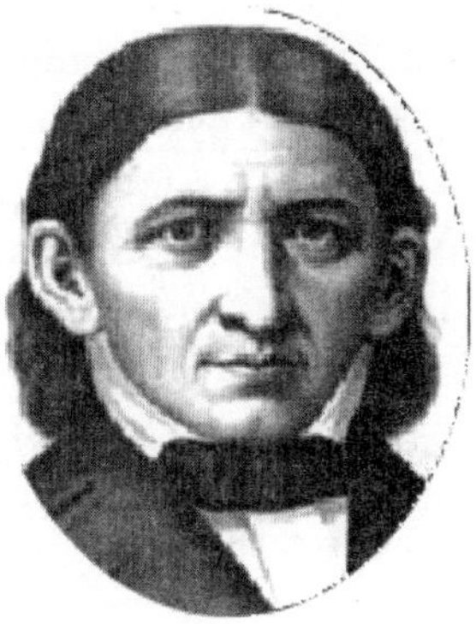

72. **(b)** Sir Thomas Watson

1792-11 December 1882: Sir Thomas Watson—A British physician who is known for describing the water hammer pulse, found in aortic regurgitation. This sign is also known as Watson's pulse. (St. Louis courier of medicine.Courier of Medicine Co. 1883, p. 190. Retrieved, 22 May 2012)

73. **(c)** Edward Jenner

First smallpox vaccine was developed by Edward Jenner. (Stefan Riedel-2005 Jan.18. Baylor univ. medical center, pp. 21-25)

74. **(b)** Thomas Hodgkin

1798 August 17-1866 April 5: Thomas Hodgkin— A British physician, who was first to describe, a form of lymphoma and blood disease, which bears his name as "Hodgkin's lymphoma". (Jay, Venita -2005—On a historical note: the legacy of Thomas Hodgkin. Journal of insurance medicine 37-3-248-9)

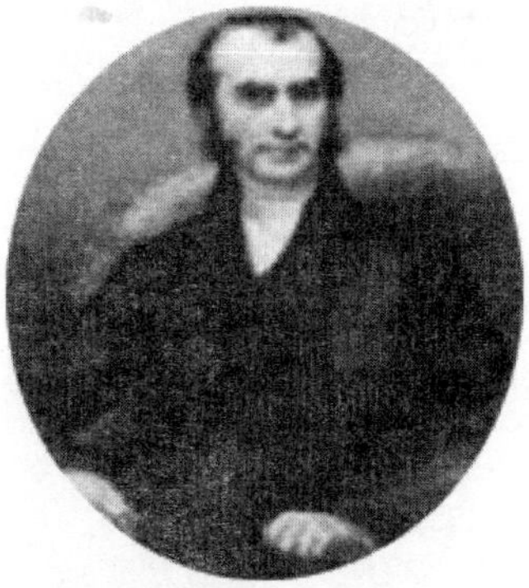

75. **(d)** Sir Dominic John Corrigan

1802 December 2—1880 February 1: Sir Dominic John Corrigan—An Irish physician who is known for his observations of the abnormal "collapsing" pulse of aortic valve insufficiency, which is named Corrigan's pulse after him. (Eoin O'Brien, Conscience and Conflict. Sir Dominic Corrigan 1802-1880, Dublin-1983)

76. **(d)** Duchenne Muscular Dystrophy

1806 September 17-1875 September 15: Guillaume-Benjamin-Amand Duchenne–He was a French-neurologist, whose greatest contribution is in the myopathies: Duchenne Muscular Dystrophy, Duchenne-Aran spinal muscular atrophy, Duchenne-Erb paralysis, Duchenne's disease (Tabes dorsalis), and Duchenne's paralysis (Progressive bulbar palsy). (Garrison, Fielding Hudson-1913–An introduction to the history of medicine. Philadelphia and London: W. B. Saunders. p. 571)

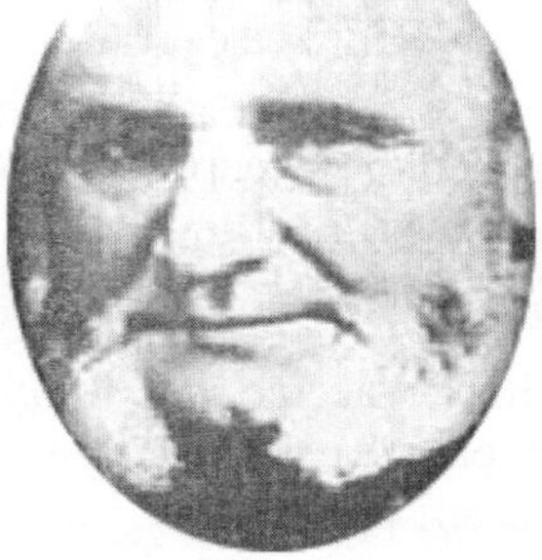

77. **(c)** Rudolf Ludwig Karl Virchow

1821 October 13–1902 September 5: Rudolf Ludwig Karl Virchow—He was first to study the Leukemia with his co-pathologist John Hughes Bennett in 1845. Because of his work he referred to as "the father of modern pathology". (Rutherford, Dr. Adam [August 2009]. "The Cell: Episode 1 the Hidden Kingdom". BBC4)

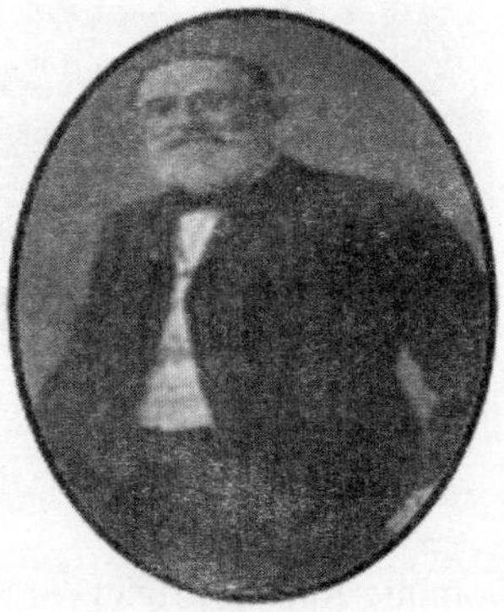

78. **(a)** Adolph Kussmaul

1822 February 22–1902 May 28: Adolph Kussmaul (Germany)—His name is honored with following things:

- Kussmaul breathing - Very deep and labored breathing with normal or reduced frequency seen in severe diabetic ketoacidosis.
- Kussmaul's sign - Paradoxical rise in the jugular venous pressure on inhalation in constrictive pericarditis or chronic obstructive pulmonary disease.
- Kussmaul disease (Also called Kussmaul-Maier disease) - Polyarteritis nodosa.
- Kussmaul's coma - Diabetic coma due to ketoacidosis.
- Kussmaul's aphasia - Selective mutism.

(Matteson EL, Kluge FJ–January 2003, Curr Opin. Rheumatol 15-1: 29–34)

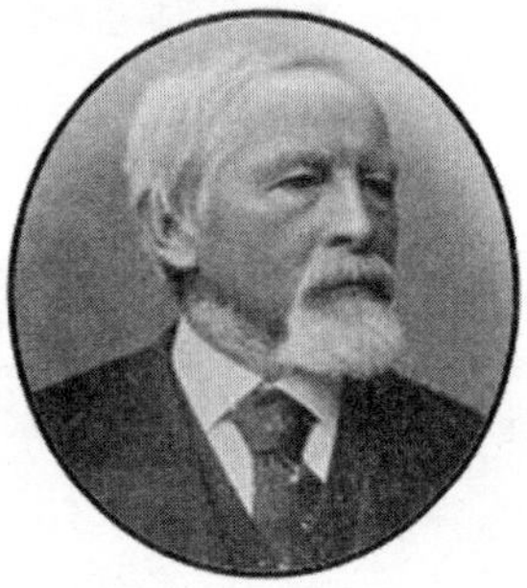

79. **(a)** Theodor Bilharz

1825 March 23–1862 May 9: Theodor Bilharz—A German physician, who was pioneer in the field of parasitology. (Edward Griffor and Craig Smorynski –Logic's Lost Genius: History of Mathematics, vol. 33)

80. **(a)** John Langdon Haydon Down

1828 November18-1896 October 7: John Langdon Haydon Down (Brittan)—He is known for his description of a genetic disorder—Down syndrome. (Janet Carr, Janet H. Carr-24 Nov 1995. Down syndrome, Cambridge Univ. Press, p1)

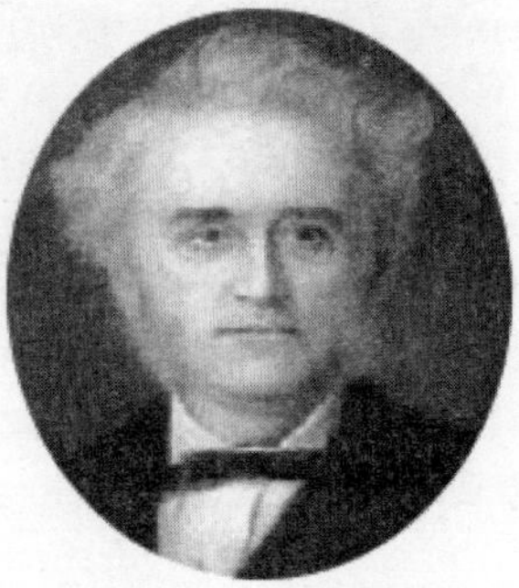

81. **(a)** Stephane Etienne Tarnier

1828 April 29 –1897 November 23: Stephane Etienne Tarnier—A French obstetrician, known as the "father of the incubator", having developed it for the thermoregulation of premature infants in a Paris maternity ward. (Dunn, PM 2002–Stephane Tarnier- the architect of perinatologye" Archives of disease in childhood. Fetal and neonatal edition 86,2–F137–9)

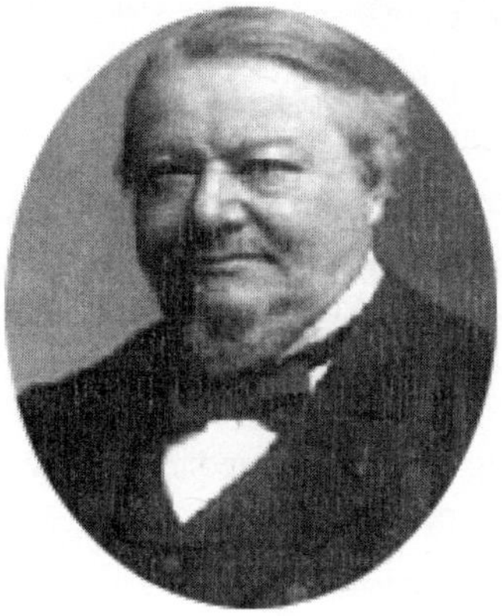

82. **(a)** Waldemar Kernig

1840–1917: Waldemar Kernig (Germany)—He named one of the important sign which is present in patients with subarachnoid hemorrhage or meningitis. It is known as positive when the thigh is bent at the hip and knee at 90 degree angles, and subsequent extension in the knee is painful. (Kernigs sign) (O'Connor, Simon; Talley, Nicholas Joseph–2001 Clinical Examination: A Systematic Guide to Physical Diagnosis. Cambridge, MA: Blackwell Publishers, p. 363)

83. **(c)** Heinrich Irenaeus Quincke

1842 August 26-1922 May 19: Heinrich Irenaeus Quincke—A German surgeon, who introduced the lumbar puncture for diagnostic and therapeutic purposes. (Quincke HI (1868). "Beobachtungen ueber Capillar- und Venenpuls" (in German). Berl klin Wochenschr 5: 337–359)

84. **(a)** Hermann Robert Koch

1843 December 11-1910 May 27: Hermann Robert Koch – A German physician, who isolated Bacillus anthraces, tuberculosis bacillus and vibrio cholerae. He was awarded the Nobel Prize in Physiology and Medicine for his tuberculosis findings in 1905. He is one of the father figure founders of microbiology. (Koch, R:1876-Cohn's Beitrage zur Biologie der Pflanzen 2: 277–310)

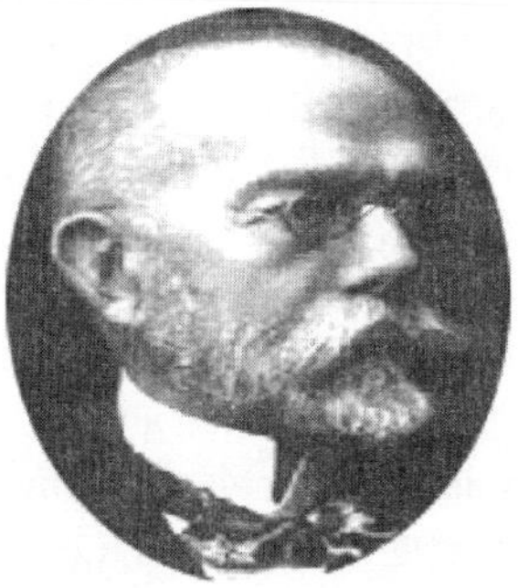

85. **(b)** Adolphe Pinard

1844–1934: Adolphe Pinard—A French obstetrician, who invented fetal stethoscope or fetoscope. It is used to hear the heart sounds of the fetus in a pregnant woman. The fetal stethoscope is also known as a Pinard's stethoscope or a pinard. (Neonatology on the Web. The History of Neonatology)

86. **(b)** Wilhelm Conrad Rontgen

1845 March 27 - 1923 February 10 :Wilhelm Conrad Rontgen – He was a German physician who discovered the electromagnetic radiation, known as X-rays or Rontgen rays on 8 November 1895. For this he was honored with the first Nobel Prize in Physics in 1901. (Glasser, Otto -1933—Wilhelm Conrad Rontgen and the Early History of the Roentgen Rays. London: John Bale, Sons and Danielsson Ltd., p. 305)

87. **(b)** Etienne-Louis Arthur Fallot

1850 September 29-1911 April 30: Etienne-Louis Arthur Fallot—A French physician, who described the anatomical defects of cyanotic congenital heart disease, which later named as, 'Tetralogy of Fallot'. (Whitworth, Judith A; Firkin, Barry G-1996-Dictionary of medical eponyms, New York: Parthenon Pub.)

88. **(a)** Joseph Jules Francois Felix Babinski

1857 November 17-1932 October 29: Joseph Jules Francois Felix Babinski—A French neurologist, who is known for his description of the Babinski sign, a pathological plantar reflex indicative of corticospinal tract damage. (Jacques Philippon, Jacques Poirer Joseph Babinski: A Biography 2008, ISBN 0-19-536975-0)

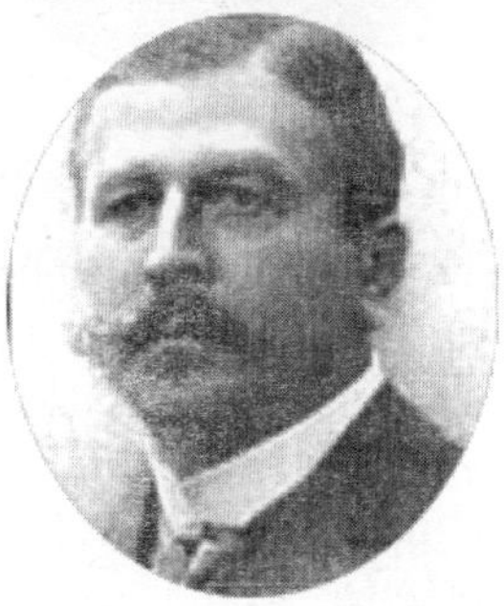

89. **(b)** Antoine Bernard-Jean Marfan

1858 June 23-1942 February 11: Antoine Bernard-Jean Marfan—He was a French pediatrician, who described a hereditary disorder of connective tissue, known as Marfan syndrome. He was also associated with Dennie-Marfan syndrome, Marfan's hyper mobility syndrome, Marfan's law, Marfan's sign, Marfan's symptom, Marfan-Madelung syndrome. (Marfan, Antoine 1896. Bulletins 3rd series: 220–226)

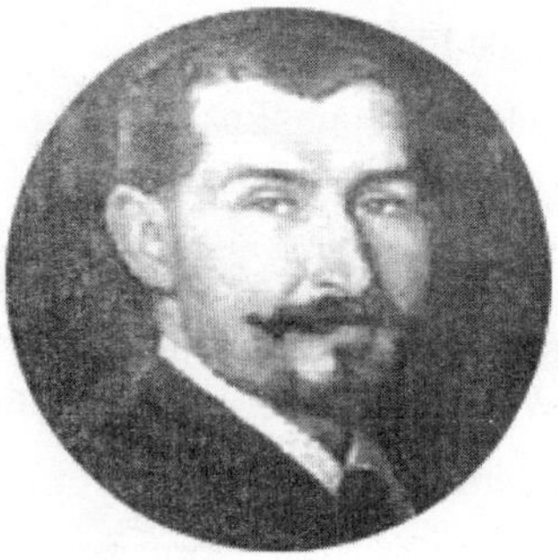

90. **(a)** Bernard Sachs

1858-1944: Bernard sachs—He was born in Baltimore and edited the Journal of Nervous and Mental Disease from1886 to 1891. He also wrote on myotonia congenital, intracerebral hemorrhage, muscular dystrophies and congenital syphilis. He wrote a number of papers on poliomyelitis and cerebral palsy. He was a pioneer of great importance in neurology's growth from adolescence to maturity and in the birth of child neurology. Because of his contribution he is known as, "the father of pediatric neurology".

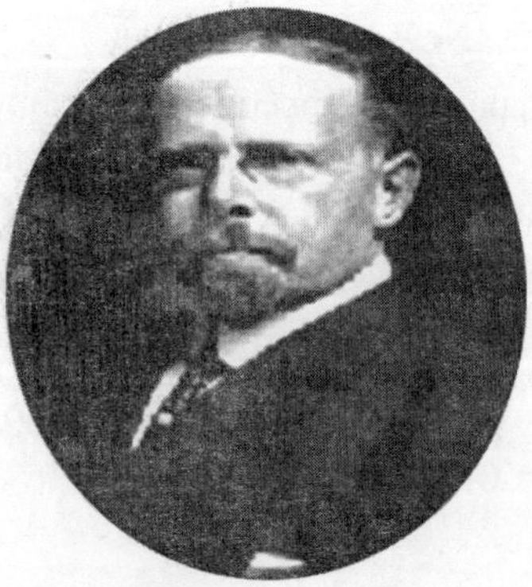

91. **(a)** Niels Ryberg Finsen

1860 December 15-1904 September 24: Niels Ryberg Finsen – An Icelandic physician and scientist, who invented the use of light–phototherapy in the treatment of neonatal jaundice. For this he was awarded the Nobel Prize in Medicine and Physiology. (Medicine 1903 at nobelprize.org.)

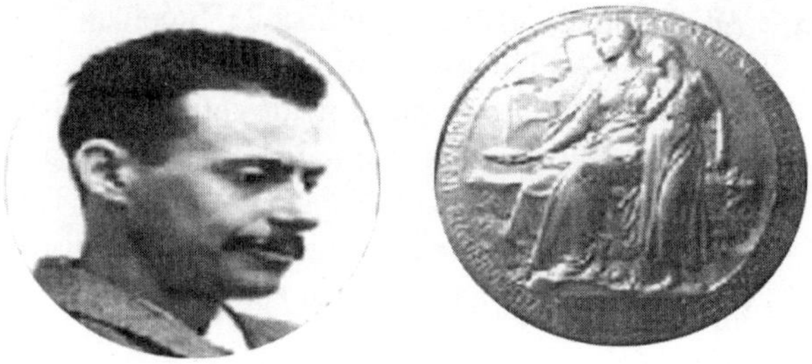

92. **(a)** William John Little

1860–William John Little—An English surgeon who was first to describe the spastic diplegia in children. That's why spastic diplegia was known as, 'Little's Disease'. Also he was the founder of the Royal Orthopedic Hospital of London. (Historical Vignette Little big man: Orthopedic Review 1988; Nov. 17 - 11-1156, pp. 1161–6).

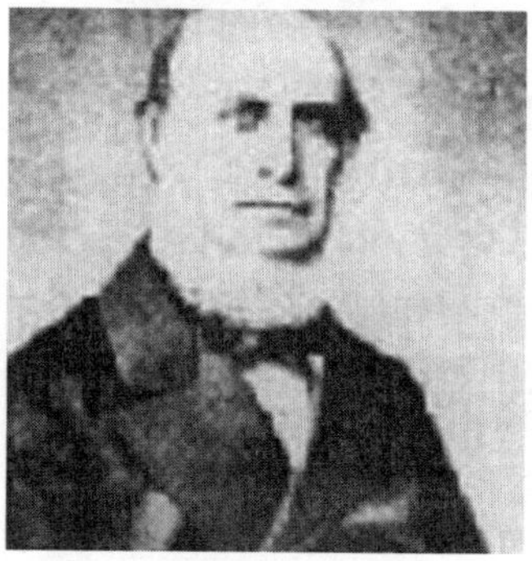

93. **(c)** Leon Charles Albert Calmette

1863 July 12-1933 October 29: Leon Charles Albert Calmette—Hc was a French physician, who discovered the Bacillus Chalmette-Guerin, an attenuated form of Mycobacterium used in the BCG vaccineagainst tuberculosis. He also developed the first antivenin for snake venom—the Chalmette's serum. ("**Leon Charles Albert Calmette**, 1863-1933". Obituary Notices of Fellows of the Royal Society 1 -3- 315)

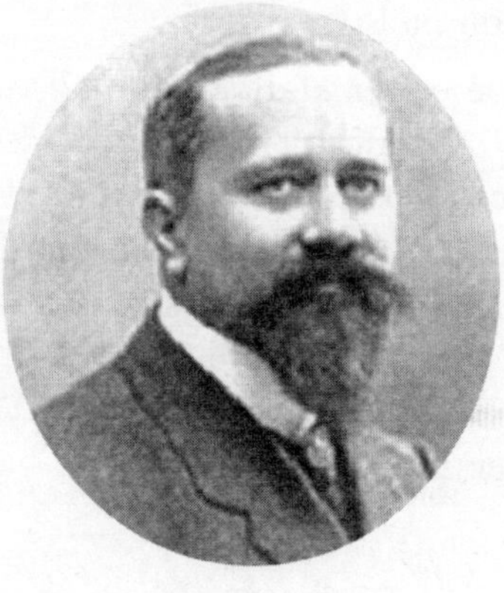

94. **(a)** Anton Ghon

1866 January 01-1936 April 23: Anton Ghon—An Austrian pathologist who was known for his work on meningitis and tuberculosis. Ghon focus–a primary infection associated with tuberculosis, as well as Ghon's complex—when the aforementioned infection involves surrounding lymph nodes, were named after him. He studied the childhood tuberculosis and its treatment in depth. (Wikipedia, the free encyclopedia)

95. **(d)** Montessori Schools

1870 August 31–1952 May 6: Maria Montessori—She was the Italian physician and educator, known for childhood education which bears her name—Montessori Schools. Her educational method is in use today in public and private schools throughout the world. (Hainstock, Elizabeth -1978—The Essential Montessori, New York: The New American Library)

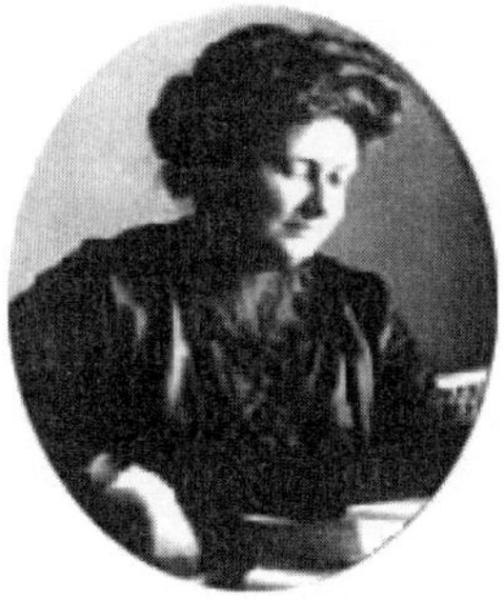

96. **(a)** Moro reflex

1874 December 08 -1951: Ernst Moro – He was an Austrian pediatrician, who discovered the neonatal reflex which was named after him as "Moro reflex". He is also known for the following: (1) Developed the Moro test (percutaneous tuberculin reaction) (2) Invented "Moro's milk", an infant-feeding formula composed by full cream milk with added 3% flour, 5% butter and 5-7% sugar. (Weirich A, Hoffmann GF. "Ernst Moro", European Journal of Pediatrics, 2005 Oct; 164-10-599-606, Pub Med)

97. **(c)** Friedrich Schatz

1875: Friedrich Schatz (Germany)—He was first to describe 'Twin-to-twin transfusion syndrome'. It is related with differences in birth weight and cord hemoglobin at the time of delivery. (Johnson, A and Moise, K, J. "Improving Survival in Twin-Twin Transfusion Syndrome" Contemporary OB/GYN December 2)

98. **(b)** Johannes Orth

1875: Johannes Orth – He was first to describe Kernicterus. He postulated that jaundice might have hematologic origins. (Web)

99. **(c)** Samuel Alexander Kinnier Wilson

1878 December 6–1937 May 12: Samuel Alexander Kinnier Wilson—A British neurologist who was the first to describe Wilson's disease. (Ala A, Walker AP, Ashkan K, Dooley JS, Schilsky ML-2007, "Wilson's disease". Lancet 369-9559:397–408.)

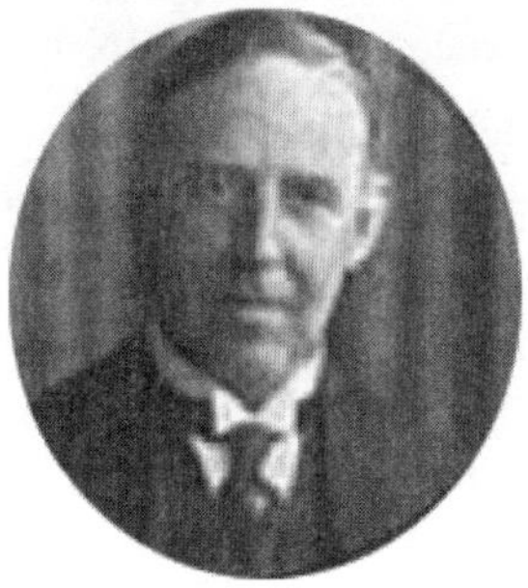

100. **(d)** Bidhan Chandra Roy

1882 July 1-1962 July 1: Bidhan Chandra Roy—He was the second Chief Minister of West Bengal in India and one who completed both F.R.C.S. and M.R.C.P. simultaneously within only two years and three months. In India, the National Doctor's Day is celebrated on the date of his birth (and death) July 1 every year. (Choudhary, Valmiki (1984). Dr. Rajendra Prasad, Correspondence and Select Documents: 1934-1937. Allied Publishers, pp. 368)

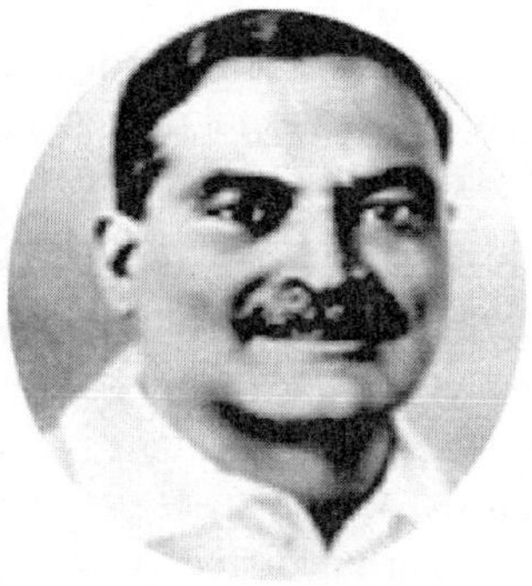

101. **(c)** Louis Wendlin Sauer

1885-1980: Louis Wendlin Sauer—A pediatrician, who invented a vaccine against pertussis (whooping cough). This has saved a countless lives around the world. (Patel SS, Wagstaff A, 1996—Acellular pertussis vaccine—A review of its immunogenicity. Drugs 52 2-254–275)

102. **(a)** Helena Kagan

1889-1978: Helena Kagan—She was the first pediatrician of Israel. She opened a clinic at her home and founded institutions to improve the health of Jerusalem children. (PMID:18653833, PubMed - indexed for MEDLINE)

103. **(c)** Henry H. Turner

1892 August 28-1970 August 4: Henry H. Turner—An American endocrinologist, who made the description of Turner Syndrome in 1938. (Sperling, M. 2008, "15". Pediatric endocrinology. Elsevier Health Sciences, p. 615. ISBN 1-4160-4090-0)

104. **(c)** Dr. Cicely Williams

1893-1992: Dr. Cicely Williams – She has diagnosed and labeled more common and fatal condition, known as kwashiorkor—a protein energy malnutrition in Africa, which focused the attention of the medical world. (Williams, Cicelyd, 1935, "Kwashiorkor". The Lancet 226-5855-1151)

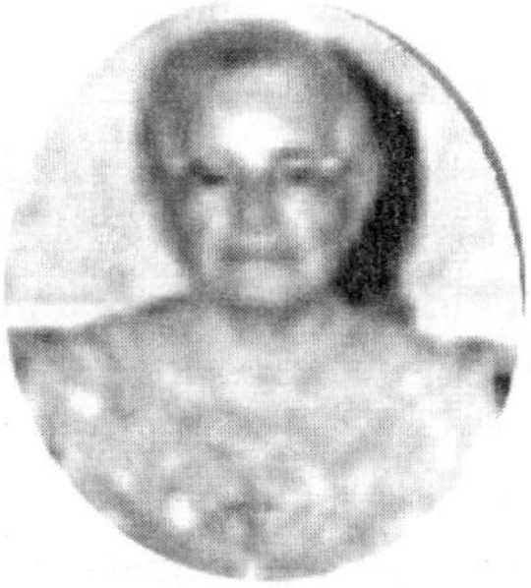

105. **(c)** Almroth Edward Wright

1896: Almroth Edward Wright—He invented inactivated whole-cell typhoid vaccine. (Fraser, Abigail, ed. "Vaccines for preventing typhoid fever", Cochrane Database Syst Rev.3)

106. **(d)** Charles Monteux

1877-1947: Charles Monteux—A French physician, who invented the diagnostic tool for tuberculosis and is named after him as Monteux test. (Starke J -1996- "Tuberculosis Skin Testing: New Schools of Thought". Journal of the American Academy of Pediatrics 98: 123–125)

107. **(a)** Sidney Farber

1903–1973: Sidney Farber–He was a pediatric pathologist, regarded as, "the father of modern chemotherapy". (Miller, Denis R. [July 2006], "A tribute to Sidney Farber – the father of modern chemotherapy", British Journal of Haematology 134, Issue 1: 20–26)

108. **(d)** Frank D. Costenbader

1905-1978: Frank D. Costenbader— American physician, who was the world's first pediatric ophthalmologist. (Marshall MM. "The History of the Costenbader Society: Costenbader's Challenges", March 19, 2000)

109. **(c)** Albert Bruce Sabin

1906 August 26-1993 March 3: Albert Bruce Sabin —An American medical researcher known for invention of an oral polio vaccine. (Smith, Derek R; Leggat Peter A 2005. "Pioneering figures in medicine: Albert Bruce Sabin"—The Kurume medical journal 52:111)

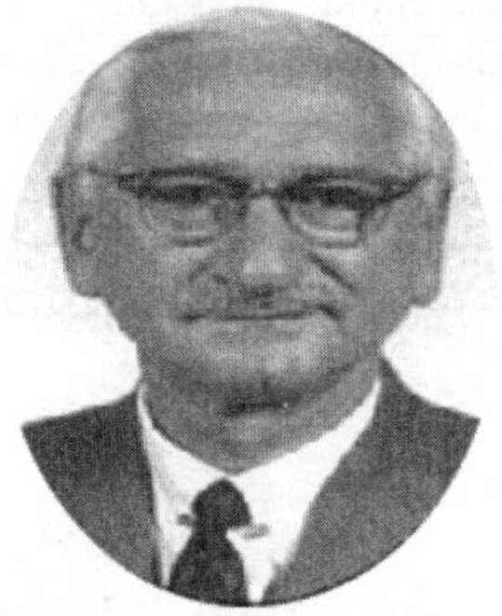

110. **(b)** Mary Mallon

1907: Mary Mallon—She was the most notorious carrier of typhoid fever, also called as Typhoid Mary. She was the first American carrier to be identified and traced. She was a cook in New York. She was detained and quarantined after another typhoid outbreak. She died of pneumonia after 26 years in quarantine. ("Nova: The Most Dangerous Woman in America")

111. **(b)** Virginia Apgar

1909-1974: Virginia Apgar—An American pediatric anesthesiologist, who was the founder of the field of neonatology. She developed the Apgar score, a method of assessing the health of newborn babies that has drastically reduced infant mortality over the world. (Finster M; Wood M. April 2005, Anesthesiology 102 4: 855–857)

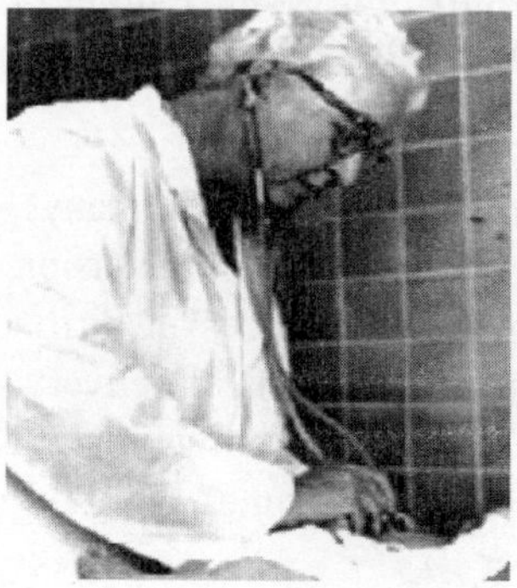

112. **(a)** Harry Fitch Klinefelter Jr.

1912 March 20-1990 February 20: Harry Fitch Klinefelter Jr.—An American endocrinologist, who studied the syndrome, which later was named as Klinefelter's syndrome. (47, XXY, or XXY syndrome) (Klinefelter, HF Jr; Reifenstein, EC Jr; Albright, F. 1942 J. Clin. Endocrinol Metab. 2:11-615–624)

113. **(a)** Jonas Edward Salk

1914 October 28-1995 June 23: Jonas Edward Salk—An American virologist, who discovered the first safe and effective polio vaccine. (Bookchin, Debbie, and Schumacher, Jim. The Virus and the Vaccine, Macmillan 2004 ISBN 0312342721)

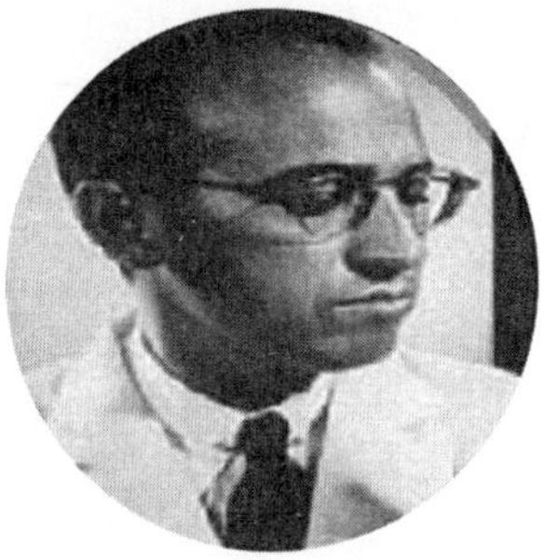

114. **(a)** Johann Sussmann Galant

1917: Johann Sussmann Galant—He described the deep abdominal reflex in newborn. In this reflex there is a contraction of the abdominal muscles on tapping the anterior superior iliac spine or touching the skin along spine from shoulder to hip. It is physiologically present until about the sixth month and after that age, it is always pathological. This reflex is named after him. (S. Galant Doctoral dissertation, Basel: Basler, 191)

115. **(a)** Lawson Wilkins

1918-1963: Lawson Wilkins—He was founder of the first pediatric endocrine clinic in the world at the Harriet Lane Home in Baltimore in 1935. He discontinued his private practice of 25 years to devote all of his time to research and teaching pediatric endocrinology. His book, 'The Diagnosis and Treatment of Endocrine Disorders in Childhood and Adolescence', is internationally accepted as the authoritative text in its field. (Web)

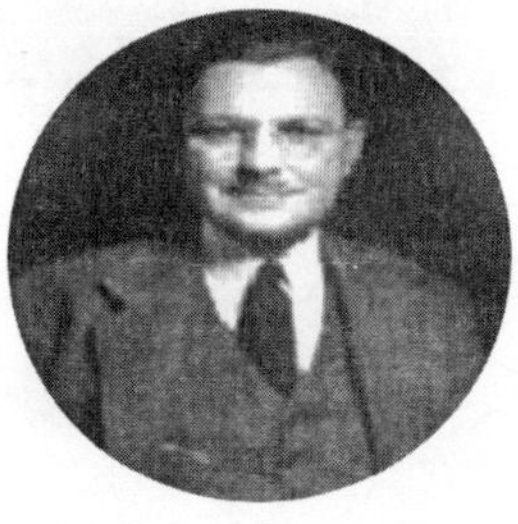

116. **(b)** Thomas Berry Brazelton

1918 May 10: Thomas Berry Brazelton (United States)—He was a pioneer in the psychology of children, regarding effect of young children's behavior, activity states and emotional expressions on the ways their parents react and thereby affect them.

He evaluated one new theory of assessment of the physical and neurological responses of newborns, also their emotional wellbeing and individual differences. This evaluation theory was known as, "Brazelton Neonatal Behavioral Assessment Scale". (Arnold Sameroff, ed. Organization and Stability in Newborn Behavior. Monograph of the Society for Research in Child Development, 1978, Vol. 43, No. 177)

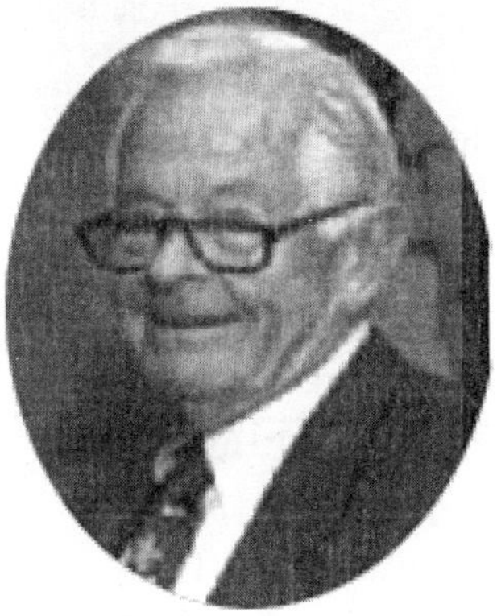

117. **(b)** J. B. Sidbury

1919: J. B. Sidbury–He was first to give blood transfusion through the Umbilical Vein in the New-born. (Web)

118. **(b)** James Mourilyan Tanner

1920 August 01- 2010 August 11: James Mourilyan Tanner—A British pediatric endocrinologist who was known for his development of the Tanner scale, which measures the stages of sexual development during puberty, which is called as Tanners score. (Jones, Steve; Martin, Robert D; Pilbeam, David R,Editors-1994, "Contributors". The Cambridge Encyclopedia of Human evolution, Cambridge University Press. P.x.)

119. **(b)** Thomas Chalmers Peebles

1921 June 5- 2010 July 8: Thomas Chalmers Peebles – He was an American physician, who first isolated the measles virus. He also stated that tetanus vaccine could be given once every 10 years, rather than annually as had been the widespread practice. (Martin, Douglas. "Dr. Thomas C. Peebles, Who Identified Measles Virus, Dies at 89", The New York Times, August 4, 2010)

120. **(d)** Rohrer

1921: Rohrer—He was first to propose Ponderal Index, which was used to measure of leanness of a person calculated as a relationship between mass and height. (Web)

121. **(d)** David Cornelius Morley

1923 June 15: David Cornelius Morley (Northampton) – A pediatrician, who designed first growth charts useful for children's progress of growth. (The independent—London: News-Tuesday 01 September 2009)

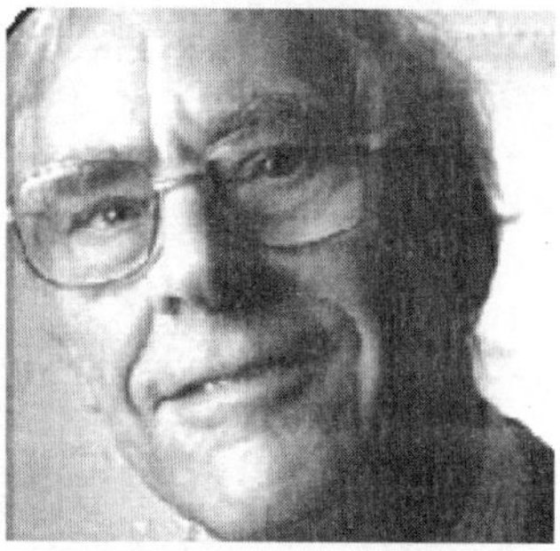

122. **(a)** Professor Wong Hock

1923 March 25-2008 December 28: Professor Wong Hock—He was the first professor of pediatrics in 1962, when he founded the department of Pediatrics in the National University of Singapore. He held the post until 1988.He had encyclopedic knowledge. He didn't even need notes while taking lectures. Those who knew him described him as a 'man of few words with a great depth of knowledge' He is often regarded as, 'the father of pediatrics in Singapore'.

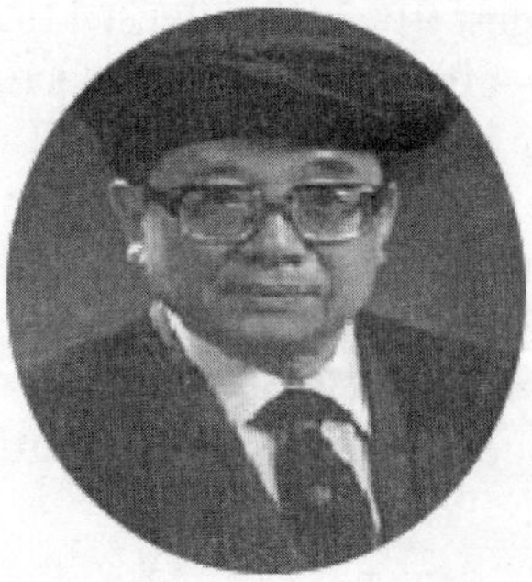

123. **(d)** 1st June

1925: International Children's Day – World Conference for the Wellbeing of Children in Geneva, Switzerland, proclaimed that June 1 will be the International Children's Day. It is usually marked with speeches on children's rights and wellbeing, children TV programs dedicated to children, families etc. ("June 1 International Children's Day". Diyifanwen.com. Retrieved 2009-08-16)

124. **(a)** Sir Robert Geoffrey Edwards

1925 September 27: Sir Robert Geoffrey Edwards—A British physiologist, who along with Patrick Steptoe, successfully pioneered conception through IVF, which led to the birth of the first test-tube baby, Louise Brown, on 25 July 1978. He was awarded the 2010 Nobel Prize in Physiology and Medicine "for the development of in vitro fertilization". (Barfield, N. -2004- "Sir George Robert Edwards OM CBE. 9 July 1908 — 2 March 2003: Elected F.R.S. 1968". Biographical Memoirs of Fellows of the Royal Society 50: 73)

125. **(a)** Baruch Samuel

1925 July 28–2011 April 5: Baruch Samuel (America)—He identified the Hepatitis B virus and later developed its diagnostic test and vaccine. For his research work he received the Nobel Prize. (Roger Highfield–6 April 2011 "The life and times of a vaccine pioneer", New Scientist, retrieved 21 April 2011)

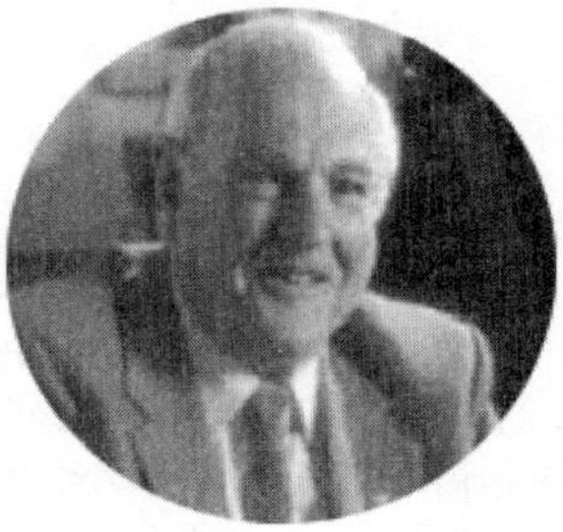

126. **(b)** Dharmendra Kumar Tyagi

1928–1969: Dharmendra Kumar Tyagi—He was an Assistant Commissioner for the Indian Family Planning program and early pioneer of family planning in India. He invented the "Red Triangle" symbol as a branding effort to familiarize and popularize the idea of family planning. (Avabai Bomanji Wadia, the light is ours: memoirs and movements, International Planned Parenthood Federation, 2001, ISBN 978-0-86089-125-3)

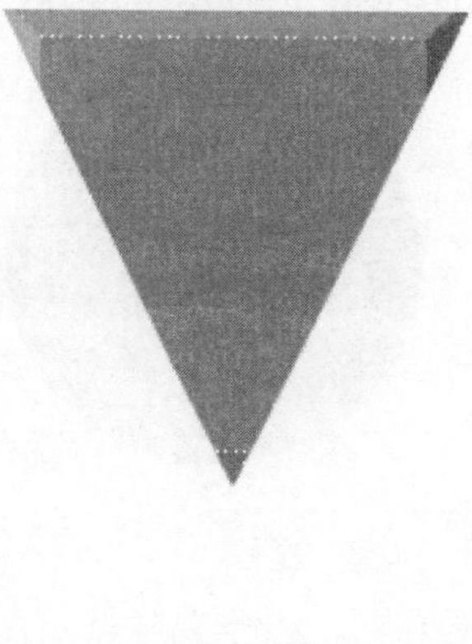

127. **(b)** Edwin Carlyle Carl Wood

1929 May 28-2011 September 23: Edwin Carlyle Carl Wood—He was an Australian gynecologist, known for his pioneering work developing the technique of in-vitro fertilization. He is best known as, "father of in-vitro fertilization". (I.V.F. In Vitro Fertilization, by Professor Carl Wood and Robyn Riley, New Edition, 1992)

128. **(b)** Subhash Mukhopadhyay

1931 January 16 - 1981 June 19: Subhash Mukhopadhyay – He was a physician from Kolkata (India) who created the world's second and India's first child named Durga alias Kanupriya Agarwal by in-vitro fertilization on October 3, 1978. This baby was born 67 days after the first IVF baby in United Kingdom. Unfortunately, he was not allowed to share his achievements with the international scientific community. Later he committed suicide. ("Subhash Mukhopadhyay—the unlucky doctor behind India's first test-tube baby". Sify.com. Oct 04, 2010)

129. **(b)** Dilip Mahalanabis

1934 November 12: Dilip Mahalanabis—He was the director of International Centre for Diarrheal Disease Research, Bangladesh at the time of the Bangladesh War. He discovered the inexpensive methods of oral rehydration therapy (ORT) for the treatment of diarrhea and cholera. It was an alternative to intravenous rehydration therapy where IVT is not available or feasible. (Guerrant, RL; Carneiro-Filho, BA; Dillingham, RA–August 2003– "Cholera, Diarrhea, and Oral Rehydration Therapy: Triumph and Indictment". Clinical Infectious Diseases 37- 3- 398–405. Retrieved -2008-07-15)

130. **(a)** Dr. Mukherjee

1938: Dr. Mukherjee—He reported the first case of beta thalassemia in India. (Pediatric on call– Dr. M. R. Lokeshwar)

131. **(c)** Louis K. Diamond

1942: Louis K. Diamond—He was the pioneer for doing exchange transfusion via umbilical vein as treatment for erythroblastosis fetalis. He established link between Rh isoimmunization and erythroblastosis fetalis. (Web)

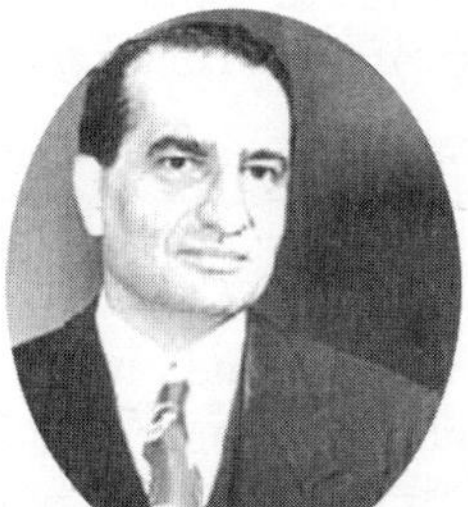

132. **(d)** 7th April

1948: World Health Day—World Health Organization held the First World Health Assembly, in which it was decided to celebrate World Health Day on 7th April of each year. It is an opportunity to draw the worldwide attention to a subject of major importance to global health each year. (World Health Organization: World Health Accessed 16 March 2011)

133. **(a)** Prof. C. C. de Silva

1949-66: Prof. C. C. de Silva—He was pioneer in the establishment of the Department of Pediatrics at the University of Ceylon in 1949. He was the first professor of pediatrics in Shri Lanka. He worked in the nutritional disorders, haemoglobinopathies and infective diarrheas. (Web)

134. **(c)** 14th November

1954: Children's Day—In India, it is celebrated on 14th November, the birthday of our first Prime Minister Jawaharlal Nehru. He was called Chacha Nehru by the kids. He emphasized the importance of giving love and affection to children, in whom he saw the bright future of India. ("National Children's Day website", 2007-03-14)

135. **(a)** Goran Haglund

1955: Goran Haglund—He was a pediatric anesthetist, who opened the first "Pediatric Emergency Ward (Pediatric Intensive Care Unit) with 7 beds at the Children's Hospital in Goteburg, Sweden. The next PICU's were established in 1961 by pediatric anesthetist Hans Feychting at St. Goran's Hospital in Stockholm and in 1963 by neonatologists G. H'Uault and J.B. Joly at Hospital St. Vincent de Paul in Paris. Also in 1963, pediatric anesthetists J.G. Stocks and I.H. McDonald opened the first Australian PICU at Melbourn's Royal Children's Hospital. The renowned G. Jackson Rees founded the first PICU in the U.K. in 1964, a sophisticated 13-bed facility, at the Alder Hey Children's Hospital, Liverpool. (G Haglund *et al.*: Pediatric emergency ward. In Stetson JB *et al.*: Neonatal Intensive Care, W H Green, 1976)

136. **(c)** Miss Sister Jean Ward

1956: Miss Sister Jean Ward – She was working at the premature unit at Rochford General Hospital at Essex, found the role of sunlight in neonatal jaundice. For her important observations she is often called as "Mother of phototherapy". (Cremer RJ, Perryman PW, Richards DH. Influence of light on the hyperbilirubinemia of infants. Lancet 1958; 1:1094-1097)

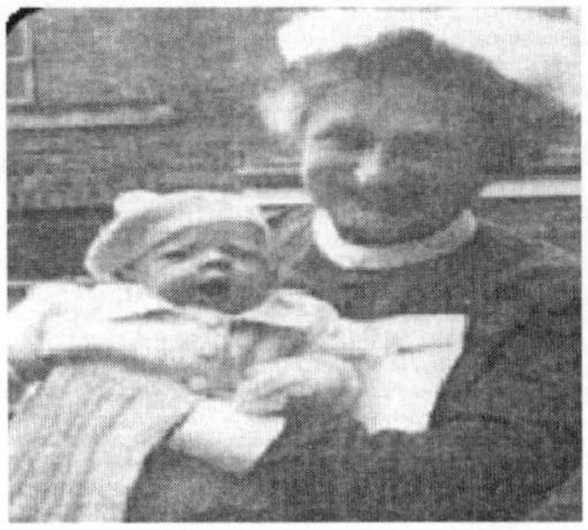

137. **(d)** 20th November

1959: Universal Children's Day—It was first declared by the United Nations General Assembly on November 20 annually. It was established to promote mutual exchange and understanding among children and promote the welfare of the world's children. It is also the anniversary of the day when the United Nations General Assembly adopted the Declaration of the Rights of the Child. (National childrens day.us.2007-03-14)

138. **(c)** Prof. Priyani Soysa

1966-1991: Prof. Priyani Soysa—She was the first pediatric woman professor in the Shri Lanka and she established the Pediatrics as a separate subject in the final year assessment. Her research included Nutrition and Infectious Diseases. She was an expert on infant feeding to the UN subcommittee on nutrition and the World Health Organization. (Web)

139. **(b)** 2nd April

1967: International Children's Literature Day – It coincides with the April 2, birthday of Hans Christian Andersen, the legendary Danish author of classic children's stories. This is a celebration of books aims to encourage children to read. (Web)

140. **(a)** Prof. Dr. Andrea Prader

1966: Prof. Dr. Andrea Prader—A pediatric endocrinologist of the University of Zurich, who developed an orchidometer—an instrument used to measure the volume of the testicles. (Prader, A. "Testicular size: Assessment and clinical importance" 1966, vol.7-240- 243)

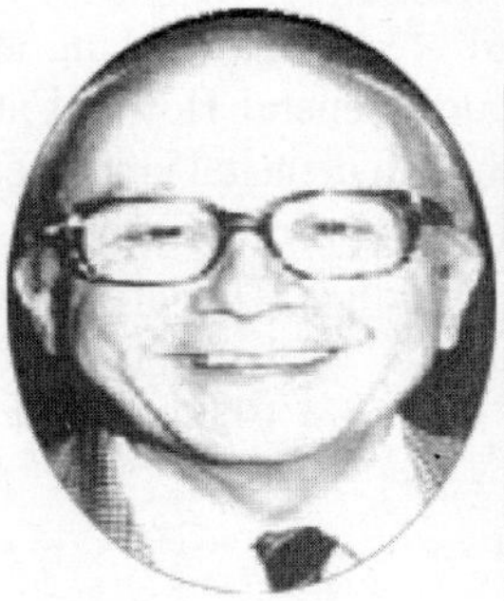

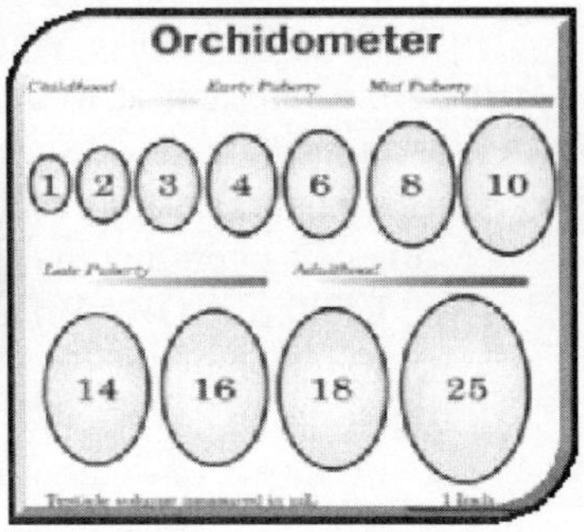

141. **(b)** Professor John Walker Smith

1968: Professor John Walker Smith—He is regarded as "father of pediatric gastroenterology" as he added new dimensions to it by discovering bowel diseases among the autistic patients at the Royal Free Hospital. (Web)

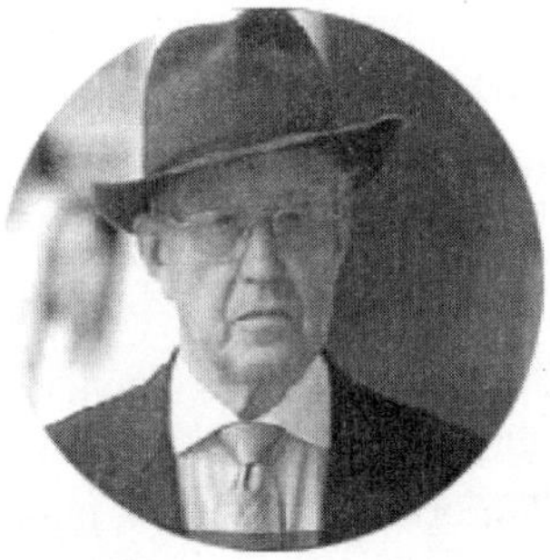

142. **(d)** Ali Maow Maalin

1977 October 26: Ali Maow Maalin (Somalia)—He was the world's last indigenous patient with smallpox on the earth. (Douglass, N.; Dumbell, K.R.; Independent evolution of monkey pox and variola viruses. J Virol, 1992; 66:7565-7)

143. **(b)** Louise Joy Brown

25 July 1978: Louise Joy Brown – He was the world's first human test tube baby born at Oldham General Hospital in England, credited to Robert Edward and Patrick Steptoe. Edward received the Nobel Prize in Medicine in 2010 for this effort. (Narayan, Pushpa October 5, 2010 "Indian lost test tube baby race to Edwards by 67 days". The Times of India. Retrieved —March 4, 2012)

144. **(a)** Dr. Edgar Rey Sanabria

1978: Dr. Edgar Rey Sanabria (Colombia)—He was the pioneer in establishing "Kangaroo Mother Care''. This had avoided the unnecessary burden in neonatal care units and alleviated the shortage of caregivers and lack of resources. He suggested that mothers have continuous skin-to-skin contact with their low birth weight babies to keep them warm and to give exclusive breastfeeding as they needed. (Charpak, N., Ruiz, J., Zupan, J.*et al.* 2005–Kangaroo mother care: 25 years after. Acta Pediatric, 94-5-514-522)

145. **(c)** 9 December 1979

1979 December 09—The global eradication of smallpox was certified, based on intense verification activities in countries and also by a commission of eminent scientists. (Fenner, Frank 2006—Nature, Nurture and Chance: The Lives of Frank and Charles Fenner. Canberra, ACT 0200: Australian National University Press, ISBN 1-920942-62-9)

146. **(a)** Child Rights and You

1979: Child Rights and You (CRY)—It is a non-profit, non-governmental organization in India, which aims to restore children's rights especially from India and works across levels from direct action to advocacy, mobilizing public opinion and policy change. It was started by Rippan Kapur, who died in 1994 at the age of 40. (CRY to focus on child rights The Hindu, April 10, 2006)

147. **(b)** Richard A. Gardner

1980: Parental alienation syndrome (PAS)—This term was coined by Richard A. Gardner. He described the disorder in which a child insults one parent without justification, due to a combination of factors, including indoctrination by the other parent. (Gardner, RA–2001 "Parental Alienation Syndrome, PAS-Sixteen Years Later". Academy Forum 45-1: 10–12. Retrieved 2009-03-31)

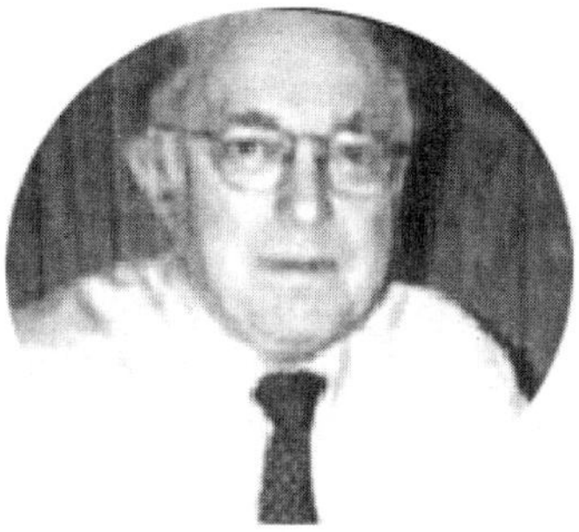

148. **(b)** 1980

1980: Over two decades fighting against smallpox, the World Health Organization had declared that the disease had been eradicated – the first disease in history to be eliminated by human effort. (Fenner, Frank, 2006–Nature, Nurture and Chance: Australian National University Press, ISBN 1-920942-62-9)

149. **(b)** 12th January

1984: National Youth Day—Government of India declared and decided to observe the birthday of Swami Vivekananda (12 January) as National Youth Day every year. (Web)

150. **(d)** Harsha

1986 August 16: Harsha—She was the first human test tube baby of the India, credited to T.C. Anand Kumar. ("Late honour for test tube pioneer". The Times of India, January 8, 2004. Retrieved, March 4, 2012)

151. **(a)** 17th April

1989: World Hemophilia Day–It is an international awareness day for hemophilia and other bleeding disorders. It is held annually on April 17, to raise funds and attract volunteers for the World Federation of Hemophilia. This is an international non-profit organization dedicated to improve the lives of people with hemophilia and other genetic bleeding disorders. (Web–hemophilia)

152. **(c)** 8th May

1994: International Thalassemia Day—It is held on the 8th of May, which is dedicated to patients with Thalassemia Major who are no longer with us but survive in our memories and to all those living, who together with their parents have joined in a long-term and difficult struggle to survive. ("Pediatric Thalassemia Treatment and Management". Medical Care, Open Publishing, 30 April 2010)

153. **(d)** 12th August

1999: International Youth Day – This was designated by the United Nations as an awareness day regarding youths and is celebrated August 12 every year. (Youth at the United Nations: 12 August–International Youth Day. Retrieved, 2008-08-12)

154. **(d)** Matt Daigle

2006: Matt Daigle—He created the International Breastfeeding Symbol in response to a contest hosted by Mothering magazine. He said his wife and son were the inspiration behind the symbol. (Mothering Magazine announces winner of International Breastfeeding Icon Design Contest, November 13, 2006)

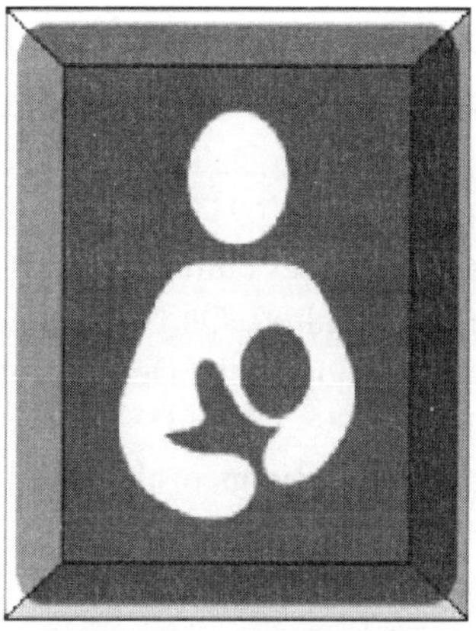

155. **(a)** 21 March

2006 March 21: World Down syndrome Day—The day and month were chosen to correspond with 21 and trisomy respectively. (Leshin, L. -2003 "Trisomy 21: The Story of Down Syndrome". Retrieved, 2006-05-21)

156. (b) 12th April

2011 April 08: International Day for Street Children—It was launched on 12th April by the Consortium for Street Children. (Web)

157. (a) 25th May

2012: International Missing Children's Day –This was declared on May 25, in order to remember those families around the world who gets their missing children. This is also remembered for those missing children who have been victims of crime and continues efforts to find out the missing children. (Web)

158. (b) Aamir Khan

2012 May 6: Satyamev Jayate–This was the show on the television debuted by Indian Bollywood actor and filmmaker Aamir Khan. It was based on female foeticide in India and through this they urged the Government of India to take action to stop illegal practice of female foeticide. This is the first programme to support national activity by private sector. ("Satyamev Jayate highlights the issue of female foeticide", IANS, Health, India, May 7, 2012)

159. (b) 14th November

In India, Children's Day is celebrated on 14 November, the birthday of the country's first Prime Minister Jawaharlal Nehru. Jawaharlal Nehru, who was fondly called Chacha Nehru (Uncle Nehru) or Chachaji (Uncle) by the kids, emphasized the importance of giving love and affection to children, whom he saw as the bright future of India.

160. (c) November 20

Universal Children's Day takes place annually on November 20. First proclaimed by the United Nations General Assembly in 1954. This day is observed to promote the objectives outlined in the Charter and for the welfare of children. On November 20, 1959 the United Nations adopted the Declaration of the Rights of the Child. The United Nations adopted the Convention on the Rights of the Child on November 20, 1989.

161. (d) 1st June

International Day for Protection of Children, observed in many countries as Children's Day on June 1 since 1950, was established by the Women's International Democratic Federation on its congress in Moscow (22 November 1949).

162. (b) 217 million

UNICEF defines child labour differently. A child, suggests UNICEF, is involved in child labour activities if between 5 and 11 years of age, he or she did at least one hour of economic activity or at least 28 hours of domestic work in a week, and in case of children between 12 to 14 years of age, he or she did at least 14 hours of economic activity or at least 42 hours of economic activity and domestic work per week.

The 2001 national census of India estimated the total number of child labour, aged 5–14, to be at 12.6 million, worldwide, about 217 million children work, many full-time. In 2001, out of a 12.6 million, about 12 million children in India were in a hazardous job.

163. (d) 14 years

The Factories Act of 1948— The Act prohibits the employment of children below the age of 14 years in any factory.

164. (d) 18 years

165. (d) 14 years

The Child Labour (Prohibition and Regulation) Act of 1986—The Act prohibits the employment of children below the age of 14 years in hazardous occupations identified in a list by the law.

166. (a) 6 to 14 years

The Right of Children to Free and Compulsory Education Act of 2009—The law mandates free and compulsory education to all children aged 6 to 14 years. This legislation also mandated that 25 percent of seats in every private school must be allocated for children from disadvantaged groups and physically challenged children.

167. (a) Education

Pratham is India's largest non-governmental organisation with the mission 'every child in school and learning well'. Founded in 1994, Pratham has aimed to reduce child labour and offer schooling to children irrespective of their gender, religion and social background.

168. (c) A male 21 or a female 18

The Child Marriage Restraint Act, 1929 was passed during the tenure of British rule on pre-partition India. It forbade the marriage of a male younger than 21 or a female younger than 18 for Hindus, Buddhists, Christians and most people of India.

169. **(a)** Child marriage

The Child Marriage Restraint Act, also called the Sarda Act, was a law to restrict the practice of child marriage. It was enacted on 1 April 1930, extended across the whole nation, with the exceptions of the states of Jammu and Kashmir, and applied to every Indian citizen. Its goal was to eliminate the dangers placed on young girls who could not handle the stress of married life and avoid early deaths. This Act defined a male child as 21 years or younger, a female child as 18 years or younger, and a minor as a child of either sex 18 years or younger. The punishment for a male between 18 and 21 years marrying a child became imprisonment of up to 15 days, a fine of 1,000 rupees, or both. The punishment for a male above 21 years of age became imprisonment of up to three months and a possible fine. The punishment for anyone who performed or directed a child marriage ceremony became imprisonment of up to three months and a possible fine, unless he could prove the marriage he performed was not a child marriage. The punishment for a parent or guardian of a child taking place in the marriage became imprisonment of up to three months or a possible fine. It was amended in 1940 and 1978 to continue raising the ages of male and female children.

170. **(b)** 18 years

UNICEF defines child marriage as a formal marriage or union before 18 years of age.

171. **(a)** 2006

The Prohibition of Child Marriage Act, 2006—Supreme Court, the Government of India brought the Prohibition of Child Marriage Act (PCMA) in 2006, and it came into effect on 1 November 2007 to address and fix the shortcomings of the Child Marriage Restraint Act. The change in name was meant to reflect the prevention and prohibition of child marriage, rather than restraining it. The previous Act also made it difficult and time consuming to act against child marriages and did not focus on authorities as possible figures for preventing the marriages. This Act kept the ages of adult males and females the same but made some significant changes to further protect the children. Boys and girls forced into child marriages as minors have the option of voiding their marriage up to two years after reaching adulthood, and in certain circumstances, marriages of minors can be null and void before they reach adulthood. All valuables, money, and gifts must be returned if the marriage is nullified, and the girl must be provided with a place of residency until she marries or becomes an adult.

Children born from child marriages are considered legitimate, and the courts are expected to give parental custody with the children's best interests in mind. Any male over 18 years of age who enters into a marriage with a minor or anyone who directs or conducts a child marriage ceremony can be punished with up to two years of imprisonment or a fine.

172. **(a)** Child marriage

Apni Beti, Apna Dhan (ABAD), which translates to "Our Daughter, Our Wealth", is one of India's first conditional cash transfer programme dedicated to delaying young marriages across the nation. In 1994, the Indian government implemented this programme in the state of Haryana. On the birth of a mother's first, second, or third child, they are set to receive ₹ 500, or US$11 within the first 15 days to cover their post-delivery needs. Along with this, the government gives ₹ 2,500, or US$55, to invest in a long-term savings bond in the daughter's name, which can be later cashed for ₹ 25,000, or US$ 550, after her 18th birthday. She can only receive the money if she is not married.

173. **(a)** Child abuse

Child abuse is the physical, sexual or emotional maltreatment or neglect of a child or children.

In the United States, the Centers for Disease Control and Prevention (CDC) and the Department for Children and Families (DCF) define child maltreatment as any act or series of acts of commission or omission by a parent or other caregiver that results in harm, potential for harm, or threat of harm to a child. Child abuse can occur in a child's home, or in the organizations, schools or communities the child interacts with. There are four major categories of child abuse: neglect, physical abuse, psychological or emotional abuse, and sexual abuse.

174. **(d)** All of above

175. **(a)** One night

Chapter 2

Clinical Pediatrics

1. **As per Hindu tradition when naming of baby is usually held?**
   (a) First 12 days (b) 20 days
   (c) 1 month (d) 1 year

2. **What are parts of pediatric age group?**
   (a) Newborn
   (b) Adolescency
   (c) Infant
   (d) All of the above

3. **What is age of majority in India?**
   (a) 12 years (b) 16 years
   (c) 18 years (d) 21 years

4. **What is voting age in India?**
   (a) 12 years (b) 14 years
   (c) 16 years (d) 18 years

5. **What is age limit for motorcycle without gear?**
   (a) 12 years (b) 14 years
   (c) 16 years (d) 18 years

6. **Marriageable age—21 years for males and 18 years for females.**
   (a) 21 years for males and 18 years for females
   (b) 16 years for males and 14 years for females
   (c) 18 years for males and 21 years for females
   (d) 14 years for males and 16 years for females

7. **In which grade of consanguinity there is marriage between brother and sister?**
   (a) Grade 4 (b) Grade 3
   (c) Grade 1 (d) Grade 2

8. **How consanguity is mentioned in pedigree chart?**
   (a) Double line (b) Single line
   (c) Circle (d) Triangle

9. **In which genetic disorder there is vertical transmission (affected individual will have affected parents)?**
   (a) X linked recessive disorder
   (b) X linked dominant disorder
   (c) Autosomal recessive disorder
   (d) Autosomal dominant disorder

10. **In which genetic disorder there is horizontal transmission (parents normal and siblings are affected)?**
    (a) X linked recessive disorder
    (b) X linked dominant disorder
    (c) Autosomal recessive disorder
    (d) Autosomal dominant disorder

11. **What is not feature of X- linked recessive disorder?**
    (a) Only males are affected
    (b) Both male and females are affected
    (c) Girls are carriers
    (d) Daughters are carriers

12. **What is visit pattern after 36th week till delivery (delivery at week 38-40) in ANC mother?**
    (a) Monthly (b) Weekly
    (c) Daily (d) Annually

13. **What is effect of advanced age of mother on foetus?**
    (a) Down syndrome (b) Dizygotic twins
    (c) Premature labour (d) All of the above

14. **Effect of advanced age of father on foetus?**
    (a) Osteogenesis imperfecta
    (b) Congenital deafness
    (c) Congenital heart diseases
    (d) All of the above

15. **Maternal diabetes mellitus is associated with which cardiac problems in baby?**
(a) Transposition of great vessels
(b) VSD
(c) PDA
(d) All of the above

16. **What are teratogenic effects of thalidomide?**
(a) TOF (b) Truncusarteriosus
(c) Limb anomalies (d) All of the above

17. **What is duration second stage of labor in primipara?**
(a) 1 hour (b) 2 hours
(c) 3 hours (d) 4 hours

18. **What is the duration of postnatal period?**
(a) 7 days (b) 28 days
(c) 42 days (d) 30 days

19. **Children are defined as living in overcrowded dwellings when there is a ratio of more than______ people per room.**
(a) Two (b) Three
(c) Four (d) Five

20. **After what age child is calculated as full unit?**
(a) 10 years (b) 12 years
(c) 16 years (d) 18 years

21. **What is minimum floor space area required for a married couple?**
(a) 5 sq. metre (b) 7 sq. metre
(c) 9 sq. metre (d) 11 sq. metre

22. **As per 2012 what is poverty line in urban area?**
(a) Rs. 21.75 per capita (b) Rs. 23.45 per capita
(c) Rs. 27.10 per capita (d) Rs. 28.65 per capita

23. **As per 2012 what is poverty line in rural area?**
(a) Rs 21.75 in rural areas
(b) Rs 28.65 in rural areas
(c) Rs 22.42 in rural areas
(d) Rs 29.22 in rural areas

24. **As per Prasad's classification what per capita income for poor class?**
(a) 15 rupees (b) 20 rupees
(c) 24 rupees (d) 30 rupees

25. **As per modified Prasad's classification what per capita income for high class?**
(a) 1905-3809 (b) 6350-12699
(c) 3810-6349 (d) 12700 above

26. **According to socioeconomic status what is class grading for doctors?**
(a) Class 1 (b) Class 3
(c) Class 4 (d) Class 2

27. **As per Pareekh classification for rural area is not a characteristic of it?**
(a) Pareekh classification
(b) Education of family head
(c) Housing
(d) Religion

28. **Kuppuswami's classification is based on:**
(a) Education (b) Occupation
(c) Income of family head (d) All of the above

29. **For examination of child between the age group of 3 months to 1 year which is ideal position?**
(a) Examination table
(b) Standing
(c) Female attendant or nurse should be present
(d) Mother's lap

30. **What are sites to take temperature in children?**
(a) Oral temperature
(b) Axillary temperatures
(c) Rectal temperatures
(d) All of the above

31. **What is average normal oral temperature?**
(a) 98.6°F (37°C) (b) 97.6°F
(c) 99.6°F (d) 101.6°F

32. **Which is generally thought to be the most accurate site for child's temperature?**
(a) Axillary temperatures
(b) Oral temperature
(c) Tympanic temperature
(d) Rectal temperatures

33. **By which fingers pulse is felt?**
(a) Index and ring finger (b) Index and thumb
(c) Index and middle fingers (d) None

34. **These are the sites for palpation of pulse:**
(a) Ulnar artery (b) Carotid artery
(c) Radial artery (d) All of the above

35. **For every 1 degree rise in temperature the increase in pulse rate occurs by:**
(a) 10 beats /min (b) 20 beats /min
(c) 30 beats /min (d) 40 beats /min

36. What is cause of bradycardia?
(a) Digoxin (b) Hypoxia
(c) Hypothyroidism (d) All of the above

37. Which drug causes tachycardia?
(a) Atropine (b) Digoxin
(c) Atenelol (d) Propranolol

38. Irregular regular pulse rhythm is seen in:
(a) Mitral stenosis
(b) Pulmonary stenosis
(c) Atrial tachyarrhythmia with fixed AV block
(d) Aortic prolapsed

39. Irregular regular pulse rhythm is seen in:
(a) Atrial or ventricular ectopics
(b) Atrial fibrillation
(c) Atrial tachyarrhythmia with varied AV block
(d) All of the above

40. Collapsing pulse is seen in:
(a) Aortic regurgitation
(b) Patent ductus arteriosus
(c) A.V. fistulas
(d) All of the above

41. Pulses alternans type of pulse is seen in:
(a) Right ventricular failure
(b) Right bundle branch block
(c) Left ventricular failure
(d) Left bundle branch block

42. Anacrotic pulse is seen in:
(a) Mitral stenosis (b) Aortic stenosis
(c) Pulmonary stenosis (d) Aortic regurgitation

43. Pulsus paradoxus type of pulse is seen in:
(a) Cardiac tamponade
(b) Aortic regurgitation
(c) A. V. fistulas
(d) Patent ductus arteriosus

44. What is normal pulse pressure?
(a) 10-20 mmHg (b) 30 - 60 mmHg
(c) 60-75 mmHg (d) 80 mmHg

45. Small volume pulse is seen in:
(a) Cardiac tamponade (b) A.V. fistulas
(c) Aortic regurgitation (d) Mitral stenosis

46. Large volume pulse is seen in:
(a) Cardiact amponade (b) Cardiac failure
(c) Aortic regurgitation (d) Mitral stenosis

47. Normal pulse rate in newborn is:
(a) 70-80 / min (b) 130 - 150 / min
(c) 90-110 / min (d) 110-120 / min

48. Capillary refill time is prolonged in:
(a) Arterial occlusion (b) Hypovolemic shock
(c) Hypothermia (d) All of the above

49. What is respiratory rate in premature neonate?
(a) 40-70/min (b) 35-55
(c) 30-45 (d) 25-40

50. Kussmaul breathing is seen in:
(a) Respiratory distress
(b) Pulmonary hypertension
(c) Diabetic ketoacidosis
(d) Metabolic acidosis

51. Cheyne-Stokes respiration is indicative of:
(a) Diabetic ketoacidosis
(b) Apnea
(c) Respiratory distress
(d) None

52. Biot's respiration is indicative of:
(a) Poor prognosis (b) Good prognosis
(c) Shock (d) None

53. What is grading of dyspnea for difficulty during dressing?
(a) Grade 4 (b) Grade 3
(c) Grade 2 (d) Grade 1

54. What is neonatal blood pressure cuff size?
(a) 5 cms (b) 7.5 cms
(c) 2.5 cms (d) 10 cms

55. What is infant's blood pressure cuff size?
(a) 2.5 cms (b) 5 cms
(c) 7.5 cms (d) 10 cms

56. Methods to record blood pressure:
(a) Palpatory (b) Auscultatory
(c) Flush method (d) All of the above

57. Normal systolic blood pressure in premature baby is:
(a) 65-85 mmHg (b) 55-75 mmHg
(c) 70-90 mmHg (d) 95-110 mmHg

58. Hill's sign signifies difference between the arms and the legs blood pressure of:
(a) > 20 mmHg (b) 10 mmHg
(c) 15 mmHg (d) 25 mmHg

59. In jugular venous pressure what does a wave signifies?
(a) Ventricular systole (b) Atrial systole
(c) Ventricular diastole (d) Atrial diastole

60. In jugular venous pressure what does prominent V wave signifies?
(a) Pulmonary stenosis
(b) Tricuspid regurgitation
(c) Aortic stenosis
(d) Mitral prolapsed

61. Low jugular venous pressure seen in:
(a) Hypovolemia (b) Mitral stenosis
(c) Right sided heart failure (d) None

62. Elevated jugular venous pressure is seen:
(a) Pulmonic stenosis
(b) Constrictive pericarditis
(c) Superior vena cava obstruction
(d) All of the above

63. Microcephaly is defined as head circumference below:
(a) 2SD (b) 3 SD
(c) 1 SD (d) None

64. Microcephaly is seen in:
(a) Fetal hydantoin syndrome
(b) Post natal insult
(c) Intrauterine CMV infections
(d) All of the above

65. Macrocephaly is defined as head circumference more than:
(a) 3 SD (b) 1 SD
(c) 1.5 SD (d) 2 SD

66. Macrocephaly is seen in:
(a) Achondroplasia (b) Rickets
(c) Mucopolysaccharidosis (d) All of the above

67. Normal cranium is known as:
(a) Turricocephaly (b) Mesocephaly
(c) Brachicephaly (d) Dolicocephaly

68. Short cranium is called as:
(a) Turricephaly (b) Mesocephaly
(c) Brachicephaly (d) Dolicocephaly

69. Long cranium is known as:
(a) Turricephaly (b) Mesocephaly
(c) Brachicephaly (d) Dolicocephaly

70. High peaked shape of skull is seen in:
(a) Turricephaly (b) Mesocephaly
(c) Brachicephaly (d) Dolicocephaly

71. Craniotabes is seen in:
(a) Rickets (b) Hydrocephalus
(c) Osteogenesis imperfecta (d) All of the above

72. Positive Macewan's sign is suggestive of:
(a) Raised intracranial tension
(b) Hypothyroidism
(c) Skull fracture
(d) Craniopharyngioma

73. Frontal boosting is seen in:
(a) Rickets (b) Achondroplasia
(c) Congenital syphilis (d) All of the above

74. When anterior fontanelle closes?
(a) Just after birth (b) 2-3 months
(c) 6 months (d) 9-18 months

75. Delayed closure of anterior fontanelle occurs in:
(a) Rickets
(b) Congenital hypothyroidism
(c) Down syndrome
(d) All of the above

76. Small anterior fontanelle is suggestive of:
(a) Increased intracranial tension
(b) Rickets
(c) Congenital hypothyroidism
(d) Craniosynostosis

77. Sunken anterior fontanelle is suggestive of:
(a) Increased intracranial tension
(b) Rickets
(c) Congenital hypothyroidism
(d) Dehydration

78. Bulging anterior fontanelle is suggestive of:
(a) Increased intracranial tension
(b) Rickets
(c) Congenital hypothyroidism
(d) Dehydration

79. Bruit on auscultation of skull is suggestive of:
(a) Increased intracranial tension
(b) Rickets
(c) Congenital hypothyroidism
(d) Dehydration

80. Flag sign consists of:
(a) Pigmented and depigmented hairs
(b) Lusterless hairs
(c) Easily plucable hairs
(d) All of the above

81. Flag sign is suggestive of:
(a) Malnutrition (b) Overhydration
(c) Obesity (d) Telogen

82. Increased quantity of hairs are seen in:
(a) Cushing's syndrome
(b) Congenital adrenal hyperplasia
(c) Intake of dilantin
(d) All of the above

83. Low hair line in back below C4 spine is seen in:
(a) Turner's syndrome
(b) Noonan's syndrome
(c) Hypothyroidism
(d) Treacher Collins syndrome

84. Mongoloid facies is seen in:
(a) Down's syndrome
(b) Noonan's syndrome
(c) Hypothyroidism
(d) Treacher Collins syndrome

85. Mongoloid facies means:
(a) Upward slanting of eyes
(b) Epicanthic folds
(c) Small nose with flat nasal bridge
(d) All of the above

86. Moon face is seen in:
(a) Cushing's syndrome
(b) Nephrotic syndrome
(c) Mobius syndrome
(d) Soto syndrome

87. Coarse facies is seen in:
(a) Hypothyroidism (b) Hurlers syndrome
(c) Soto syndrome (d) All of the above

88. Mask like facies seen in:
(a) Wilson's disease (b) Mobius syndrome
(c) Depression (d) All of the above

89. Triangular facies is indicative of:
(a) Russel Silver syndrome (b) Mobius syndrome
(c) Soto syndrome (d) Nephrotic syndrome

90. Upper eyelid coloboma is seen in:
(a) Goldenhar's syndrome
(b) Noonan's syndrome
(c) Hypothyroidism
(d) Treacher Collins syndrome

91. Lower eyelid coloboma is seen in:
(a) Goldenhar's syndrome
(b) Noonan's syndrome
(c) Hypothyroidism
(d) Treacher Collins syndrome

92. Ptosis is observed in conditions like:
(a) Noonan's syndrome (b) Myasthenia gravis
(c) Horner's syndrome (d) All of the above

93. Antimongoloidslantis seen in:
(a) Down's syndrome (b) Horner's syndrome
(c) Turner's syndrome (d) Noonan's syndrome

94. Proptosis is observed in:
(a) Retinoblastoma (b) Apert's syndrome
(c) Hyperthyroidism (d) All of the above

95. Epicanthal fold is seen in:
(a) Down's syndrome (b) Noonan's syndrome
(c) Turner's syndrome (d) All of the above

96. Hypertelorism is seen in:
(a) Down's syndrome (b) Noonan's syndrome
(c) Turner's syndrome (d) All of the above

97. Bitot spots is seen in:
(a) Sclera (b) Eyelid
(c) Iris (d) Conjunctiva

98. Congenital cataract is seen in:
(a) Rubella (b) Galactosemia
(c) Wilson's disease (d) All of the above

99. Blue sclera is suggestive of:
(a) Marfan's syndrome
(b) Osteogenesis imperfecta
(c) Ehler Danlos syndrome
(d) All of the above

100. On examination of fundus papilledema is seen in:
(a) Intracranial space occupying lesion
(b) Meningitis
(c) Intracranial bleed
(d) All of the above

101. Ear tag is seen in:
(a) Klinefelter's syndrome (b) Goldenhar syndrome
(c) Mobius syndrome (d) Soto syndrome

102. Deformed pinna is seen in:
(a) Fragile X syndrome
(b) Blooms syndrome
(c) Xeroderma pigmentosa
(d) Mucopolysaccharides

103. Large prominent ear is seen in:
(a) Fragile X syndrome
(b) Blooms syndrome
(c) Xeroderma pigmentosa
(d) Mucopolysaccharides

104. Low set ears is a feature of:
(a) Down's syndrome (b) Turner's syndrome
(c) Mucopolysaccharides (d) All of the above

105. Koplik's spots on buccal mucosa is diagnostic of:
(a) Chicken pox (b) Monkey pox
(c) Rubella (d) Measles

106. Delayed primary dentition seen in:
(a) Vitamin D deficiency (b) Calcium deficiency
(c) Hypothyroidism (d) All of the above

107. Swollen, spongy, bleeding gums is seen in:
(a) Scurvy (b) Rickets
(c) Chondrodysplasia (d) Hemophilia

108. Gum hyperplasia is observed with:
(a) Treatment with phenytoin
(b) Scurvy
(c) Leukemia
(d) All of the above

109. Gum blue line is observed in:
(a) Lead poisoning (b) Mercury poisoning
(c) Copper poisoning (d) Tobacco chewing

110. Macroglossia is observed with:
(a) Beckwith syndrome (b) Amyloidosis
(c) Congenital hypothyroidism (d) All of the above

111. Tongue is observed in:
(a) Typhoid fever (b) Uraemia
(c) Candidiasis (d) All of the above

112. Raw Beefy tongue is seen in:
(a) Niacin deficiency (b) Biotin deficiency
(c) Pyridoxin deficiency (d) Thiamine deficiency

113. Strawberry tongue is characteristic of:
(a) Strawberry tumour (b) Kawasaki disease
(c) Infective endocarditis (d) All of he above

114. Lip Rhagades is seen in conditions like:
(a) Congenital syphilis
(b) Riboflavin deficiency
(c) Iron deficiency
(d) All of the above

115. Central cyanosis is seen in:
(a) Respiratory distress syndrome
(b) Foreign body in respiratory tract
(c) Acute severe asthma
(d) All of the above

116. Single palmar crease is seen in:
(a) Down's syndrome (b) Turner's syndrome
(c) Burns (d) Trauma

117. Clubbing is seen in:
(a) AV fistula
(b) Intrathoracic tuberculosis
(c) Lung abscess
(d) All of the above

118. Tanner score is related to:
(a) Lymphatic growth (b) Sexual maturity
(c) Respiratory maturity (d) None

119. Adult testicular volume is:
(a) 5 ml (b) 20 ml
(c) 10ml (d) 25ml

120. Neonatal penile length is:
(a) 2cm (b) 6cm
(c) 4cm (d) 10cm

121. Glasgow coma scale consists of:
(a) Eye opening (b) Motor activity
(c) Verbal response (d) All of the above

122. What is the cause of anosmia?
(a) Meningitis (b) Refsum's disease
(c) Kallman's syndrome (d) All of the above

123. What is normal visual acuity?
(a) 6/6 (b) 3/6
(c) 6/18 (d) 20/20

124. Average field of vision at outward direction is:
(a) 100 degree (b) 75 degree
(c) 60 degree (d) 55 degree

125. **What is the cause of papilloedema?**
(a) Pseudotumor cerebri
(b) Central retinal vein thrombosis
(c) Cavernous sinus thrombosis
(d) All of the above

126. **What is the cause of nystagmus?**
(a) Optic atrophy (b) Cerebellar ataxia
(c) Friedreich's ataxia (d) All of the above

127. **What is the cause of non-paralytic squint?**
(a) Cerebral palsy
(b) Retrolental fibroplasias
(c) Optic atrophy
(d) All of the above

128. **What is the cause of ptosis?**
(a) Myesthenia gravis (b) Horner's syndrome
(c) Botulism (d) All of the above

129. **What is the cause of diplopia?**
(a) Raised intracranial tension
(b) Labyrinthine involvement
(c) 3rd cranial nerve palsy
(d) All of the above

130. **Which muscle is innervated by trochlear nerve?**
(a) Superior oblique muscle of the eye
(b) Lateral rectus
(c) Medial rectus
(d) Superior rectus

131. **Lateral rectus muscle of the eye is innervated by:**
(a) Trochlear nerve (b) Trigeminal nerve
(c) Facial nerve (d) Abducens nerve

132. **Which is the largest of the cranial nerve?**
(a) Trigeminal nerve (b) Facial nerve
(c) Trochlear nerve (d) Abducens nerve

133. **Which is the branch of trigeminal nerve?**
(a) Ophthalmic nerve (b) Maxillary nerve
(c) Mandibular nerve (d) All of the above

134. **Which cranial nerve controls the muscles of facial expression?**
(a) Facial nerve (b) Trochlear nerve
(c) Trigeminal nerve (d) Abducens nerve

135. **Which nerve gives sensory - special taste sensations on the anterior 2/3rd of tongue?**
(a) Trochlear nerve (b) Trigeminal nerve
(c) Abducens nerve (d) Facial nerve

136. **Liver span at birth is:**
(a) 5 cm (b) 5.6 to 5.9 cm
(c) 6 cm (d) 7.5 cm

137. **For positive puddle sign minimum amount of ascites fluid is:**
(a) 10-20 ml (b) 500 ml
(c) 100-120 ml (d) 1000-1500 ml

138. **Fluid thrill is present in which grades of ascites?**
(a) Grade 3 (b) Grade 2
(c) Grade 1 (d) Grade 0

139. **Which cranial nerve is responsible for transmission of equilibrium (balance) information from the inner ear to the brain?**
(a) Trochlear nerve
(b) Facial nerve
(c) Vestibulocochlear nerve
(d) Abducens nerve

140. **Which cranial nerve is responsible for sensation over posterior 1/3rd of tongue?**
(a) Facial nerve (b) Trochlear nerve
(c) Abducens nerve (d) Vagus nerve

141. **Spinal accessory cranial nerve provides motor innervations to which muscle of the neck?**
(a) Sternocleido mastoid (b) Artenoid
(c) Posterior pharyngeal (d) Trapezius muscle

142. **Which cranial nerve is responsible for protrution of tongue?**
(a) Hypoglossal nerve
(b) Facial nerve
(c) Trochlear nerve
(d) Abducens nerve

143. **Upper motor neuron is located in:**
(a) Thalamus (b) Hypothalamus
(c) Pons (d) Cerebral cortex

144. **Grade the power–Able to move against the gravity but not against resistance:**
(a) Grade 3 (b) Grade 2
(c) Grade 1 (d) Grade 0

145. **Hypertonia is caused by:**
(a) Strychnine poisoning (b) Tetanus
(c) Tetany (d) All of the above

146. **Hypotonia is caused by:**
(a) Hypothyroidism (b) Myasthenia gravis
(c) Lead poisoning (d) All of the above

147. Cremasteric reflex is absent in:
(a) Testicular torsion
(b) Upper and lower motor neuron disorders
(c) A spine injury of L1-L2
(d) All of the above

148. Absence or decreased knee reflex is known as:
(a) Chadwicks sign (b) Higashi sign
(c) Mobius sign (d) Westphal's sign

149. What is root value of knee jerk?
(a) L2- L4 (b) L1 -L2
(c) L5- S1 (d) S1-S2

150. What is root value of ankle jerk / Achilles reflex?
(a) S1-S2 (b) L1 -L2
(c) L2-L4 (d) L5- S1

151. Classically delayed Achilles reflex is seen in:
(a) Down syndrome (b) Malnutrition
(c) Hypothyroidism (d) Hepatic failure

152. Absence of triceps reflex is seen in:
(a) Poliomyelitis
(b) Myopathy
(c) Lower motor neurone lesion
(d) All of the above

153. Irregular triceps reflex is seen in:
(a) Hypothyroidism (b) Juvenile diabetes
(c) Trauma (d) Hyperthyroidism

154. Clonus is graded as:
(a) Grade 4 reflex (b) Grade 3 reflex
(c) Grade 2 reflex (d) Grade 1 reflex

155. Deep reflexes are absent in:
(a) Friedreich's ataxia
(b) Severe spastic children
(c) Down's syndrome
(d) All of the above

156. Deep reflexes are brisk in:
(a) Tetanus (b) Cerebral palsy
(c) Hysteria (d) All of the above

157. Which is the test for coordination?
(a) Dysdiadochokinesia (b) Rebound test
(c) Finger nose test (d) All of the above

158. Sensory ataxia is seen in:
(a) Temporal lobe epilepsy
(b) Hippocampal agenesis
(c) Broca's aphasia
(d) Tabes dorsalis

159. Spastic gait is seen in:
(a) Quadriplegia (b) Sepsis
(c) Hyperthyroidism (d) Cerebral palsy

160. Circumduction gait is seen:
(a) Medulloblastoma (b) Brain abscess
(c) Anticonvulsant drugs (d) Hemiplegia

161. Waddling type of gait is observed in:
(a) Distal myopathies (b) Polyneurirtis
(c) Proximal myopathies (d) Hip dislocation

162. Which is the cause of ataxia?
(a) Cerebellitis
(b) Dandy Walker's syndrome
(c) Arnold Chairi syndrome
(d) All of the above

163. Which is the involuntary movement?
(a) Myoclonus (b) Tics
(c) Ballismus (d) All of the above

164. What is cause of chorea?
(a) Rheumatic fever (b) Wilson's disease
(c) Amphetamine (d) All of the above

165. Hypertrophy of the muscle is seen in:
(a) UMN lesions
(b) Extrapyramidal lesions
(c) LMN lesions
(d) None

166. Atrophy of the muscle is seen in:
(a) UMN lesions
(b) Extrapyramidal lesions
(c) LMN lesions
(d) None

167. Which is sign of meningeal irritation?
(a) Nuchal rigidity (b) Kernig's sign
(c) Brudzinski sign (d) All of the above

168. Upper respiratory tract consists of:
(a) Nasal cavity (b) Pharynx
(c) Larynx (d) All of the above

169. Lower respiratory tract consists of:
(a) Trachea (b) Primary bronchi
(c) Lungs (d) All of the above

170. Right lung has how many lobes:
(a) Three lobes (b) Two lobes
(c) One lobe (d) Four lobes

171. Pectus excavatum means:
(a) Barrel chest
(b) Prominence of the sternum
(c) Absence of ribs
(d) Depression in the sternum

172. Pectus carinatum means:
(a) Barrel chest
(b) Prominence of the sternum
(c) Absence of ribs
(d) Depression in the sternum

173. Apex beat is obscured in:
(a) Obesity (b) Emphysema
(c) Pericardial effusion (d) All of the above

174. Increased vocal fremitus is observed in:
(a) Consolidation (b) Pleural effusion
(c) Pneumothorax (d) Bronchial obstruction

175. Decreased vocal fremitus is observed in:
(a) Pneumothorax (b) Pleural effusion
(c) Bronchial obstruction (d) All of the above

176. Hyper resonant percussion note is seen in:
(a) Consolidation (b) Bronchial obstruction
(c) Pleural effusion (d) Pneumothorax

177. Impaired percussion note is seen in:
(a) Pleural effusion (b) Bronchial obstruction
(c) Pneumothorax (d) Consolidation

178. Stony dullness percussion note is seen in:
(a) Pleural effusion
(b) Bronchial obstruction
(c) Pneumothorax
(d) Consolidation

179. Vesicular type of breath sound has following characteristic:
(a) Low pitched
(b) No pause
(c) Rustling or breezy quality
(d) All of the above

180. Bronchial type of breath sound has following characteristic:
(a) Definite pause (b) High pitched
(c) Blowing quality (d) All of the above

181. Which is a type of crepitation?
(a) Fine (b) Medium
(c) Coarse (d) All of the above

182. In which condition fine crackle is audible?
(a) Pneumonia (b) Pulmonary edema
(c) Bronchiolitis (d) All of the above

183. Increased vocal resonance is observed in:
(a) Consolidation (b) Bronchial obstruction
(c) Pleural effusion (d) Pneumothorax

184. Decreased vocal resonance is observed in:
(a) Consolidation (b) Bronchial obstruction
(c) Pleural effusion (d) Pneumothorax

185. Aortic area pulsations are observed in:
(a) Aortic regurgitation
(b) Aortic aneurysm
(c) Dilatation of ascending aorta
(d) All of the above

186. Pulmonary area pulsations are observed in:
(a) Pulmonary hypertension
(b) Aortic regurgitation
(c) Dilatation of ascending aorta
(d) Aortic aneurysm

187. Carotid area pulsations are observed in:
(a) Hyperdynamic states (b) Coarctation of aorta
(c) Aortic regurgitation (d) All of the above

188. Supra clavicular pulsations are observed in:
(a) Aortic regurgitation (b) Coarctation of aorta
(c) Tricuspid regurgitation (d) Mitral stenosis

189. Epigastric pulsations are observed in:
(a) Aortic regurgitation (b) Coarctation of aorta
(c) Tricuspid regurgitation (d) Mitral stenosis

190. Hepatic pulsations are observed in:
(a) Aortic regurgitation
(b) Tricuspid regurgitation
(c) Coarctation of aorta
(d) Mitral stenosis

191. Tapping apex beat is observed in:
(a) Aortic regurgitation
(b) Mitral stenosis
(c) Aortic stenosis
(d) Tricuspid regurgitation

192. Heaving apex beat is observed in:
(a) Aortic regurgitation
(b) Mitral stenosis
(c) Aortic stenosis
(d) Tricuspid regurgitation

193. Hyper dynamic apex beat is observed in:
(a) Mitral stenosis
(b) Atrial septal defect
(c) Mitral regurgitation
(d) Tricuspid regurgitation

194. Para sternal heave is observed in:
(a) Mitral regurgitation
(b) Mitral stenosis
(c) Atrial septal defect
(d) All of the above

195. Palpable P_2 heart sound in:
(a) Aortic stenosis
(b) Mitral stenosis
(c) Atrial septal defect
(d) Pulmonary hypertension

196. Palpable A_2 heart sound in:
(a) Aortic stenosis
(b) Mitral stenosis
(c) Atrial septal defect
(d) Pulmonary hypertension

197. Opening snap is heard in:
(a) Aortic stenosis
(b) Pulmonary hypertension
(c) Atrial septal defect
(d) Mitral stenosis

198. Thrills in carotid areas is suggestive of:
(a) Pulmonary hypertension
(b) Atrial septal defect
(c) Aortic stenosis
(d) Mitral stenosis

199. Thrills in aortic areas is suggestive of:
(a) Atrial septal defect
(b) Aortic stenosis
(c) Mitral stenosis
(d) Pulmonary hypertension

200. Thrills in pulmonary areas is suggestive of:
(a) Pulmonary stenosis (b) ASD
(c) VSD (d) All of the above

201. Continuous thrill is suggestive of:
(a) PDA (b) ASD
(c) VSD (d) Mitral stenosis

202. Apical diastolic thrill is suggestive of:
(a) Mitral regurgitation (b) VSD
(c) ASD (d) Mitral stenosis

203. Apical systolic thrill is suggestive of:
(a) Mitral regurgitation (b) VSD
(c) ASD (d) Mitral stenosis

204. Lower left para sternal thrill is suggestive of:
(a) Mitral regurgitation (b) VSD
(c) ASD (d) Mitral stenosis

205. Loud first heart sound is heard in:
(a) Normally in children (b) Mitral stenosis
(c) Tricuspid stenosis (d) All of the above

206. Soft heart sound is heard in:
(a) Pericardial effusion (b) Emphysema
(c) Tricuspid regurgitation (d) All of the above

207. Split first heart sound is heard in:
(a) RBBB (b) AV block
(c) Atrial fibrillation (d) All of the above

208. Wide second sound split is heard in:
(a) RBBB
(b) Pulmonary stenosis
(c) Ventricular septal defect
(d) All of the above

209. Reverse split sound is heard in:
(a) LBBB (b) Aortic stenosis
(c) Coarctation of arota (d) All of the above

210. Single second heart sound is heard in:
(a) Pulmonary stenosis (b) Tetralogy of Fallot
(c) Pulmonary atresia (d) All of the above

211. Third heart sound is heard in:
(a) Normally in children
(b) Myocarditis
(c) Hypertrophic cardiomyopathy
(d) All of the above

212. Loud first heart sound is heard in:
(a) Mitral stenosis (b) Tricuspid stenosis
(c) Sinus tachycardia (d) All of the above

213. Fourth heart sound is heard in:
(a) Hypertrophic cardiomyopathy
(b) Myocarditis
(c) Normally in children
(d) All of the above

214. Multiple auscultatory clicks are heard in:
(a) Hypertrophic cardiomyopathy
(b) Ebstein's anomaly
(c) Sinus tachycardia
(d) Myocarditis

215. Nada's major criteria includes:
(a) Systolic murmur with thrill
(b) Cyanosis
(c) Diastolic murmur
(d) All of the above

216. Pathological murmur is associated with:
(a) Murmur associated with thrill
(b) All diastolic murmurs
(c) With abnormal heart sound
(d) All of the above

217. Ejection systolic murmur is heard in:
(a) Aortic stenosis (b) Pulmonary stenosis
(c) Atrial septal defect (d) All of the above

218. Pan systolic murmur is heard in:
(a) Ventricular septal defect (b) Mitral regurgitation
(c) Tricuspid regurgitation (d) All of the above

219. Late systolic murmur is heard in:
(a) Mitral valve prolapse
(b) Ventricular septal defect
(c) Tricuspid regurgitation
(d) Aortic regurgitation

220. Diastolic murmur with thrill is graded as:
(a) Grade 4 (b) Grade 3
(c) Grade 2 (d) Grade 1

221. Early diastolic murmur is observed in:
(a) Atrial septal defect (b) Aortic stenosis
(c) Aortic regurgitation (d) Mitral stenosis

222. Mid diastolic murmur is observed in:
(a) Atrial septal defect (b) Aortic stenosis
(c) Mitral stenosis (d) Aortic regurgitation

223. Which is the functional diastolic murmur?
(a) Graham Steel (b) Carey Coombs
(c) Austin Flint (d) All of the above

224. Wide fixed split of second heart sound occurs in
(a) Atrial septal defect
(b) Aortic stenosis
(c) Patent ductus arteriosus
(d) Severe AS

225. Paradoxical split of second heart sound occurs in:
(a) LBBB
(b) Severe AS
(c) Severe LV dysfunction
(d) All of the above

226. Continuous murmur is heard in:
(a) Patent Ductus Arteriosus
(b) Aortic Stenosis+Aortic Regurgitation
(c) VSD+ Aortic Regurgitation
(d) All of the above

227. Which is the method for palpation of spleen?
(a) Shot's manoeuvre (b) Castell's method
(c) Dipping method (d) All of the above

228. What is moderate grade splenomegaly?
(a) 4-7 cms (b) <3 cms
(c) 5 cms (d) >7 cms

229. What is moderate grade splenomegaly?(below costal margin)
(a) <4 cm (b) 5 cm
(c) 5 to 7 cm (d) >7 cm

230. Murphy's sign is indicative of:
(a) Inflamed gallbladder (b) Appendix
(c) Worm infestation (d) Kidney stone

231. For percussion pleximeter is:
(a) Left hand middle finger
(b) Right hand middle finger
(c) Left hand index finger
(d) Right hand index finger

Answers

1. **(a)** First 12 days

Naming a baby in Hindu tradition usually held after the first 12 days of a baby's delivery. In Maharashtra, the paternal aunt has the honor of naming her brother's child. In Muslims tradition they removes the baby's hair and to observe the aqeeqah and to name the child on the seventh day after birth. Gold or silver equivalent to the weight of the removed hair may be given as charity to the poor. Sikhs often selects a name for a child by opening the Sikh holy book, the guru granath sahib to a random page and choosing a name that begins with the first letter of the first word on the page.

2. **(d)** All of the above

Age

- **Pediatric age**–From birth to 12 years in developing countries and upto 14 years in developed countries. Adolescent children are also part of Pediatrics.

Child	
Newborn	Birth-28 days
Infant	28 days-1 year
Toddler	1-3 years
Preschool age	3-6 years
Preschool age	6-12 years
Adolescency	12-18 years

3. **(c)** 18 years

Age of majority–It is the chronological moment when minors cease to legally be considered children and assume control over their persons, actions, and decisions, thereby terminating the legal control and legal responsibilities of their parents or guardian over and for them. Most countries it is set at majority at 18 years.

Age of majority (years)	Countries
14	Albania.
15	Indonesia (for females), Iraq, Iran.
16	Cuba, Kyrgyzstan, United Kingdom–England, Scotland, Wales.
17	North Korea, Tajikistan.
18	Afghanistan, Albania, American Samoa, United States, Austria, Australia, Bangladesh, Brazil, China, Germany, India, Italy, Nepal, Pakistan, Saudi Arabia, Sri Lanka, United Kingdom, Zimbabwe.
19	South Korea, United States – Alabama, Nebraska.
20	New Zealand, Taiwan (Republic of China), Thailand, Tunisia.
21	United States, Swaziland, Singapore, Egypt.

4. **(d)** 18 years.
5. **(c)** 16 years.
6. **(a)** Marriageable age–21 years for males and 18 years for females.
7. **(c)** Grade 1

- Consanguinity:

Grade 1: Marriage between brother and sister.

Grade 2: Marriage with the fathers own sister or mothers own brother.

Grade 3: Marriage with father's sister's son or daughter or mother's brother's son or daughter.

Grade 4: Marriage with distant relatives.

8. **(a)** Double line

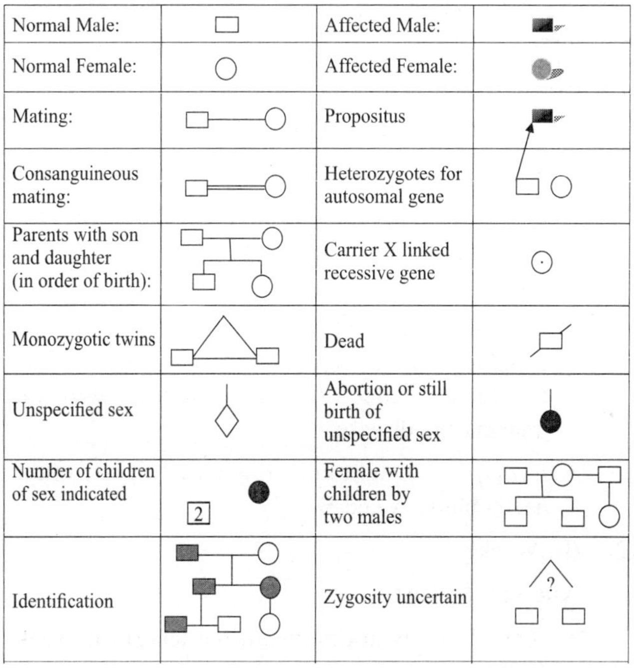

9. **(d)** Autosomal Dominant Disorder

Autosomal Dominant Disorder

- Male and female are affected with equal frequency.
- Vertical transmission (affected individual will have affected parents).
- Fifty percent risk for offspring's of affected individual at each pregnancy although it may be nonpenetrant).

- Unaffected children of affected parents will have unaffected children (unless the gene is nonpenetrant).
- Unaffected children of affected parents will have unaffected children (unless the gene is nonpenetrant).

Example: Achondroplasia, Marfan's syndrome, neurofibromatosis, tuberous sclerosis, von Willebrand's Disease (some types) osteogenesis imperfecta some types retinoblastoma.

10. **(c)** Autosomal recessive disorder

Autosomal Recessive (AR) Disorder

- Male and female are affected with equal frequency.
- Horizontal transmission (parents normal and siblings are affected).
- Twenty five percent risk at each pregnancy for the offsprings.
- If both parents are affected, then all siblings will be affected.
- Consanguinity of parents is common.

Example: Thalassaemia, Wilson's disease, congenital adrenal hyperplasia, albinism, Werdnig-Hoffmann disease.

11. **(b)** Both male and females are affected

X-Linked Recessive (XLR) Disorder

- Principally, males are affected.
- There is a 50 percent risk of getting the disease for boys and 50 percent risk of being carriers for girls if the mother is carrying the gene.
- Sons of an affected male are unaffected. All the daughters of an affected male are carriers. The unaffected males of a carrier mother will not transmit the disease.
- *Example:* Duchenne muscular dystrophy, haemophilia A and B.

12. **(b)** Weekly

Antenatal Visits

- Monthly visits in first two trimesters (from week 1–28).
- Fortnightly visits from 28th week to 36th week of pregnancy.
- Weekly visits after 36th week till delivery (delivery at week 38–40).

13. **(d)** All of the above

Effect of Advanced Age of Mother on Foetus—Down Syndrome, Dizygotic Twins, Premature Labour, Mental Subnormality.

14. **(d)** All of the above

Effect of Advanced Age of Father on Foetus—Marfan's Syndrome, Alport's Syndrome, Achondroplasia, Osteogenesis Imperfecta, Congenital Deafeness, Congenital Heart Diseases.

15. **(d)** All of the above

Maternal Conditions and Associated Cardiac Problems in Child

1. Diabetes mellitus—Transposition of great vessels, VSD, PDA.
2. SLE—Congenital heart block.
3. Phenylketonurea—TOF, VSD, ASD, PDA, COA.
4. Rubella—Pulmonary artery stenosis, PDA, VSD, ASD.
5. Mumps—Endocardial fibroelastosis.

16. **(d)** All of the above

Teratogenic Drugs—Effect on Baby

Drug	Cardiac anomalies	Other features
Sodium valproate	Hypoplastic left heart AS, PA,VSD	Facial dysmorphism, learning disability
Hydantoin	PS, VSD, ASD, PDA, COA	Growth retardation
Alcohol	VSD, PDA, ASD, TOF	Growth retardation, mental retardation, microcephaly
Oestrogen	VSD,TOF,TGA	Ambiguous genitalias
Progestrone	TOF	Ambiguous genitalias
Vit. D	Supravalvular AS	Craniosynostosis
Vit. A	Conotruncal anomalies, TOF, TGA, Truncus arteriosus	Abnormal facies, neural and renal anomalies
Indomethacin	Intrauterine closure of ductus arteriosus	Renal dysfunction
Thalidomide	TOF, VSD, ASD, Truncus arteriosus	Limb anomalies, duodenal/ anal atresia

17. **(a)** 1 hour

Duration Stage of Labor

Gravida	1st Stage	2nd Stage
Primi	16 hours	1 hour
Multi	8 hours	30 minutes

18. **(c)** 42 days

Postnatal history – Related with mother in 42 days after birth (postnatal period).

19. **(a)** Two

20. **(a)** 10 years

Overcrowding–Children are defined as living in overcrowded dwellings when there is a ratio of more than two people per room (excluding bathrooms but including kitchen and living room). The overcrowding ratio is obtained by dividing the total number of household members by the total number of rooms occupied by the household. Children between 1 to 10 years are counted as half a unit.

21. **(d)** 11 sq. metre

Floor Space—The WHO accepted standards for floor space are:

Area (in sq. metre)	No. of persons
11 or more	2 persons
9 to 10	1.5 persons
7 to 9	1 person
5 to 7	0.5 person
Under 5	Nil

22. **(d)** Rs. 28.65 per capita

23. **(c)** Rs 22.42 in rural areas

Per capita income = Total income of the family/ No. of family members

- Poverty line-2012-Planning Commission on further reduced poverty line to Rs. 28.65 per capita daily consumption in cities and Rs 22.42 in rural areas.

24. **(a)** 15 rupees

25. **(b)** 6350-12699

Prasad Classification

Social Class	Income per capita (Rupees) Prasad's Classification	Income per capita (Rupees) Modified Classification July 2008
Upper High	100 above	12700 above
High	50-99	6350-12699
Upper Middle	30-49	3810-6349
Lower Middle	15-29	1905-3809
Poor	Below 15	Below 1904

26. **(d)** Class 2

Socioeconomic status:

- Class 1 - Executives, judges and collectors
- Class 2 - Professionals such as doctors
- Class 3 - Trained workers
- Class 4 - Untrained workers
- Class 5 - Street dwellers.

27. **(d)** Religion

Rural areas, Pareekh classification based on nine characteristics namely:

1. Caste
2. Occupation of family head
3. Education of family head
4. Level of social participation of family head
5. Landholding
6. Housing
7. Farm power
8. Material possessions
9. Type of family.

28. **(d)** All of the above

Kuppuswami's Classification

Based on Education, Occupation and Income of Family Head.

(a) Education **(c) Per capita Income (Rs. in month)**

Professional degree, PG and above	7	1500 or above	12
Graduate	6	750-1499	10
Intermediate of past high school diploma	5	565-749	6
High school certificate	4	375-564	4
Middle school completion	3	225-374	3
Primary school or illiterate	2	75-224	2
Illiterate	1	Below 75	1

(b) Occupation

Profession	10
Semi Profession	6
Clerk, Shop Owner, Farm Owner	5
Skilled Workers	4
Semi Skilled Workers	3
Unskilled	2
Unemployed	1

The score is graded as follows:

Upper	26–29
Upper Middle	16–25
Lower Middle	11–15
Upper lower	5–10
Lower	5

29. **(d)** Mother's lap.

Position for Examination.

- 0 – 3 months – examination table.
- 3 months to 1 year – mother's lap.
- 1 – 3 year – standing or mother's lap.
- After 3 years – examination table.
- Adolescent girl – female attendant or nurse should be present at the time of examination.

30. **(d)** All of the above

TEMPERATURE:

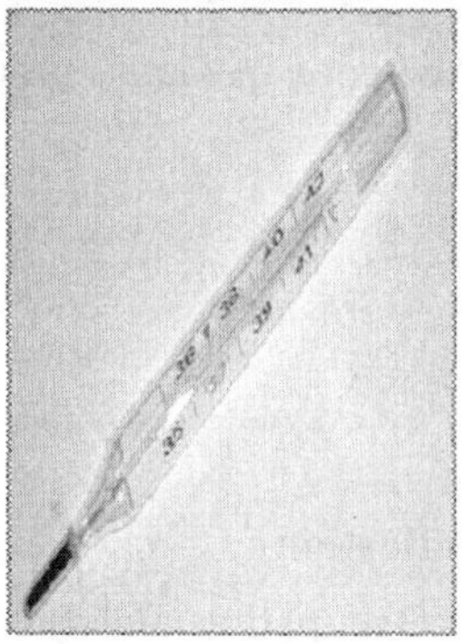

Axillary thermometer

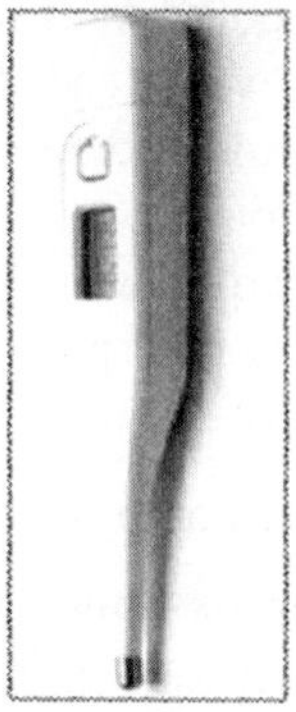

Digital thermometer

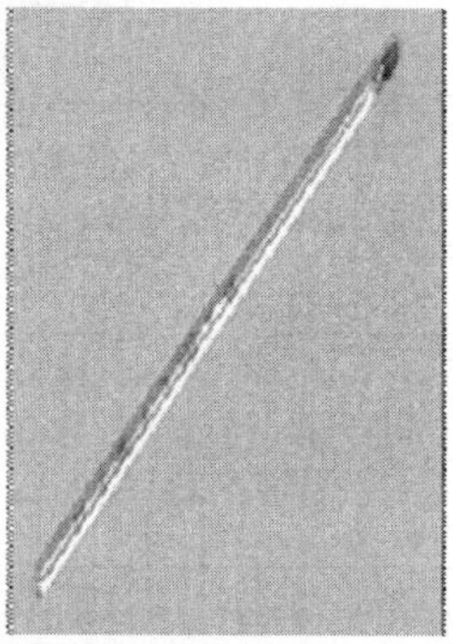

Rectal thermometer

Rectal Temperatures

- Put child on stomach on lap, then put thermometer gently into the anus for about 1 inch. If child is less than 6 months old, put it in only about 1/2 inch.
- Hold child still and leave the thermometer in 2 minutes with a glass thermometer.
- Fever if the rectal temperature is above 100.4° F (38° C).

Axillary Temperatures

- Put the tip of the thermometer in an armpit.Then close the armpit by holding the elbow against the chest for 4 or 5 minutes. The tip of the thermometer must be covered by skin.
- Fever if the armpit temperature is above 99.0° F (37.2° C).

Oral Temperatures

- Child should not have a cold or hot drink in the last 30 minutes.
- Keep tip of the thermometer under one side of the tongue and toward the back.
- Hold the thermometer in place with his lips and fingers (not teeth) for 3 minutes.
- Fever if the temperature is above 100° F (37.8° C).
- Body temperature - Lowest levels around 4 a.m. and the highest in the late afternoon, between 4:00 and 6:00 p.m.

31. **(a)** 98.6°F (37°C)

The average normal oral temperature is 98.6°F (37°C). An oral temperature is 0.5°F (0.3°C) to 1°F (0.6°C) lower than a rectal or ear (tympanic) temperature.

32. **(d)** Rectal temperatures

33. **(c)** Index and middle fingers

34. **(d)** All of the above

The sites for palpation of pulse are:

- Ventral aspect of the wrist on the side of the thumb (radial artery).
- Ulnar artery.
- Neck (carotid artery).
- Inner side of the elbow, or under the biceps muscle (brachial artery).
- Groin (femoral artery).
- Behind the medial malleolus on the feet (posterior tibial artery).
- Middle of dorsum of the foot (dorsalispedis).
- Behind the knee (popliteal artery).
- Over the abdomen (abdominal aorta).
- Chest (apex of the heart), which can be felt with one's hand or fingers.
- Temple (superficial temporal artery).
- Lateral edge of the mandible (facial artery).
- Near the ear (basilar artery).

35. **(a)** 10 beats /min

36. **(d)** All of the above

Bradycardia

- Physiological–Sleep, Athletes.
- Pathological–Hypoxia/Hypothermia/Hypothyroidism/Heart block/Drugs—β blockers, Digoxin.

37. **(a)** Atropine

Tachycardia

- Physiological—Exertion, Crying, Anxiety.
- Pathological—High output states – Anemia, Thyrotoxicosis, Hypovolemia, Hypotension, Drugs – Atropine, Nifedepine.

38. **(c)** Atrial tachyarrhythmia with fixed AV block

39. **(d)** All of the above

40. **(d)** All of the above

41. **(c)** Left ventricular failure

42. **(b)** Aortic stenosis

43. **(a)** Cardiac tamponade

Pulse – Character

1. Collapsing pulse (water hammer pulse) jerky pulse with full expansion followed by sudden collapse (Aortic Regurgitation, Patent Ductus Arteriosus, A-V fistulas, pregnancy, Paget's disease, thyrotoxicosis, anemia).
2. Alternating pulse (pulses alternans) - Regular rate, amplitude varies from beat to beat seen in Left Ventricular Failure.
3. Pulses bisferiens two strong systolic peaks separated by a midsystolic dip seen in Aortic Stenosis, Aortic Incompetence.
4. Anacrotic pulse slow rising pulse in aortic stenosis.
5. Diacrotic pulse, two systolic and diastolic peaks (sepsis, hypovolemic, cardiogenic shock).
6. Pulsus paradoxus (amplitude decreases with inspiration and increases during expiration) seen in cardiac tamponade, COPD, massive P.E.

44. **(b)** 30 – 60 mmHg

45. **(a)** Cardiac tamponade

46. **(c)** Aortic regurgitation

Pulse – Volume

- Pulse Pressure – Difference between systolic and diastolic blood pressure.
- Normal: 30 – 60 mmHg.
- Small volume – cardiac tamponade / failure.
- Large volume – PDA, Aortic regurgitation.

47. **(b)**130 – 150 / min

Normal pulse rate:

Age	Pulse rate / min
Newborn	130 - 150
1 month to 1 year	110 - 130
1 - 2 years	100 - 120
2 - 4 years	110
4 - 6 years	100
6 - 8 years	90 - 100
8 - 10 years	90
10 - 12 years	80 - 90
> 12 years	80

48. **(d)** All of the above

Capillary Refill—Blanch the nail bed with sustained pressure for several seconds on a toe nail or finger nail, release the pressure, observe the time elapsed before the nail regains full color.

- Should occur almost instantly – in less than 2 seconds.
- Longer than 2 seconds implies circulatory system compromise (i.e.: arterial occlusion, hypovolemic shock, hypothermia).

49. **(a)** 40-70/min

Normal Respirations

Age	Pulse rate / min
Premature	40-70
0-3 months	35-55
3-6 months	30-45
6-12 months	25-40
1-3 years	20-30
3-6 years	20-25
6-12 years	14-22
Over age 12	12-18

50. **(c)** Diabetic ketoacidosis

Kussmaul breathing is a deep and labored breathing pattern often associated with severe metabolic acidosis, particularly diabetic ketoacidosis.

51. **(b)** Apnea

Cheyne–Stokes respiration is characterized by progressively deeper and sometimes faster breathing, followed by a gradual decrease that results in a temporary stop in breathing called an apnea. The pattern repeats, with each cycle.

52. **(a)** Poor prognosis

Biot's respiration (ataxic respiration) characterized by groups of quick, shallow inspirations followed by regular or irregular periods of apnea. It indicates a poor prognosis.

53. **(a)** Grade 4

Dyspnea Scale (MMRC)

Grade	Description of Breathlessness
0	Breathless with strenuous exercise.
1	Short of breath when hurrying on level ground or walking up a slight hill.
2	On ground level walks slower than people of the same age because of breathlessness, or have to stop for breath when walking at my own pace.
3	Stops for breath after walking about 100 yards or after a few minutes on level ground.
4	Too breathless to leave the house or I am breathless when dressing.

54. **(c)** 2.5 cms

55. **(b)** 5 cms

Blood Pressure is the pressure exerted by circulating blood upon the walls of blood vessels.

Age	Cuff size
Newborn	2.5 cm
Infant	5 cm
1 – 8 years	9 cm
>8 years	12.5 cm

56. **(d)** All of the above

• Palpatory	• Auscultatory
• Flush method	• Oscillometry
• Non-invasive Doppler	

Recording Blood Pressure—Cuff applied directly over skin and not through clothes. A clothes artificially raises Blood Pressure. The bladder should cover 2/3rd circumference of upper arm. Center inflatable bladder should be over brachial artery. Position lower cuff border 2.5 cm above antecubital area. Patient's arm should be slightly flexed at elbow. Position stethoscope bell over brachial artery. Wait 5 minutes of rest before checking blood pressure. Check blood pressure in right arm, while seated. Take blood pressure at heart level. Inflate cuff rapidly to level above suspected systolic BP. Deflate cuff slowly at a rate of 2-3 mmHg per second. In coarctation of aorta all 4 limbs BP recorded listen for auditory vibrations from artery (Korotkoff).

Systolic Blood Pressure: Onset of consecutive sounds.

Diastolic Blood Pressure: Disappearance of sounds.

Formulas for Systolic Blood Pressure Estimate (for over age 1 year)

1. Median Systolic BP = 90 mmHg + (2 × Age in years).
2. Minimum Systolic BP = 70 mmHg + (2 × Age in years).

57. **(b)** 55-75 mmHg

Normal Blood Pressures

Age	Systolic B.P.	Diastolic B.P.
Premature	55-75	35-45
0-3 months	65-85	45-55
3-6 months	70-90	50-65
6-12 months	80-100	55-65
1-3 years	90-105	55-70
3-6 years	95-110	60-75
6-12 years	100-120	60-75
Over age 12	110-135	65-85

58. **(a)** > 20 mmHg

Relationship Between Blood Pressure in the Legs and Arms:

- To measure the blood pressure in the legs, place the cuff around the thigh and listen or palpate over the popliteal artery.
- Indirect measurement – the SBP in the legs is 10 – 15 mmHg higher than in the arms.
- Direct measurement – no difference.
- Hill's sign – > 20 mmHg difference between the arms and the legs (AR).
- Coarctation of the aorta – BP in legs is much less than in the arms.

59. **(b)** Atrial systole

60. **(b)** Tricuspid regurgitation

61. **(a)** Hypovolemia

62. **(d)** All of the above

Jugular Venous Pressure

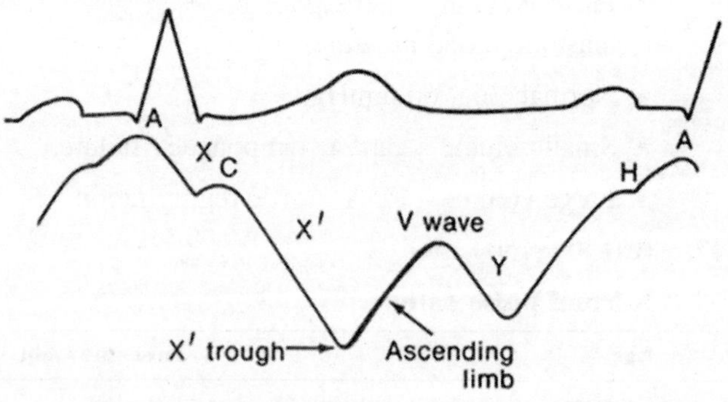

- a wave – atrial systole.
- c wave – movement of tricuspid valve ring into right atrium.
- v wave – peak pressure in right atrium.
- a-x descent – atrial relaxation.
- v-y descent – ventricular filling.

JVP – Measurement

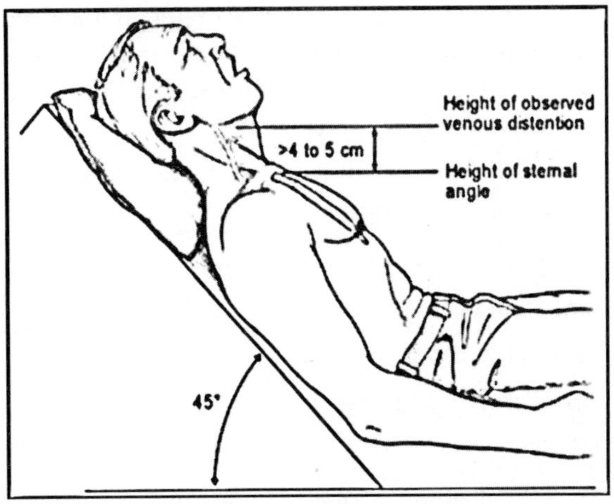

- Place child in supine position initially to engorge jugular veins.
- Gradually raise head of bed until jugular venous pulsations become evident between angle of jaw and clavicle.
- Palpating contralateral carotid pulse will help identify venous pulsations.
- Place the end of a ruler in the mid axillary line at level of nipple, with ruler extended vertically.
- Using another ruler, place it horizontally to intersect the vertical ruler and the meniscus of the JVD. The value on the vertical ruler should be less than 9 cm H_2O.

  Abnormalities of jugular venous pulse:

  a wave : absent (AF), prominent (PS, PHT, TS), cannon waves : (Arrhythmias).

  v wave : prominent – TR.

  x descent : prominent - constrictive pericarditis.

  y descent : slow (TS), fast (TR), Absent (cardiac tamponade).

  Low jugular venous pressure: Hypovolemia.
- Elevated jugular venous pressure:
  - Intravascular volume overload conditions due to valvular disease (tricuspid or pulmonic stenosis or regurgitation), right ventricular ischemia or infarction, cardiomyopathy or secondary to left heart failure (mitral stenosis/ regurgitation, aortic stenosis/regurgitation, cardiomyopathy, myocardial ischaemia/ infarction).
  - Right ventricular failure.
  - Constrictive pericarditis.
  - Pericardial effusion with tamponade physiology.
  - Obstructive atrial myxoma.
  - Superior vena cava obstruction.

63. **(b)** 3 SD

64. **(d)** All of the above

Head Size

- Microcephaly: HC < 3 SD below normal
  - Primary → Primary asymptomatic / Primary symptomatic
  - Secondary
- Intrauterine infections
  - CMV, rubella, toxoplasmosis.
- Intrauterine toxin
  - Fetal alcohol syndrome.
  - Fetal hydantoin syndrome.
- Perinatal / post natal insult
  - Meningitis, encephalitis, ICH.

65. **(d)** 2 SD

66. **(d)** All of the above

Macrocephaly:HC> 2 SD.

- Familial, Hydrocephalus, Achondroplasia, Cerebral gigantism, Fragile X syndrome, Muco-polysaccharidosis, Rickets, Thalassemia.

67. **(d)** Mesocephaly

68. **(c)** Brachicephaly

69. **(d)** Dolicocephaly

70. **(a)** Turricephaly

Shape

Cephalic index (length-width or length-breath index) = maximum cranial width/maximum cranial length multiplied by 100

Type of skull	Appearance	Length-width index
Turricephaly	High peaked	>85
Oxicephaly	High and slopping	>85
Brachycephaly	Short cranium	80-85
Mesocephaly	Normal cranium	60-75
Dolicocephaly	Long cranium	70-75
Scaphocephaly	Canoeoshaped	<70

- Brachycephaly – decreased antero posterior diameter due to fusion of coronal sutures.

- Dolichocephaly – increased anteroposterior diameter due to fusion of sagittal sutures.

71. **(d)** All of the above

Craniotabes: It is elicited by applying pressure on the scalp behind and above the ears. Presence of a snapping sound on pressure is indicative of craniotabes.

Causes:

Physiological	Osteogenesis Imperfecta
Rickets	Lacunar skull and craniofenestria
Congenital syphilis	Hypervitaminosis A
Hydrocephalus	Mandibulofacial dysostosis

72. **(a)** Raised intracranial tension

Macewan's sign–It should be elicited after the closure of anterior fontanelle. The skull is percussed with the fingers and cracked–pot sound is heard. It is positive in cases with raised intracranial tension due to separation of sutures.

73. **(d)** All of the above

Bossing / Prominence

- Frontal bone is involved it is called frontal bossing or both central parts of frontal and parietal bone is involved.
  - Rickets, Hydrocephalus, Congenital syphilis, Thalassemia, Achondroplasia.

74. **(d)** 9 – 18 months

75. **(d)** All of the above

76. **(d)** Craniosynostosis

77. **(d)** Dehydration

78. **(a)** Increased intracranial tension

Anterior Fontanel—2.5 × 2.5 cm, closes between 9 – 18 months

- Delayed closure / large fontanel–Rickets, Hydrocephalus, Congenital Hypothyroidism, Achondroplasia, Osteogenesisimperfecta, Down syndrome.
- Small AF : Craniosynostosis, Variation of normal.
- Sunken AF : Dehydration.
- Bulging AF : Increased intracranial tension / hydrocephalus.

79. **(a)** Raised intracranial pressure

Abnormal translucency is seen in:

Transillumination of Skull—Should be done with a torch in a dark room over the frontal and occipital regions. In frontal region: if translucency exceeds 1 inch it is abnormal. In occipital region: if translucency exceeds half an inch it is abnormal. Abnormal translucency is seen in hydrocephalus, subdural effusion and hematoma.

Auscultation of skull for bruit in patients with raised intracranial pressure.

80. **(d)** All of the above

81. **(a)** Malnutrition

82. **(d)** All of the above

83. **(a)** Turner's syndrome

Hair

- Malnutrition : Sparse straight, thin, pluckable, lack luster with alternate areas of pigmented and depigmented hair (Flag sign).
- Alopecia: Congenital ectodermal dysplasia, Alopecia areata, Treatment for malignancy.
- Hypertrichosis: Increased quantity of hair : Cushing's syndrome, Precocious puberty e.g.: Congenital adrenal hyperplasia, Drugs like dilantin.
- Hair Line
  a. Low hair line in back below C4 spine – Turner's syndrome.
  b. Low hair line in front – Hypothyroidism.
  c. Excess projection of hair into cheek – Treacher Collins syndrome.

84. **(a)** Down's syndrome

85. **(d)** All of the above

86. **(a)** Cushing's syndrome

87. **(d)** All of the above

88. **(d)** All of the above

89. **(a)** Russel Silver syndrome

Face

- **Down's syndrome**–Upward slanting of eyes, epicanthic folds, small nose with flat nasal bridge, narrow short palate, furrowed protruding tongue, small dysplastic ears, facial grimace on crying.
- Moon face – Cushing's syndrome.
- Puffy face – Nephrotic syndrome.
- Coarse facies – Hypothyroidism, Hurlers syndrome, Soto syndrome.
- Mask like facies – Wilson's disease, Mobius syndrome, Depression.
- Mongoloid facies – Down's syndrome.
- Triangular facies – Russel Silver syndrome.

90. **(a)** Goldenhar's syndrome

91. **(d)** Treacher Collin's syndrome

92. **(d)** All of the above

93. **(d)** Noonan's syndrome

94. **(d)** All of the above

95. **(d)** All of the above

96. **(d)** All of the above

97. **(d)** Conjunctiva

98. **(d)** All of the above

99. **(d)** All of the above

100. **(d)** All of the above

101. **(b)** Goldenhar syndrome

102. **(a)** Fragile X syndrome

103. **(a)** Fragile X syndrome

104. **(d)** All of the above

105. **(d)** Measles

106. **(d)** All of the above

107. **(a)** Scurvy

108. **(d)** All of the above

109. **(a)** Lead poisoning

110. **(d)** All of the of above

Macroglossia: Beckwith syndrome, Amyloidosis, Lymphangiomas, Angioneurotic edema, Mucopolysaccharidosis, Down's syndrome, Pompe's disease, Congential hypothyroidism, Hurlers syndrome, Duchenne muscular dystrophy and physiological.

111. **(d)** All of the above

112. **(a)** Niacin deficiency

113. **(b)** Kawasaki disease

114. **(d)** All of the above

115. **(d)** All of the above

Cyanosis–Bluish or violet discoloration of the skin or mucus membrane due to excess amount of deoxygenated haemogoblin (>5gm/dl) in the peripheral blood vessels associated with inadequate oxygenation of the systemic tissue.

Types – Peripheral and Central

Peripheral Cyanosis–is due to excessive extraction of oxygen from the blood when the circulation is impaired.

Central cyanosis–is due to oxygen undersaturation of the arterial blood from poor gaseous exchange in the lungs resulting from respiratory failure or pulmonary edema or when there is right to left shunt. E.g., Respiratory Distress Syndrome, Foreign body, Tension Pneumothorax, Acute severe asthma, Pulmonary embolism.

Difference between Central and Peripheral Cyanosis

Central	Peripheral
Visible in warm areas and skin	Skin
Venous admixture and defective ventilation, perfusion/diffusion	Vasoconstriction, low cardiac output
Dec arterial oxy sat	Increased arteriovenous oxygen difference
Deoxy Hb >5 gm/dl	Normal
Clubbing present	Absent

116. **(a)** Down's syndrome

117. **(d)** All of the above

Clubbing–Bulbous enlargement of soft parts of the terminal phalanges with both transverse and longitudinal curving of the nails. It is due to interstitial edema and dilation of the arterioles and capillaries.

Grading:

1. Softening of nail bed.
2. Obliteration of the angle of nail bed.
3. Swelling of the subcutaneous tissue over the base of nail.
4. Swelling of fingers in all dimensions hypertrophic pulmonary osteoarthropathy.

Causes: Bronchiectasis, Lung abscess, Empyema, Intrathoracic tuberculosis, AV fistula.

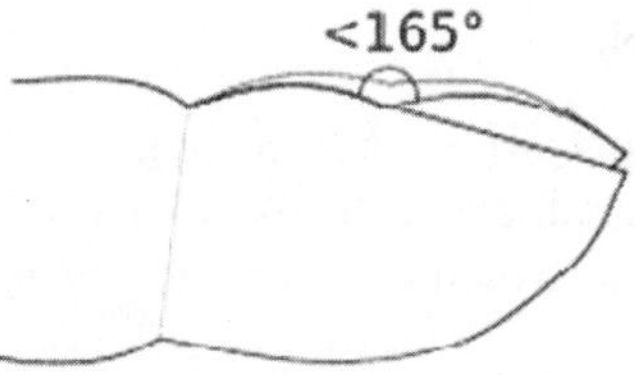

118. **(b)** Sexual maturity

119. **(b)** 20 ml

120. **(c)** 4 cm

EXTERNAL GENITALIA

Tanner Staging Sexual Maturity Score

Pubic Hair (both male and female)

1. Tanner I — No pubic hair at all [10 and under] (prepubertal state).

2. Tanner II — Small amount of long, downy hair with slight pigmentation at the base of the penis and scrotum (males) or on the labia majora [10-11] (female).
3. Tanner III — Hair becomes more coarse and curly, and begins to extend laterally [12-14].
4. Tanner IV—Adult-like hair quality, extending across pubis but sparing medial thighs [13-15].
5. Tanner V — Hair extends to medial surface of the thighs [16+].

Genitals (male)

1. Tanner I — prepubertal (testicular volume less than 1.5 ml; small penis of 3 cm or less).
2. Tanner II — Testicular volume between 1.6 and 6 ml; skin on scrotum thins, reddens and enlarges; penis length unchanged.
3. Tanner III — Testicular volume between 6 and 12 ml; scrotum enlarges further; penis begins to lengthen to about 6 cm.
4. Tanner IV — Testicular volume between 12 and 20 ml; scrotum enlarges further and darkens; penis increases in length to 10 cm and circumference.
5. Tanner V — Testicular volume greater than 20 ml; adult scrotum and penis of 15 cm in length.

Breasts (female)

1. Tanner I — No glandular tissue; areola follows the skin contours of the chest (prepubertal).
2. Tanner II — Breast bud forms, with small area of surrounding glandular tissue; areola begins to widen.
3. Tanner III — Breast begins to become more elevated, and extends beyond the borders of the areola, which continues to widen but remains in contour with surrounding breast.
4. Tanner IV — Increased breast size and elevation; areola and papilla form a secondary mound projecting from the contour of the surrounding breast.
5. Tanner V — Breast reaches final adult size; areola returns to contour of the surrounding breast, with a projecting central papilla.

Penile length

Birth-4 cms	4 years-5 cms
11 years-6 cms	Adolescent-12 cms

121. (d) All of the above

Glasgow Coma Scale

Eye opening	Motor activity	Verbal response
Spontaneous – 4	Follows commands – 6	Oriented – 5
Verbal stimuli – 3	Localises pain – 5	Confused – 2
Pain – 2	Withdraws to pain – 4	Inappropriate word – 3
None – 1	Flexion to pain – 3	Nonspecific sounds – 2
	Extension to pain – 2	None – 1
	None – 1	

122. (d) All of the above

Cranial Nerve 1. Olfactory nerve:

- Sensory nerve for sense of smell.
- Originates on the olfactory mucosa in the anterosuperior nasal cavity and travels down the olfactory tract until it reaches the olfactory bulb, where the fascicles of the olfactory nerve pass through foramina on the cribriform plate, which resides on the roof of the nasal cavity.
- Causes of anosmia
  - Chronic rhinitis.
  - Trauma.
  - Subarachnoid haemorrhage.
  - Meningitis.
  - Refsum's disease.
  - Zinc deficiency.
  - Kallman's syndrome.

123. (a) 6/6

124. (a) 100 degree

125. (d) All of the above

126. (d) All of the above

Cranial Nerve 2. Optic nerve:

- Transmits visual information from the retina to the brain.
- Visual acuity, color vision, field of vision, fundus.

Interpretation of Snellen's chart:

- 6/6- normal vision 6/5- superior vision
- 6/18- moderately poor 6/60- poor visual acuity

Average field of vision- Outward-100 degree, Upward and inward-60 degree, Downward -75 degree.

Causes of Papilloedema:

Increased intracranial tension	Malignant hypertension
Central retinal vein thrombosis	Cavernous sinous thrombosis
GB syndrome	Pseudo-tumor cerebri
Leukemia	

Nystagmus:

Physilogical	Optic atrophy
Congenital	Labyrinthine cause
Cerebellar ataxia	Cerebellar tumor
Hydrocephalus	Friedreich's ataxia
Diphenyl hydantoin sodium	Aspirin

127. **(d)** All of the above

128 **(d)** All of the above

129. **(d)** All of the above

Cranial Nerve 3. Oculomotor nerve:

- Derived from the basal plate of the embryonic midbrain.
- Enters the orbit via the superior orbital fissure and controls most of the eye's movements, including constriction of the pupil and maintaining an open eyelid by innervating the levator palpebrae superioris muscle.

Causes of Squint:

Non-paralytic—concomitant	Paralytic non-concomitant
• Hereditary	• Congenital
• Refractory	• Juvenile
• Cataract	
• Cerebral palsy	
• Retrolental fibroplasias	
• Optic atrophy, retinal detachment	

Ptosis:

3rd cranial nerve palsy	Horner's syndrome
Myesthenia gravis	Congenital syphilis
Progressive ocular myopathy	Beriberi
Botulism	

Diplopia:

Raised intracranial tension	Squint
Head injury	Labyrinthine involvement
8th nerve involvement	Myesthenia gravis
3rd cranial nerve palsy	

130. **(a)** Superior oblique muscle of the eye

131. **(d)** Abducens nerve

132. **(a)** Trigeminal nerve

133. **(d)** All of the above

Cranial nerve 6. Trigeminal nerve:

- Largest of the cranial nerves.
- Sensation in the face and certain motor functions such as biting and chewing.
- Three major branches: The ophthalmic nerve (V_1), the maxillary nerve (V_2), and the mandibular nerve (V_3).
- The ophthalmic and maxillary nerves are purely sensory. The mandibular nerve has both sensory and motor functions.

134. **(a)** Facial nerve

135. **(d)** Facial nerve

Cranial Nerve 7. Facial nerve:

- Emerges from the brainstem between the pons and the medulla.
- Controls the muscles of facial expression.
- Also supplies preganglionic parasympathetic fibers to several head and neck ganglia.
- Sensory – Special taste sensations on the anterior 2/3rd of tongue.

Testing by:

– 5% glucose solution–Sweet.
– 3% sodium solution–Salt.
– 1% citric acid–Sour
– Quinine hydrochloride–Bitter

- Motor Muscles of face - Ask the child to show his teeth, Frowning, Whistling, Blowing of the mouth, close his eyes tightly.

136. **(b)** 5.6 to 5.9 cm

Liver Span: Form the point of dullness to the lower margin

Birth	5.6 to 5.9 cm
2 months	5 cm
1 year	6 cm
2 years	6.5 cm
3 years	7 cm
4 years	7.5 cm
5 years	8 cm
12 years	9 cm

137. **(c)** 100-120 ml

Ascites–Minimum amount of fluid for (ml)

Diagnostic tap	10-20
Puddle sign	100-120
Shifting dullness	500
Fluid thrill	1000-1500
USG	100
CT Scan	100

138. **(a)** Grade 3

Grade	Severity	Findings
1	Mild	Puddle sign present, USG shows fluid
2	Moderate	Shifting dullness present, no fluid thrill
3	Severe	Fluid thrill present, tense ascites

139. **(c)** Vestibulo-cochlear nerve

140. **(d)** Vagus nerve

Cranial Nerve 10. Vagus nerve:

- Innervations of the viscera.
- Conveys sensory information about the state of the body's organs to the central nervous system. 80-90% of the nerve fibers in the vagus nerve are afferent (sensory) nerves communicating the state of the viscera to the brain.
- Sensation over posterior 1/3rd of tongue.

141. **(d)** Trapezius muscle

Cranial Nerve 11. Spinal accessory:

- Provides motor innervations from the central nervous system to two muscles of the neck: The sternocleidomastoid muscle and the trapezius muscle. The sternocleidomastoid muscle tilts and rotates the head, while the trapezius muscle has several actions on the scapula, including shoulder elevation and adduction of the scapula.
- Shrugging of shoulders against resistance, rotate the chin against resistance

142. **(a)** Hypoglossal nerve

143. **(d)** Cerebral cortex

Motor impulses from cerebral cortex reach the musculature by two neurons.

First - Upper motor neuron is in the cerebral cortex.

Second - Lower motor neuron located in motor nuclei of cranial nerves in the brainstem and in the anterior grey column cells of the spinal cord.

144. **(a)** Grade 3

Movement and Strength

- Medical research council grading of muscle weakness:

Grade	Features
0	No power. Complete paralysis
1	Visible or palpable flicer
2	Able to move eliminating the gravity
3	Able to move against the gravity but not against resistance
4	Able to move against partial resistance
5	Normal power

145. **(d)** All of the above

146. **(d)** All of the above

Causes:

- **Nonparalytic:** Prematurity, scurvy, rickets, hypothyroidism, birthasphyxia, cerebral palsy, mental retardation, down's syndrome.
- **Paralytic:** Spinalcordtrauma,poliomyelitis, Guillain-Barré syndrome, lead poisoning, myesthenia gravis, DMD, polymyositis.
- Cerebellar lesion.
- Neuronal shock.
- LMN lesion.
- Rheumatic chorea.

147. **(d)** All of the above

Cremasteric Reflex:

- Elicited by lightly stroking the superior and medial part of the thigh.
- Normal response is an immediate contraction of the cremaster muscle that pulls up the testis on the side stroked (and only on that side).
- Sensory and motor fibers of the genitofemoral nerve formed by fibers from both the L1 and L2 spinal nerves.
- In boys, this reflex may be exaggerated which can occasionally lead to a misdiagnosis of cryptorchidism.
- Absent with testicular torsion, upper and lower motor neuron disorders, as well as a spine injury of L1-L2. It can also occur if the ilioinguinal nerve has accidentally been cut during a hernia repair.

148. **(d)** Westphal's sign

149. **(a)** L2-L4

150. **(a)** S1-S2

151. **(c)** Hypothyroidism

152. **(d)** All of the above

153. **(d)** Hyperthyroidism

154. **(a)** Grade 4 reflex

Reflex	Grading
0	Absent
1	Present
2	Brisk
3	Very brisk
4	Clonus

155. **(d)** All of the above

156. **(d)** All of the above

157. **(d)** All of the above

158. **(d)** Tabesdorsalis

159. **(d)** Cerebral palsy

160. **(d)** Hemiplegia

161. **(c)** Proximal myopathies

162. **(d)** All of the above

Causes of ataxia:

Cerebellitis	Brain abscess
Medulloblastoma	Tuberculoma
Ataxia telangiectasia	Arnold Chiari syndrome
Dandy-Walkers syndrome	Anticonvulsant drugs
Chickenpox	Measles

163. **(d)** All of the above

164. **(d)** All of the above

165. **(a)** UMN lesions

166. **(c)** LMN lesions

Difference Between UMN and LMN

UMN Lesions	LMN Lesions
Loss of voluntary movements	Loss of voluntary movements
Increased tone and rigidity	Loss of muscle tone
Exaggerated tendon reflexes	Absence of tendon reflexes
Hypertrophy of the muscle	Atrophy of the muscle

- **Nuchal rigidity** is the inability to flex the neck forward due to rigidity of the neck muscles.
- **Kernig's sign** is positive when the thigh is bent at the hip and knee at 90 degree angles, and subsequent extension in the knee is painful (leading to resistance) this may indicate subarachnoid hemorrhage or meningitis. Patients may also show opisthotonus—spasm of the whole body that leads to legs and head being bent back and body bowed backwards.
- **Brudzinski sign:**

  Brudzinski's cheek phenomenon–A pressure on the cheek elicits a reflex rise and flexion of the forearm. It is found in patients with meningitis.

  Brudzinski symphyseal sign–Which pressure on the pubic symphysis, elicits a reflex flexion of the hip and knee and abduction of the leg. It is found in patients with meningitis.

  Brudzinski neck sign–Which forced flexion of the neck elicits a reflex flexion of the hips. It is found in patients with meningitis, subarachnoid haemorrhage and possibly encephalitis.

166. **(d)** All of the above

167. **(d)** All of the above

169. **(d)** All of the above

Respiratory System

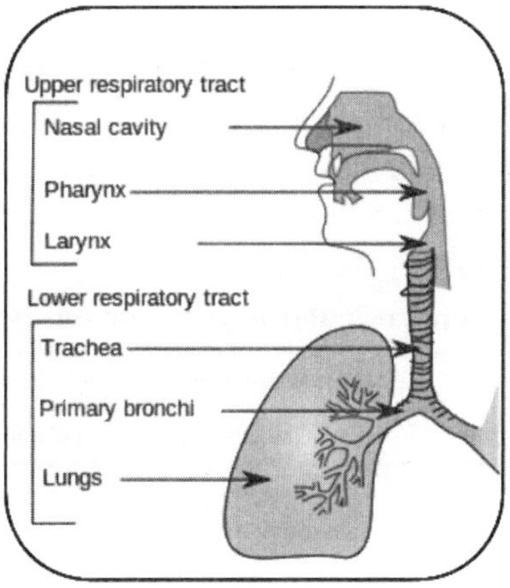

170. **(a)** Three lobes

Anatomy:

Bronchopulmonary segment is a wedge of the lung tissue, supplied by a single bronchus and corresponding pulmonary artery and vein.

Right lung has three lobes:

Upper Lobe: 1. Apical, 2. Anterior, 3. Posterior

Middle Lobe: 1. Lateral, 2. Medial

Lower Lobe: 1. Apical, 2. Antenior basal, 3. Post basal, 4. Lateral basal, 5. Medial basal

Left lung two lobes:

Upper Lobe: 1. Apical, 2. Anterior, 3. Posterior, 4. Superior lingual, 5. Inferior lingual

Lower Lobe: 1. Apical, 2. Anterior basal, 3. Posterior basal, 4. Lateral basal

171. **(d)** Depression in the sternum

172. **(b)** Prominence of the sternum

173. **(d)** All of the above

174. **(a)** Consolidation

175. **(d)** All of the above

176. **(d)** Pneumothorax

177 **(d)** Consolidation

178. **(a)** Pleural effusion

179. **(d)** All of the above

180. **(d)** All of the above

Breath Sounds

- **Vesicular** sounds are low pitched, low intensity sounds heard over the healthy lung tissue. This is characterised by active inspiration due to inflow of the air into bronchi and alveoli, followed by shorter expiration due to elastic recoil of the alveoli without a pause between inspiration and expiration.
- **Bronchial breath:** The inspiration is low in intensity while the expiration is high pitched, loud and prolonged ≥ the duration of inspiration. There will be a pause in between.

Difference between Vesicular and Bronchial Breathing

Vesicular	Bronchial
Normal breath sounds	Can be normal or abnormal
Heard all over the chest except over larynx, trachea	Normally heard all over the larynx, trachea
Rustling or breezy quality	Blowing quality
Low pitched	High pitched
Inspiration > Expiration	Expiratory phase = > inspiration
No pause	Definite pause

181. **(d)** All of the above
182. **(d)** All of the above
183. **(a)** Consolidation
184. **(d)** All of the above
185. **(d)** All of the above
186. **(a)** Pulmonary hypertension
187. **(d)** All of the above
188. **(a)** Aortic regurgitation
189. **(a)** Aortic regurgitation
190. **(b)** Tricuspid regurgitation
191. **(b)** Mitral stenosis
192. **(c)** Aortic stenosis
193. **(c)** Mitral regurgitation
194. **(d)** All of the above
195. **(d)** Pulmonary hypertension
196. **(a)** Aortic stenosis
197. **(d)** Mitral stenosis
198. **(c)** Aortic stenosis
199. **(b)** Aortic stenosis
200. **(d)** All of the above
201. **(a)** PDA
202. **(d)** Mitral stenosis
203. **(a)** Mitral regurgitation
204. **(b)** VSD
205. **(d)** All of the above
206. **(d)** All of the above
207. **(d)** All of the above
208. **(d)** All of the above
209. **(d)** All of the above
210. **(d)** All of the above
211. **(d)** All of the above
212. **(d)** All of the above
213. **(a)** Hypertrophic cardiomyopathy
214. **(b)** Ebstein's anomaly
215. **(d)** All of the above

Nadas' Criteria:

MAJOR

1. Systolic murmur with thrill.
2. Any diastolic murmur.
3. Cyanosis.
4. Congestive cardiac failure.

MINOR

1. Systolic murmur without thrill.
2. Abnormal P2.
3. Abnormal BP.
4. Abnormal CXR.
5. Abnormal ECG.

1. Major or 2. Minor Criteria indicates Presence of Congenital Heart Disease.

216. **(d)** All of the above
217. **(d)** All of the above
218. **(d)** All of the above
219. **(a)** Mitral valve prolapse
220. **(a)** Grade 4

Diastolic Murmurs

Grading I - IV

1. Very Soft.
2. Soft.
3. Loud.
4. Loud with thrill.

221. **(c)** Aortic regurgitation
222. **(c)** Mitral stenosis
223. **(d)** All of the above

224. **(a)** Atrial septal defect

225. **(d)** All of the above

226. **(d)** All of the above

227. **(d)** All of the above

228. **(a)** 4-7 cms

Grades of splenomegaly:

Grade	Palpable spleen below left costal margin (cms)
Mild	<3
Moderate	4-7
Massive	>7

229. **(c)** 5 to 7 cm

Grades of hepatomegaly:

Grade	Hepatomegaly below right costal margin (cms)
Mild	<4
Moderate	5-7
Massive	>7

230. **(a)** Inflamed gallbladder

Murphy's Sign: Can be elicited by asking the child to breath deeply while palpating for the gallbladder. At the height of inspiration the breath is arrested with a gasp as the inflamed gallbladder is felt.

231. **(a)** Left hand middle finger

Chapter 3

Growth and Development

1. **As per definition of a runaway is a youth younger than __________ who is gone for at least 1 night from his or her home without parental permission.**
   (a) 14 years (b) 16 years
   (c) 18 years (d) 20 years

2. **The brain comprises __________ neurons at birth.**
   (a) 50 billion (b) 100 billion
   (c) 150 billion (d) 200 billion

3. **At what age child follows moving object 180 degrees?**
   (a) 2 months (b) 4 months
   (c) 6 months (d) 8 months

4. **What is the age of "hatching" socially (becoming interested in a wider world)?**
   (a) 4 months (b) 6 months
   (c) 8 months (d) 12 months

5. **At what age the first stage of personality development comes?**
   (a) 1 month (b) 2 months
   (c) 4 months (d) 6 months

6. **Object permanence (constancy) appears at what age?**
   (a) 2 months (b) 4 months
   (c) 7 months (d) 9 months

7. **At what age infant adept at nonverbal communication (expressing a range of emotion)?**
   (a) 7 months (b) 9 months
   (c) 12 months (d) 14 months

8. **At what age child makes a tower of 3 cubes?**
   (a) 12 months (b) 13 months
   (c) 15 months (d) 18 months

9. **At what age child goes up stairs on alternating feets?**
   (a) 30 months (b) 36 months
   (c) 42 months (d) 48 months

10. **At what age child knows full name?**
    (a) 24 months (b) 30 months
    (c) 36 months (d) 42 months

11. **At what age child rides tricycle?**
    (a) 12 months (b) 20 months
    (c) 24 months (d) 30 months

12. **At what age child stands momentarily on one foot?**
    (a) 30 months (b) 3 months
    (c) 42 months (d) 48 months

13. **At what age child knows age and sex?**
    (a) 22 months (b) 25 months
    (c) 30 months (d) 34 months

14. **At what age child goes to toilet alone?**
    (a) 36 months (b) 48 months
    (c) 52 months (d) 55 months

15. **At what age child draws triangle from copy?**
    (a) 48 months (b) 60 months
    (c) 70 months (d) 80 months

16. **At what age child dresses and undresses?**
    (a) 36 months (b) 48 months
    (c) 60 months (d) 76 months

17. **At what age children are about ½ of their ultimate adult height?**
    (a) 12 months (b) 18 months
    (c) 24 months (d) 36 months

18. At what age children's visual acuity reaches 20/30?
(a) 1 year (b) 2 years
(c) 3 years (d) 4 years

19. At what age children's visual acuity reaches 20/20?
(a) 6 years (b) 4 years
(c) 2 years (d) 1 year

20. At what age children have all 20 primary teeths erupted?
(a) 1 year (b) 2 years
(c) 3 years (d) 4 years

21. Handedness is usually established by the age of:
(a) 3rd year (b) 4 years
(c) 6 years (d) 8 years

22. Bed-wetting is normal in girls up to age of:
(a) 2 years (b) 4 years
(c) 6 years (d) 8 years

23. Bed-wetting is normal in boys up to age of:
(a) 1year (b) 3 years
(c) 5 years (d) 8 years

24. In girls, what is the first visible sign of puberty?
(a) Appearance of breast buds
(b) Menarche
(c) Pubarche
(d) Axillary hair growth

25. In boys, what is the first visible sign of puberty?
(a) Breast buds
(b) Testicular enlargement
(c) Axillary hair
(d) Harshness of voice

26. At what age gender identity is established?
(a) 9 months (b) 12 months
(c) 15 months (d) 18 months

27. At what age gender stablity is established?
(a) 6- 9 months
(b) Between 18 and 30 months
(c) 30- 36 months
(d) 40-44 months

28. At what age gender constancy is established?
(a) 12 months (b) 24 months
(c) 30 months (d) 48 months

29. At what age ratio of upper body segment to lower body segment equals approximately 1.7?
(a) 1 year (b) Birth
(c) 3 years (d) 7 years

30. At what age ratio of upper body segment to lower body segment equals approximately 1.3?
(a) 3 years (b) Birth
(c) 1 year (d) 7 years

31. At what age ratio of upper body segment to lower body segment equals approximately 1.0?
(a) 3 years (b) 5 years
(c) 7 years (d) Birth

32. Higher upper/lower body ratios are characteristic of:
(a) Rickets (b) Achondroplasia
(c) Chondrodysplasia (d) None

33. Delayed eruption of teeth is usually considered when there are no teeth approximately by the age of:
(a) 13 months (b) 15 months
(c) 18 months (d) 20 months

34. Delayed eruption of teeth is seen in:
(a) Hypothyroidism
(b) Hypoparathyroidism
(c) Familial
(d) All of the above

35. The Individuals with Disabilities Education Act (IDEA) is concerned with:
(a) To identify sick children
(b) To locate and treat children
(c) To determine burden of disability
(d) All of the above

36. The hallmark of rumination disorder is:
(a) Weight loss
(b) Failure to gain
(c) Repeated regurgitation of food without associated gastrointestinal illness
(d) All of the above

37. Upto what age thumb sucking is considered normal?
(a) 9 months-1year (b) 1-2 years
(c) 2-4 years (d) 4-5 years

Answers

1. **(c)** 18 years
2. **(b)** 100 billion
3. **(a)** 2 months
4. **(a)** 4 months
5. **(c)** 4 months
6. **(d)** 9 months
7. **(a)** 7 months
8. **(c)** 15 months
9. **(a)** 30 months
10. **(b)** 30 months
11. **(d)** 30 months
12. **(a)** 30 months
13. **(c)** 30 months
14. **(b)** 48 months
15. **(b)** 60 months
16. **(c)** 60 months
17. **(c)** 24 months
18. **(c)** 3 years
19. **(b)** 4 years
20. **(c)** 3 years
21. **(a)** 3 years
22. **(b)** 4 years
23. **(c)** 5 years
24. **(a)** Appearance of breast buds
25. **(b)** Testicular enlargement
26. **(d)** 18 months
27. **(b)** Between 18 and 30 months
28. **(c)** 30 months
29. **(b)** Birth
30. **(a)** 3 years
31. **(c)** 7 years
32. **(a)** Rickets
33. **(a)** 13 months
34. **(d)** All of the above
35. **(b)** To locate and treat children
36. **(d)** All of the above
37. **(d)** 4–5 years

Chapter 4

Neonatology

1. **What is neonatal period?**
   (a) Birth to first 28 days of life
   (b) First 7 days of life
   (c) 7- 28 days of life
   (d) After 1 month

2. **Early neonate is:**
   (a) 7 to 28 days (b) Birth to 7 days
   (c) Birth to 28 days (d) After 1 month

3. **Late neonate:**
   (a) Birth to 7 days (b) Birth to 28 days
   (c) 7th to 28th day (d) After 1 month

4. **Perinatal period is from:**
   (a) 28th week of gestation to 7th day of life
   (b) 24th week of gestation to 14th day of life
   (c) 7th week of gestation to 28th day of life
   (d) 14th week of gestation to 24th day of life

5. **Extended perinatal period is from:**
   (a) 28th week of gestation to 7th day of life
   (b) 24th week of gestation to 14th day of life
   (c) 14th week of gestation to 24th day of life
   (d) 22nd week of gestation to 7th day of life

6. **Full term baby is:**
   (a) Between 37 to 42 weeks of pregnancy
   (b) 32-36 weeks
   (c) 40-42 weeks
   (d) None

7. **Preterm babies:**
   (a) 42-45 weeks (b) 40-42 weeks
   (c) 37-40 weeks (d) Born before 37 weeks

8. **Post term baby is:**
   (a) After 45 weeks (b) Born after 42 weeks
   (c) 37-40 weeks (d) Born before 37 weeks

9. **Low birth weight means:**
   (a) Birth weight less than 2500 gm
   (b) Birth weight less than 1000 gm
   (c) Birth weight less than 600 gm
   (d) Birth weight less than 1500 gm

10. **Very low birth weight means:**
   (a) Birth weight less than 2500 gm
   (b) Birth weight less than 1000 gm
   (c) Birth weight less than 600 gm
   (d) Birth weight less than 1500 gm

11. **Extremely low birth weight means:**
   (a) Birth weight less than 2500 gm
   (b) Birth weight less than 1000 gm
   (c) Birth weight less than 600 gm
   (d) Birth weight less than 1500 gm

12. **Small for gestational age or small for date means:**
   (a) Birth weight less than 10th percentile for that period of gestation
   (b) Birth weight less than 5th percentile for that period of gestation
   (c) Birth weight less than 3rd percentile for that period of gestation
   (d) Birth weight less than 50th percentile for that period of gestation

13. **Large for gestational age or large for date means:**
   (a) Birth weight more than 90th percentile for that period of gestation
   (b) Birth weight more than 75th percentile for that period of gestation
   (c) Birth weight more than 50th percentile for that period of gestation
   (d) Birth weight more than 25th percentile for that period of gestation

14. Appropriate for gestational age means:
(a) Birth weight between 10th and 90th percentile for that period of gestation
(b) Birth weight more than 90th percentile for that period of gestation
(c) Birth weight less than 10th percentile for that period of gestation
(d) Birth weight less than 50th percentile for that period of gestation

15. Which is the component of APGAR SCORE?
(a) Breathing (b) Muscle tone
(c) Reflex response (d) All of the above

16. Neuromuscular maturity components of modified Ballard score:
(a) Posture (b) Square window
(c) Arm recoil (d) All of the above

17. Which is a criterion for Parkin score?
(a) Skin texture (b) Breast size
(c) Ear firmness (d) All of the above

18. Silverman Anderson score includes:
(a) Audible grunt (b) Nasal flare
(c) Xiphoid retraction (d) All of the above

19. Downe's score have following parameter:
(a) Respiratory rate (b) Cyanosis
(c) Retractions (d) All of the above

20. Downe's score indicates:
(a) Need of surfactant
(b) Prematurity
(c) Impending respiratory failure
(d) None

21. Conditions to anticipate neonatal birth asphyxia:
(a) Mother more than 35 years age
(b) Meconium stained liquor
(c) Decrease fetal activity
(d) All of the above

22. Prerequisites for birth of newborn:
(a) Switch on warmer/ bulb (100 watt)
(b) Prewarm the sheets
(c) Cheque suction machine
(d) All of the above

23. Step in attending birth of newborn baby:
(a) Dry the baby
(b) Remove the wet sheet
(c) Suction the mouth first and then nose
(d) All of the above

24. Components of warm chain:
(a) Breastfeeding
(b) Warm resuscitation
(c) Skin-to-skin contact
(d) All of the above

25. Foetal weight gain in third trimester is due to:
(a) Increase in the number of cells
(b) Increase in the number and size of cells
(c) Increase in the size of cells
(d) All of the above

26. Prelacteal feeds includes:
(a) Sugar water (b) Honey
(c) Dextrose saline (d) All of the above

27. Galactogogues includes:
(a) Metoclopramide (b) Alfalfa
(c) Anise (d) All of the above

28. Because of immature circulation, a newborn who has been lying on his or her side will appear red on the dependent side of the body and pale on the upper side is a:
(a) Harlequin sign (b) Chadwick's sign
(c) Mottling (d) None

29. Which is a type of haemangiomas?
(a) Nevus flames (b) Strawberry
(c) Cavernous (d) All of the above

30. A white creamy cheese like substance that serves as a skin lubricant is usually noticeable on a newborn's skin folds at birth in a term neonate is known as:
(a) Vernix caseousa (b) Brown fat
(c) Epstein pearl (d) Lanugo

31. The fine hair that covers the newborn shoulders, back and upper arms is known as:
(a) Vernix caseousa (b) Brown fat
(c) Epstein pearl (d) Lanugo

32. A pinpoint papule can be found on the cheek or across the bridge of the nose is known as:
(a) Milia (b) Erythema toxicum
(c) Epstein pearl (d) None

33. A newborn rash that usually appears in the first to 4th day of life but may disappear up to 2 weeks of age is known as:
(a) Erythema toxicum (b) Milia
(c) Epstein pearl (d) Lanugo

34. A newborn's head appears disproportionately large because it is about ---------- of the total length.
(a) 1/8th (b) 1/4th
(c) 1/2nd (d) None

35. Anterior fontanelle normally closes with bone when the baby is between:
(a) 5-6 months
(b) 12 and 18 months
(c) 18-24 months
(d) After 24 months

36. Posterior fontanelle closes by:
(a) 2-3 weeks (b) 3-4 weeks
(c) 5-6 weeks (d) 6 to 8 weeks

37. Swelling on top of the head or throughout the scalp due to fluid squeezed into the scalp during the birth process is known as:
(a) Caput succedaneum (b) Hydrocephalus
(c) Cephalohematoma (d) Lipoma

38. Collection of blood on the outer surface of the skull is known as:
(a) Caput succedaneum (b) Hydrocephalus
(c) Cephalohematoma (d) Lipoma

39. Tongue-tie should be operated before:
(a) True speech develops (b) 8 months
(c) 6 months (d) 4 months

40. Little white-colored cysts can occur along the gum line or on the hard palate is called as:
(a) Erythema toxicum (b) Epstein pearls
(c) Lanugo (d) Milia

41. Reason for swollen breasts are present during the first week of life in many female and male babies:
(a) Congenital gynaecomastia
(b) Passage of female hormones across the mother's placenta
(c) Mastitis
(d) None

42. Normally how much liver palpable below the right costal region?
(a) 2 cm (b) 4 cm
(c) 6 cm (d) 8 cm

43. Normally how much spleen is palpable below the left costal region?
(a) 5 mm (b) 1 cm
(c) 1-2 cm (d) 3-4 cm

44. Umbilical cord has:
(a) Two veins, one artery
(b) Two arteries and one vein
(c) One artery and one vein
(d) None

45. Vaginal discharge in neonate is due to:
(a) Vulvutis (b) Maternal hormones
(c) Perinatal infections (d) Diabetes

46. What percentage of undescended testicle in full-term newborn?
(a) 0.5% (b) 1%
(c) 2% (d) About 4%

47. In India, normal term newborn at birth weight is:
(a) 2-2.5 kg (b) 2.5-2.8 kg
(c) 1.5-2 kg (d) 2.5-3.9 kg

48. Normal newborn loses how much of birth weight during the first few days after birth?
(a) 2-3% (b) 5-10%
(c) 15-20% (d) 25%

49. In India, length of normal term newborn is:
(a) 42 cms (b) 45 cms
(c) 50 cms (d) 55 cms

50. In India, normal term newborns head circumference is:
(a) 28-30 cms (b) 34- 35 cms
(c) 35-38 cms (d) 40-42 cms

51. Approximately neonatal blood pressure is:
(a) 58/44 mmHg (b) 70/55 mmHg
(c) 85/65 mmHg (d) 100/60 mmHg

52. Non-shivering thermogenesis is done by:
(a) Yellow fat (b) Brown fat
(c) Shivering (d) Proteins

53. Brown fat is found at:
(a) Nape of the neck (b) Axillae
(c) Around the kidneys (d) All of the above

54. Co-ordinated sucking in neonate occurs at:
(a) 32 weeks (b) 34 weeks
(c) 38 weeks (d) 40 weeks

55. Preterm milk is rich in:
(a) Protein (b) Minerals
(c) Immunoglobulins (d) All of the above

56. Colostrum is very rich in:
(a) Proteins (b) Vitamin A
(c) Sodium chloride (d) All of the above

57. **Colostrum is known to contain antibodies called immunoglobulins such as:**
(a) IgA (b) IgG
(c) IgM (d) All of the above

58. **Foremilk is rich in:**
(a) Carbohydrates (b) Protein
(c) Vitamins (d) All of the above

59. **Hind milk is rich in:**
(a) Water (b) Protein
(c) Fat (d) Micronutrients

60. **Alarm signals in neonate:**
(a) Poor feeding (b) Lethargy
(c) Excessive cry (d) All of the above

61. **Prolactin is secreted by:**
(a) Anterior pituitary (b) Posterior pituitary
(c) Thalamus (d) Hypothalamus

62. **Role of prolactin on the breast:**
(a) Contracts myocyte to eject the milk
(b) Inhibit let down reflex
(c) Hypertrophy of breasts
(d) Acts on the milk secreting cells to produce milk

63. **Prolactin production is enhanced by:**
(a) Early suck of the baby
(b) Often and how long the baby suckled
(c) How strongly and how well the baby is attached at the breast
(d) All of the above

64. **Prolactin production inhibited by:**
(a) Delayed initiation of breast feeds
(b) Prelacteal feeds
(c) Bottles
(d) All of the above

65. **Milk ejection reflex is initiated by:**
(a) Prolactin (b) Oxytocin
(c) ADH (d) Somatostatin

66. **Oxytocin is secreted by:**
(a) Post pituitary (b) Anterior pituitary
(c) Hypothalamus (d) Thalamus

67. **Oxytocin reflex is stimulated by:**
(a) Loving thought of baby (b) Sound of baby
(c) Confidence (d) All of the above

68. **Oxytocin reflex is inhibited by:**
(a) Worry (b) Stress
(c) Pain (d) All of the above

69. **Rooting reflex is stimulated by touching a finger to baby's:**
(a) Forehead
(b) Upper lip
(c) Cheek or the corner of the mouth
(d) Ear

70. **Repetitive tapping on the forehead of neonate there is blink response to the first several taps but if the blinking persists it is known as:**
(a) Myerson's sign (b) Herlequin sign
(c) Macevan's sign (d) Glabellar tap

71. **Moro's reflex appears at:**
(a) 24 weeks of gestation (b) 28 weeks of gestation
(c) 4 weeks after birth (d) 3 months after birth

72. **Persistence of Moro's reflex in the neonate is suggestive of:**
(a) Quadriplegia (b) Fracture clavicle
(c) Brachial plexus injury (d) Neurological damage

73. **An asymmetrical Moro's reflex response indicates:**
(a) Fractured clavicle (b) Quadriplegia
(c) Neurological damage (d) Frontal lobe damage

74. **Stepping reflex disappear approximately at:**
(a) Just after birth (b) 1 month
(c) 3 months (d) 2 months

75. **Palmar reflex disappears around:**
(a) 2 months (b) 4 months
(c) 8 months (d) Sixth month

76. **Kangaroo-mother care is helpful in:**
(a) Maintain the temperature of infant
(b) Facilitates breastfeeding
(c) Improves mother infant bonding
(d) All of the above

77. **First day fluid requirement in neonate is:**
(a) 60 - 80 ml /kg/day (b) 20-40 ml /kg/day
(c) 80-100 ml /kg/day (d) 100-120 ml /kg/day

78. **How much extra fluid is given to neonate receiving phototherapy?**
(a) 10 ml/kg (b) 15 ml / kg
(c) 20 ml/kg (d) 25 ml/kg

79. **How you will test 5th cranial nerve?**
(a) Uvula position (b) Moro reflex
(c) Rooting reflex (d) Position of scapula

80. **How you will test 7th cranial nerve?**
(a) Rooting reflex (b) Grimace of crying
(c) Sucking (d) Uvula position

81. How you will test 12th cranial nerve?
(a) Rooting reflex (b) Grimace of crying
(c) Vigorous sucking (d) Uvula position

82. Total calorie content of human breast milk is:
(a) 52 kcal/100 ml (b) 58 kcal/100 ml
(c) 67 kcal/100 ml (d) 75 kcal/100 ml

83. Maximum storage time of expressed breast milk at room temperaturre (25°C) is:
(a) Six to eight hours
(b) Ten to twelve hours
(c) Fifteen to twenty-four hours
(d) More than 24 hours

84. Maximum storage time of expressed breast milk in a refrigerator (4°C) is:
(a) Up to 24 hours (b) Up to five days
(c) Up to 7 days (d) More than ten days

85. Maximum storage time of expressed breast milk in chest or upright manual defrost deep freezer (-20°C) is:
(a) 2-4 months (b) Four to six months
(c) Six to twelve months (d) More than 12 months

86. At what age weaning is started?
(a) 6 months (b) 4 months
(c) 3 months (d) 2 months

87. What is incidence of neonatal hyperbilirubinemia in full term neonates?
(a) 20% (b) 40%
(c) 45% (d) 60%

88. What is incidence of neonatal hyperbilirubinemia in pre term neonates?
(a) 25% (b) 50%
(c) 66% (d) 80%

89. Breastfeeding jaundice in neonate appears at what age?
(a) 3-4 days (b) 4 to 7 days
(c) 7 to 10 days (d) 10 to 12 days

90. Breast milk jaundice in neonate appears at what age?
(a) 4 to 7 days (b) 3-4 days
(c) 7 to 10 days (d) 10 to 12 days

91. Physiological jaundice appears in:
(a) Before 24 hours
(b) After 72 hours
(c) On 7th day
(d) 24-72 hours

92. Who is father of phototherapy?
(a) David Clark (b) R Paludetto
(c) Niels Ryberg Finsen (d) Manual

93. Who is mother of phototherapy?
(a) Miss Sister Jean Ward
(b) Elizabeth M Williamson
(c) Angelo A Izzo
(d) Jenna Jamson

94. Which light is commonly used in phototherapy?
(a) Blue (b) White
(c) Red (d) Yellow

95. What is the maximal surface area of naked baby exposed distance from tube light in phototherapy?
(a) 60 cm (b) 45 cm
(c) 30 cm (d) 15 cm

96. Adverse effects of phototherapy:
(a) Bronze Baby syndrome
(b) Loose green stools
(c) Riboflavin deficiency
(d) All of the above

97. Who is father of the incubator?
(a) Stephane Etienne Tarnier
(b) Jonathan Nelson
(c) Professor René Chamussy
(d) Berytech

98. Specific risks for the preterm neonate:
(a) Apnea of prematurity
(b) Hypoxic-ischemic encephalopathy
(c) Patent ductus arteriosus
(d) All of the above

99. Sarnat and Sarnat scoring for hypoxic ischemic encephalopathy includes:
(a) Moro reflex (b) Seizures
(c) EEG (d) All of the above

Answers

1. **(a)** Birth to first 28 days of life
2. **(b)** Birth to 7 days
3. **(c)** 7th to 28th days
4. **(a)** 28th week of gestation to 7th day of life
5. **(d)** 22nd week of gestation to 7th day of life
6. **(a)** Between 37 to 42 weeks of pregnancy
7. **(d)** Born before 37 weeks
8. **(b)** Born after 42 weeks
9. **(a)** Birth weight less than 2500 gm
10. **(d)** Birth weight less than 1500 gm
11. **(b)** Birth weight less than 1000 gm
12. **(a)** Birth weight less than 10th percentile for that period of gestation
13. **(a)** Birth weight more than 90th percentile for that period of gestation
14. **(a)** Birth weight between 10th and 90th percentile for that period of gestation
15. **(d)** All of the above

Apgar Score:

Criteria	0	1	2
Breathing	Nil	Slow, gasping	Crying
Heart rate/min	Nil	Upto 100	More than100
Muscle tone	Flaccid	Inbetween	Flexed
Reflex response	Nil	Grimace	Cry
Color	Pale or blue	Peripheral cyanosis	Pink

16. **(d)** All of the above

GESTATIONAL AGE ASSESSMENT:

Modified Ballard Score

1. Neuromuscluar maturity:

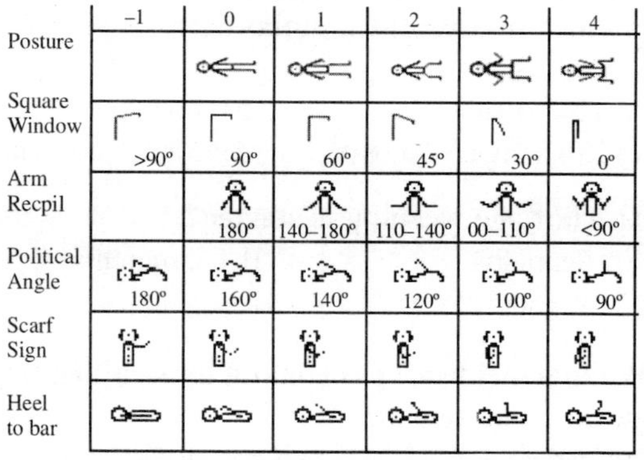

2. Physical maturity (shown in the Table given below):

Sign	Score							Sign score
	-1	0	1	2	3	4	5	
Skin	Sticky, friable, transparent	Gelatinous, red, translucent	Smooth pink, visible veins	Superficial peeling and/or rash, few veins	Cracking, pale areas, rare veins	Parchment, deep cracking, no vessels	Leathery, cracked, wrinkled	
Lanugo	None	Sparse	Abundant	Thinning	Bald areas	Mostly bald		
Plantar surface	Heel-toe 40-50 mm: -1 <40 mm: -2	>50 mm No crease	Faint red marks	Anterior transverse crease only	Creases over anterior two-thirds	Creases over entire sole		
Breast	Imperceptible	Barely perceptible	Flat areola No bud	Stippled areola 1-2 mm bud	Raised areola 3-4 mm bud	Full areola 5-10 mm bud		
Eye/ear	Lids fused. Loosely: -1 Tightly: -2	Lids open. Pinna flat; stays folded	Sl. Curved pinna; soft; slow recoil	Well-curved pinna; soft but ready to recoil	Formed and firm; instant recoil	Thick cartilage; ear stiff		
Genitals (male)	Scrotum flat; smooth	Scrotum empty; faint rugae	Testes in upper canal; rare rugae	Testes descending; few rugae	Testes down; good rugae	Testes pendulous; deep rugae		
Genitals (female)	Clitoris prominent and labia flat	Prominent clitoris and small labia minora	Prominent clitoris and enlarging minora	Majora and minora equally prominent	Majora large, minora small	Majora cover clitoris and minora		
						Total physical maturity score		

Total score	Weeks
–10	20
–5	22
0	24
5	26
10	28
15	30
20	32
25	34
30	36
35	38
40	40
45	42
50	44

17. **(d)** All of the above

Parkin Score:

Score	Skin texture	Skin color	Breast size	Ear firmness
0	Very thin	Dark red	No breast tissue palpable	Pinna soft and folded without springing back position
1	Thin smooth	Uniformally pink	Not more than 0.5 cm	Pinna soft along edge and easy to fold but returns slowly back
2	Smooth and med thickness	Pale pink	0.5-1 cms diameter	Cartilage thin but felt
3	Stiff feeling	Pale	>1cm diameter	Pinna firm
4	Thick and parchment like			

Maturity Score:

Parkin score	Age in weeks
1	26
2	30
3	33
4	34
5	35
6	36
7	37
8	38
9	39
10	40
11	41
12	42

18. **(d)** All of the above

A score of 7 or more indicates impending respiratory failure

Score	Upper chest	Lower chest retraction	Xiphoid retraction	Nasal flare	Grunt audible
0	Sync	None	None	None	None
1	Lag on insp	Just visible	Just visible	Minimal	Steth only
2	See-saw	Marked	Marked	Marked	Naked ear

19. **(d)** All of the above

20. **(c)** Impending respiratory failure

A score of 7 or more indicates impending respiratory failure

Score	Resp Rate/ min	Cyanosis	Air entry	Retractions	Grunt
0	<60	None	Good	None	None
1	60-80	In air	Diminished	Mild	Steth only
2	>80 or apneic	In 40% O_2	Barely audible	Moderate/ severe	Naked ear

21. **(d)** All of the above

Conditions to Anticipate Neonatal Birth Asphyxia– Mother more than 35 years age, Diabetes, PIH, Hydramnios, Anemia/Isoimmunisat., P.R.O.M. /PPROM, Multiple Gestation, Fetal Malformation, Decrease Fetal Activity, Preterm, SGA, Post term, Prolonged 2nd stage, Abnormal presentation, Premature labour, Precipitous labour, Non-reassuring fetal heart, APH Cord prolapsed, Meconium stained liquor, Emergency LSCS.

22. **(d)** All of the above

23. **(d)** All of the above

24. **(d)** All of the above

Ten Commandant of Warm Chain

1. Warm delivery room.
2. Immediate drying.
3. Skin-to-skin contact.
4. Breastfeeding.
5. Bathing and weighing postponed.
6. Appropriate clothing and bedding.
7. Mother and baby together.
8. Warm transportation.
9. Warm resuscitation.
10. Training/awareness raising.

25. **(c)** Increase in the size of cells

Foetal Weight Gain:

1st trimester – Increase in the number of cells.

2nd trimester – Increase in the number and size of cells.

3rd trimester – Increase in the size of cells.

26. **(d)** All of the above

Prelacteal feeds - Feed other than breast milk given to baby immediately after birth is called as prelacteal feeds.

1. Sugar water.
2. Milk mixed with jaggery.
3. Hot water mixed with sugar or jaggery.
4. Honey.
5. Milk mixed with sugar.
6. Dextrose saline.
7. Ghuty.
8. Suvarnajal.

27. **(d)** All of the above

Galactogogues – A substance that promotes lactation in a lactating mother.

Asparagus racemosus	Fenugreek
Brewer's yeast	Blessed thistle
Alfalfa	Anise
Astragalus root	Bermuda grass
Boza	Burdock
Nettle	Fennel
Goat's rue	Torbangun
Flax	Pumpkin seeds
Oatmeal	Red raspberry leaf
Quinoa	Soapwort
Vervainmarshmallow (althaea) root	
Domperidone	Metoclopramide.

28. **(a)** Harlequin sign

29. **(d)** All of the above

30. **(a)** Vernixcaseousa

31. **(d)** Lanugo

The newborn of 37-39 weeks gestational age has more lanugo than the 40 week old infant.

32. **(a)** Milia

Newborn sebaceous glands are immature. At least one pinpoint papule can be found on the cheek or across the bridge of the nose. It disappears by 2-4 weeks of age as the sebaceous glands mature and drain.

33. **(a)** Erythema toxicum

34. **(b)** 1/4th

35. **(b)** 12 and 18 months

The anterior fontanelle is at the junction of the two parietal bones and the two fused frontal bones. It is diamond-shaped and covered by a thick fibrous layer. It measures 2-3 cm in width and 3-4 cm in length. It normally closes with bone when the baby is between 12 and 18 months of age.

36. **(d)** 6 to 8 weeks

The posterior fontanelle is at the junction of the parietal bone and occipital bone. It is triangular and measures about 1cm in length. It closes by 6 to 8 weeks.

37. **(a)** Caput succedaneum

Caput succedaneum: This refers to swelling on top of the head or throughout the scalp due to fluid squeezed into the scalp during the birth process. Caput is present at birth and clears in a few days.

38. **(c)** Cephalohematoma

Cephalohematoma: This is a collection of blood on the outer surface of the skull. It is due to friction between the infant's skull and the mother's pelvic bones during the birth process. The lump is usually confined to one side of the head. It first appears on the second day of life and may grow larger for up to 5 days. It doesn't resolve completely until the baby is 2 or 3 months of age.

39. **(a)** True speech developes

40. **(b)** Epstein pearls

Epstein pearls: Little white-colored cysts can occur along the gum line or on the hard palate. These are a result of blockage of normal mucous glands. They disappear after 1 to 2 months.

41. **(b)** Passage of female hormones across the mother's placenta

42. **(a)** 2 cm

43. **(c)** 1-2 cm

44. **(b)** Two arteries and one vein

45. **(b)** Maternal hormones

Vaginal discharge in neonate: As the maternal hormones decline in the baby's blood, a clear or white discharge can flow from the vagina during the latter part of the first week of life. Occasionally the discharge will become pink or blood-tinged (false menstruation). This normal discharge should not last more than 2 to 3 days.

46. **(d)** About 4%

47. **(d)** 2.5-3.9 kg

48. **(b)** 5-10%

49. **(c)** 50 cms

50. **(b)** 34- 35 cms

51. **(a)** 58/44 mmHg

52. **(b)** Brown fat

53. **(d)** All of the above

54. **(a)** 32 weeks

55. (d) All of the above
56. (d) All of the above
57. (d) All of the above
58. (d) All of the above
59. (c) Fat
60. (d) All of the above
61. (a) Anterior pituitary
62. (d) Acts on the milk secreting cells to produce milk
63. (d) All of the above
64. (d) All of the above
65. (b) Oxytocin
66. (a) Post pituitary
67. (d) All of the above
68. (d) All of the above
69. (c) Cheek or the corner of the mouth

Rooting reflex is stimulated by touching a finger to baby's cheek or the corner of the mouth. The neonate responds by turning the head toward the stimulus, opening the mouth and searching for the stimulus. This is a necessary reflex triggered by the mother's nipple during breastfeeding. It is usually inhibited by the third to fourth month.

70. (a) Myerson's sign
71. (b) 28 weeks of gestation
72. (d) Neurological damage
73. (a) Fractured clavicle

The Moro reflex occurs when an infant is lying in a supine position and is stimulated by allowing head to fall backwards momentarily and immediate support by examiner's hand. This stimulus results in a symmetrical extension of the infant's extremities while forming a C shape with the thumb and forefinger. This is followed by a return to a flexed position with extremities against the body. Inhibition of this reflex occurs from the third to the sixth month. An asymmetrical response with this reflex may indicate a fractured clavicle or a birth injury to the nerves of the arm. Absence of this reflex in the neonate is an ominous implication of underlying neurological damage.

74. (d) 2 months

Stepping reflex is observed by holding the infant in an upright position and touching one foot lightly to a flat surface, such as the bed. The infant responds by making walking motions with both feet. This reflex will disappear at approximately two months of age.

75. (d) Sixth months

Plantar and palmar grasp: Grasping reflex occurs as the palmar reflex when a finger is placed in the neonate's palm and the neonate grasps the finger. The palmar reflex disappears around the sixth month. Similarly, the plantar reflex occurs by placing a finger against the base of the neonate's toes and the toes curl downward to grasp the finger. This reflex becomes inhibited around the ninth to tenth month.

76. (d) All of the above

- A non-conventional method of caring for low birth weight and preterm newborns after initial stabilization.
- Assists in maintaining the temperature of infant.
- Facilitates breastfeeding.
- Helps to increase the duration of breastfeeding.
- Improves mother infant bonding.
- Promotes physical growth and extra-uterine adaptation, and increases the mother's confidence, ability and involvement in the care of her small newborn.
- Dress the baby with a cap, socks, kurta and napkin.
- Place the newborn in a prone and upright (diagonal) position between the mother's breasts, covered with the mother's clothes and shawl/blanket (A loose blouse, sweater or wrap tied at the waist holds the baby).
- Let baby suckle at breasts as often as he wants, at least every 2 hourly.
- Advise the mother to sleep in propped up position so that the baby stays upright.
- Make sure the baby stays warm at all times.
- Dress the baby with extra clothing if environmental temperature is low, and cover his head.
- Ask the father or another family member to 'kangaroo' the baby when mother wants to bathe or rest, or wrap infant in several layers of warm clothing, covered with blankets and keep in a warm place.

77. (a) 60 - 80 ml /kg/day
78. (b) 15 ml / kg

Guidelines for Fluid Requirement:

- First day 60 - 80 ml/kg/day.
- Daily increment 15 ml/kg till day 7.
- Add extra 20 - 30 ml/kg for infants under radiant warmer and 15 ml/kg for those receiving phototherapy.

79. (c) Rooting reflex
80. (b) Grimace of crying
81. (c) Vigorous sucking

Examination of Cranial Nerves in Newborn

2nd	Turns to the diffuse light
8th	Optokinetic nystagmus is elicited by holding the baby on the back on outstreched arms hand supporting the occiput and gently turning slowly in clockwise
3rd, 4th, 6th	Both rotates in the same direction
3rd, 4th, 6th	Dolls eye response in the turning of the eyes in an opposite direction
2nd	Ptosis and pupillary reaction
5th	Rooting reflex
7th	Grimace of crying
8th	Startle to hand clap
9th, 10th	Gag reflex
12th	Vigorous sucking and striping action by tongue

82. **(c)** 67 kcal/100 ml

83. **(a)** Six to eight hours

84. **(b)** Up to five days

85. **(c)** Six to twelve months

Storage of Expressed Breast Milk

Place of storage	Temperature		Maximum storage time
In a room	25°C	77°F	Six to eight hours
Insulated thermal bag with ice packs			Up to 24 hours
In a refrigerator	4°C	39°F	Up to five days
Freezer compartment inside a refrigerator	–15°C	5°F	Two weeks
A combined refrigerator and freezer with separate doors	–18°C	0°F	Three to six months
Chest or upright manual defrost deep freezer	–20°C	–4°F	Six to twelve months

86. **(a)** 6 months

Weaning:

- *6 to 7 Months:* Cereals like rice, oatmeal and barley because they are the least likely to be allergenic along with breast milk.
- *6 to 8 Months:* Add strained/mashed vegetables and fruits with breast milk.
- *7 to 9 Months:* Meats, dry cereal, crackers, bagels, cooked vegetables, soft fruits with breast milk.
- *8 to 12 Months:* Mashed or finely chopped food with breast milk. This is the perfect time for the baby to join the family at the table.
- *After one year:* Eggs, fish, peanut butter.

87. **(d)** 60%

88. **(d)** 80%

89. **(a)** 3-4 days

90. **(a)** 4 to 7 days

91. **(d)** 24-72 hours

92. **(c)** Niels Ryberg Finsen

93. **(a)** Miss Sister Jean Ward

94. **(a)** Blue

95. **(b)** 45 cm

96. **(d)** All of the above

PHOTOTHERAPY:

Father of phototherapy

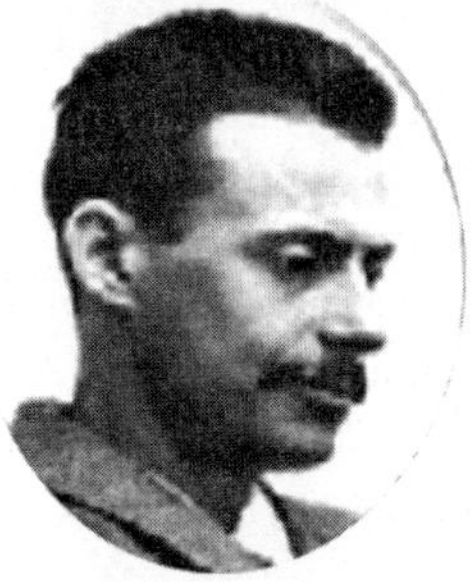

Niels Ryberg Finsen

Mother of phototherapy

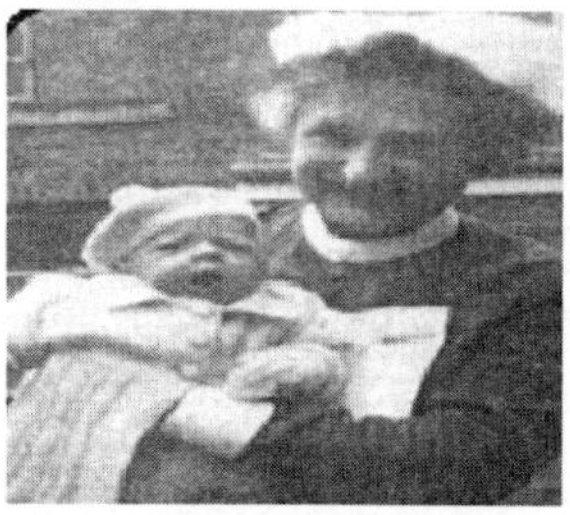

Miss Sister Jean Ward

Phototherapy: Unconjugated bilirubin → conjugated photoproducts → bile → stool and urine.

- Blue light → 450-460 nm wavelength and irradiance of 6-12μW/cm^2/nm.
- The maximal surface area of naked baby exposed distance - 45 cm.
- The eyes and genitalia covered.
- Feeding every 2 hours and frequent change of posture are necessary.
- Ideally double surface.
- The baby is turned every 2 hours or after each feed.
- Temp is monitored every 2-4 hours.
- Weight is taken daily.
- More frequent breast feeds or 10-20% extra IV fluids are provided.
- Serum total bilirubin is measured every 12 hours.
- Phototherapy is discontinued if two serum total Bilirubin values are less than 10 mg/dl.

Adverse Effects:

- Increased insensible water loss.
- Loose green stools.
- Hyperthermia / Hypothermia.

- Rashes (erythema).
- Oxidative injury.
- UV light irradiation.
- Bronze baby syndrome.
- Riboflavin deficiency.

97. **(a)** Stephane Etienne Tarnier

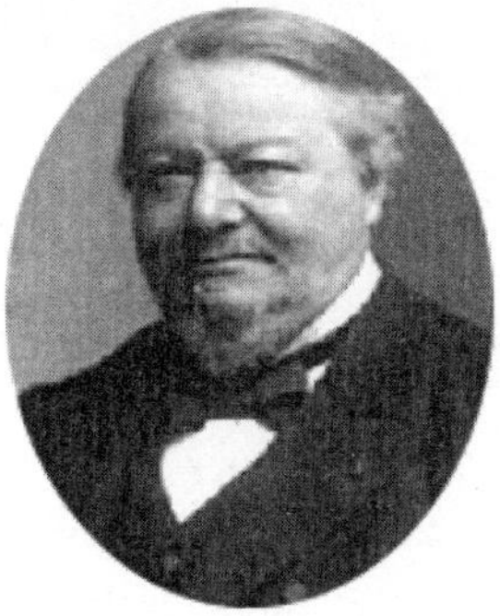

Stephane Etienne Tarnier
"Father of the incubator"

98. **(d)** All of the above

- Specific risks for the preterm neonate–Apnea of prematurity, hypoxic-ischemic encephalopathy (HIE), retinopathy of prematurity (ROP), developmental disability, cerebral palsy intraventricular hemorrhage, patent ductus arteriosus, respiratory distress syndrome. Chronic lung disease – Bronchopulmonary dysplasia or BPD, hypoglycemia, feeding difficulties, rickets of prematurity, hypocalcemia, inguinal hernia, and necrotizing enterocolitis (NEC), anemia of prematurity, thrombocytopenia, hyperbilirubinemia lead to kernicterus. Infection–Sepsis, pneumonia and urinary tract infection.

99. **(d)** All of the above

Sarnat and Sarnat Scoring for hypoxic ishemic encephalopathy:

Sign	**Stage 1**	**Stage 2**	**Stage 3**
Level of consciousness	Hyper alert	Lethargic	Stuporous/coma
Muscle tone	Normal	Hypotonic	Flaccid
Posture	Normal	Flexion	Decerebrate
Tendon reflex	Hyperactive	Hyperactive	Absent
Myoclonus	Present	Present	Absent
Moro reflex	Strong	Weak	Absent
Pupils	Mydriasis	Miosis	Unequal
Seizures	None	Common	Decerebration
EEG	Normal	Low voltage changing to seizure activity	Early periodic pattern, later isopotential
Duration	<24 hours	2-14 days	Days to week
Outcome	Good	Variable	Death/ severe deficits

Chapter 5

Adolescency

1. **Which of the following is 1st sign of puberty in female?**
   (a) Development of breast
   (b) Development of pubic hair
   (c) Development of axillary hair
   (d) Menarche

2. **In boys, the first visible sign of puberty:**
   (a) Testicular enlargement
   (b) Penile growth
   (c) Development of axillary hair
   (d) Voice change

3. **Stereotypical adolescence is:**
   (a) Early adolescent (b) Middle adolescent
   (c) Late adolescent (d) None

4. **20 years healthy male assumes himself as female, this is:**
   (a) Transvestism (b) Trans-sexualism
   (c) Homosexualism (d) Schizophrenia

5. **The final stages of breast, penile, pubic hair development occur by:**
   (a) 15-16 years (b) 16-17 years
   (c) 17-18 years (d) 18-19 years

6. **Leading causes of adolescent morbidity and mortality is:**
   (a) Unintended pregnancy
   (b) Sexually transmitted infections
   (c) Automobile and motorcycle accidents
   (d) Substance use and abuse

7. **Approximate retension time of alcohol in urine is:**
   (a) 7-10 hours
   (b) 10-13 hours
   (c) 16-18 hours
   (d) 24 hours

8. **Approximate retension time of alcohol in blood is:**
   (a) 7-10 hours
   (b) 10-13 hours
   (c) 24 hours
   (d) 48 hours

9. **Elbow fuses in boys at the age of:**
   (a) 13-13.5 years (b) 15-15.5 years
   (c) 16-16.5 years (d) 18-19 years

10. **Period of early adolescence:**
    (a) 10-13 years (b) 13-16 years
    (c) 16-19 years (d) 8-12 years

Answers

1. **(a)** Development of breast
(Nelson Textbook of Pediatrics, 18th ed.)
In girls, the first visible sign of puberty and the hallmark of SMR2 is the appearance of breast buds, between 8 and 12 years of age. Menses typically begins 2-2½ years later, during SMR3-4 (median age, 12 years; normal range, 9-16 years), around the peak height velocity. Less obvious changes include enlargement of the ovaries, uterus, labia and clitoris, and thickening of the endometrium and vaginal mucosa.

2. **(a)** Testicular enlargement
(Nelson Textbook of Pediatrics, 18th ed.)
In boys, the first visible sign of puberty and the hallmark of SMR2 is testicular enlargement, beginning as early as 9½ years. This is followed by penile growth during SMR3. Peak growth occurs when testis volumes reach approximately 9-10 cm^3 during SMR4. Under the influence of LH and testosterone, the seminiferous tubules, epididymis, seminal vesicles, and prostate enlarge.

3. **(b)** Middle adolescent
(Nelson Textbook of Pediatrics, 18th ed.)
Middle adolescence refers to "stereotypical adolescence". Relationships with parents become more strained and distant due to redirected energies toward peer relationships and separation from the family. Dating can become a lightning rod for parent-child battles, in which the real issue may be the separation from parents rather than the particulars of "with whom" or "how late". The majority of teenagers progress through adolescence with minimal difficulties rather than experiencing the stereotypical "storm and stress". It is the large minority of adolescents (approximately 20-30%) who do experience stress and struggle through this period who require support. Adolescents with visible differences are also at risk for problems, such as not developing adequate social skills and confidence and having more difficulty establishing satisfying relationships.

4. **(b)** Trans-sexualism
(Nelson Textbook of Pediatrics, 18th ed.)
Trans-sexualism is the conviction by a person who is biologically a member of one gender that he or she is a member of the other gender. Trans-sexual adolescents (transpersons) feel discomfort and a sense of inappropriateness about their assigned sex. Trans-sexuals usually have a difficult time with social and occupational functioning. Concurrent psychopathologic conditions and depression are common, as is societal consternation. The natural history of trans-sexualism is not well understood. A preponderance of adult trans-sexuals had gender identity disorders as children and adolescents.Extreme femininity in boys is a predisposing factor. Some remember being confused about gender identity as early as 2 years of age. Which particular effeminate boys will later show trans-sexual behavior cannot be accurately predicted.

5. **(a)** 17-18 years
(Nelson Textbook of Pediatrics, 18th ed.)
The final stages of breast, penile and pubic hair development occur by 17-18 years of age in 95% of males and females.

6. **(a)** Automobile and motorcycle accidents
(Nelson Textbook of Pediatrics, 18th ed.)
The health conditions having the greatest impact on the status of adolescent health are early unintended pregnancy, sexually transmitted infections, mental disorders, injuries, and substance use and abuse. Automobile and motorcycle accidents are the leading causes of adolescent morbidity and mortality. Alcohol is a factor in approximately one third of the fatal accidents involving adolescents. In addition, other factors such as driver error, less frequent use of seat belts, and the presence of other teen passengers increases the severity of crashes involving teen drivers.

7. **(b)** 10-13 hours

(Nelson Textbook of Pediatrics, 18th ed.)

Urine Screening for Drugs Commonly Abused by Adolescents

Drug	Major metabolite	Initial	First confirmation	Second confirmation	Approximate retention time
Alcohol (blood)	Acetaldehyde	GC	IA		7–10 hours
Alcohol (urine)	Acetaldehyde	GC	IA		10–13 hours
Amphetamines		TLC	IA	GC, GC/MS	48 hours
Barbiturates		IA	TLC	GC, GC/MS	Short-acting (24 hours); long-acting (2–3 weeks)
Benzodiazepines		IA	TLC	GC, GC/MS	3 days
Cannabinoids	Carboxy- and hydroxyl-metabolites	IA	TLC	GC/MS	3–10 days (occasional user); 1–2 months (chronic user)
Cocaine	Benzoyl ecgonine	IA	TLC	GC/MS	2–4 days
Methaqualone Opiates	Hydroxylated metabolites	TLC	IA	GC/MS	2 week
Heroin	Morphine Glucuronide	IA	TLC	GC, GC/MS	2 days
Morphine	Morphine Glucuronide	IA	TLC	GC, GC/MS	2 days
Codeine	Morphine Glucuronide	IA	T LC	GC, GC/MS	2 days
Phencyclidine		TLC	IA	GC, GC/MS	8 days

8. **(a)** 7-10 hours

(Nelson Textbook of Pediatrics, 18th ed.)

Refer as above.

9. **(a)** 13-13.5 years

(Nelson Textbook of Pediatrics, 18th ed.)

Boys Modal Age Between (Yr)	Area	Girls Modal Age Between (Yr)
Elbow		
13.0–13.5	Onset in humerus	11.0–11.5
15.0–15.5	Complete in ulna	12.5–13.0
Foot and Ankle		
14.0–14.5	Onset in great toe	12.5–13.0
15.5–16.0	Complete in tibia, fibula	14.0–14.5
Hand and Wrist		
15.0–15.5	Onset in distal phalanges	13.0–13.5
17.5–18.0	Complete in radius	16.0–16.5
Knee		
15.0-15.5	Onset in tibial tuberosity	13.5-14.0
17.5-18.0	Complete in fibula	16.0-16.5
Hip and Pelvis		
15.5-16.0	Onset in greater trochanter	14.0-14.5
After 18.0	Complete in symphysis	17.5-18.0
Shoulder and Clavicle		
15.5-16.0	Onset in greater tubercle of humerus	14.0-14.5
After 18.0	Complete in clavicle	17.5-18.0

10. **(a)** 10-13 years

(Nelson Textbook of Pediatrics, 18th ed.)

Central Issues in Early, Middle and Late Adolescence

Variable	Early adolescence	Middle adolescence	Late adolescence
Age (yr)	10–13	14–16	17–20 and beyond
Sexual maturity rating[*]	1–2	3–5	5
Somatic	Secondary sex characteristics	Height growth peaks	Physically mature
	Beginning of rapid growth	Body shape and composition change	Slower growth
	Awkward appearance	Acne and odor	
		Menarche/spermarche	
Cognitive and moral	Concrete operations	Emergence of abstract thought (formal operations)	Future-oriented with sense of perspective
	Unable to perceive long-term outcome of current decision-making	May perceive future implications, but may not apply in decision-making	Idealism; absolutism
	Conventional morality	Questioning mores	Able to think things through independently
Self-concept/ identity formation	Preoccupied with changing body	Concern with attractiveness	More stable body image
	Self-consciousness about appearance and attractiveness	Increasing introspection	Attractiveness may still be of concern
	Fantasy and present-oriented	"Stereotypical adolescent"	Emancipation complete
			Firmer identity
Family	Increased need for privacy	Conflicts over control and independence	Emotional and physical separation from family
	Increased bid for independence	Struggle for acceptance of greater autonomy	Increased autonomy
Peers	Seeks same-sex peer affiliation to counter instability	Intense peer group involvement	Peer group and values recede in importance
		Preoccupation with peer culture	Intimacy/possible commitment takes precedence
		Peers provide behavioural example	
Sexual	Increased interest in sexual anatomy	Testing ability to attract partner	Consolidation of sexual identity
	Anxieties and questions about genital changes, size	Initiation of relationships and sexual activity	Focus on intimacy and formation of stable relationships
	Limited dating and intimacy	Questions of sexual orientation	Planning for future and commitment
Relationship to society	Middle school adjustment	Gauging skills and opportunities	Career decisions (e.g., college, work)

Chapter 6

Nutrition (1)

1. **Routine perinatal administration of vitamin K is recommended as prophylaxis against:**
   (a) Infective hepatitis
   (b) Hemorrhagic disease of the newborn
   (c) Cirrhosis
   (d) None

2. **Human milk contains relatively high concentrations of:**
   (a) Secretory immunoglobulin A
   (b) IgM antibodies
   (c) Kinins
   (d) Prostaglandins

3. **Which virus have been demonstrated in breast milk ?**
   (a) Cytomegalovirus (CMV)
   (b) Human T-cell lymphotropic virus type 1
   (c) Rubella virus
   (d) All of the above

4. **Which hormone release stimulates milk secretion by the cuboidal cells in the acini or alveoli of the breast?**
   (a) Prolactin (b) Oxytocin
   (c) Thyroxine (d) GH

5. **Which factor decides adequacy of breast milk supply to baby?**
   (a) After feed baby sleeps 2-4 hours
   (b) Passes urine 5-6 times in 24 hours
   (c) Gains weight adequately
   (d) All of the above

6. **Contraindication for breastfeeding:**
   (a) Mother on anti thyroid drugs
   (b) Mother on anti malignancy drugs
   (c) Child having galactosemia
   (d) All of the above

7. **Which is the first predictor of overweight?**
   (a) Low birth weight (b) High birth weight
   (c) Maternal steroid levels (d) None

8. **Disease associated with childhood obesity:**
   (a) Bardet-Biedl syndrome (b) Cushing syndrome
   (c) Cohen syndrome (d) All of the above

9. **Night blindness occurs because of absence of retinal in the visual pigment:**
   (a) Cone pigment (b) Melanin
   (c) Rhodopsin (d) None

10. **The range of normal vitamin A levels is:**
    (a) 10-20 g/Dl (b) 20-60 g/Dl
    (c) 80-100 g/Dl (d) 100-120 g/Dl

11. **At what age rickets of prematurity presents?**
    (a) 1-4 months (b) 4-8 months
    (c) 8-12 months (d) 1- 2 years

12. **What are features of rickets of prematurity presents?**
    (a) Nontraumatic fractures (b) Traumatic fractures
    (c) Bowing of legs (d) CTEV

13. **Which is vitamin K dependent clotting factor?**
    (a) II (b) VII
    (c) IX (d) X
    (e) All of the above

14. **How much daily maintenance fluid volume requirement for child of 0-10 kg?**
    (a) 50 mL/kg (b) 100 mL/kg
    (c) 150 mL/kg (d) 200 mL/kg

15. **A normal plasma osmolality is:**
    (a) 230-245 mOsm/kg (b) 250-265 mOsm/kg
    (c) 285-295 mOsm/kg (d) 315-325 mOsm/kg

16. **5% dextrose provides how much calories?**
    (a) 17 calories/100 ml (b) 24 calories/100 ml
    (c) 50 calories/100 ml (d) 75 calories/100 ml

Answers

1. **(b)** Hemorrhagic disease of the newborn
2. **(a)** Secretory immunoglobulin A
3. **(a)** Cytomegalovirus (CMV)
4. **(a)** Prolactin
5. **(d)** All of the above
6. **(d)** All of the above
7. **(b)** High birth weight
8. **(d)** All of the above

Diseases Associated with Childhood Obesity

Syndrome	Manifestation
Alström syndrome	Hypogonadism, retinal degeneration, deafness, diabetes mellitus
Bardet-Biedl syndrome	Retinal degeneration, syndactyly, polydactyly, hypogonadism, mental retardation, autosomal recessive
Carpenter syndrome	Polydactyly, syndactyly, cranial synostosis, mental retardation
Cohen syndrome	Midchildhood-onset obesity, short stature, prominent maxillary incisors, hypotonia, mental retardation, microcephaly, decreased visual activity
Cushing syndrome	Adrenal hyperplasia or pituitary tumor
Deletion 9q 34	Early-onset obesity, mental retardation, brachycephaly, synophrys, prognathism, behavior and sleep disturbances
ENPP1 gene mutations	Insulin resistance, childhood obesity, chromosome 6q
Fröhlich syndrome	Hypothalamic tumor
Hyperinsulinism	Nesidioblastosis, pancreatic adenoma, hypoglycemia, Mauriac syndrome (poor diabetic control)
Leptin or leptin receptor gene mutation	Early-onset severe obesity, infertility (hypogonadotropic hypogonadism); uncommon; leptin deficiency treatable with recombinant leptin
Melanocortin 4 receptor gene mutation	Early-onset severe obesity, increased linear growth, hyperphagia, hyperinsulinemia; homozygous worse than heterozygous; common genetic cause of obesity
Muscular dystrophy	Late-onset obesity due in part to inactivity
Myelodysplasia	Spina bifida due in part to inactivity
Prader-Willi syndrome	Neonatal hypotonia, normal growth immediately after birth, small hands and feet, mental retardation, hypogonadism; some have partial deletion of chromosome 15 and loss of paternally expressed genes; hyperphagia leading to severe childhood obesity; ghrelin paradoxically elevated
Pro-opiomelanocortin deficiency	Obesity, red hair, adrenal insufficiency, hyperproinsulinemia
Pseudohypopara-thyroidism	Variable hypocalcemia, cutaneous calcifications
Turner syndrome	Ovarian dysgenesis, lymphedema, web neck, XO chromosome

Contd.

Contd.

9. **(c)** Rhodopsin
10. **(b)** 20–60 g/Dl
11. **(a)** 1–4 months
12. **(a)** Nontraumatic fractures
13. **(e)** All of the above
14. **(b)** 100 mL/kg

Body Weight Method for Calculating Daily Maintenance Fluid Volume

Body weight	Fluid per day
0–10 kg	100 mL/kg
11–20 kg	1,000 mL + 50 mL/kg for each kg > 10 kg
>20 kg	1,500 mL + 20 mL/kg for each kg > 20 kg[*]

15. **(c)** 285-295 mOsm/kg
16. **(a)** 17 calories/100 mL

Chapter 7

Nutrition (2)

1. **EER (Estimated Energy Requirement) for normal infant as compared to normal adult is approximately:**
   (a) Is equal to normal adult
   (b) Is half of normal adult
   (c) Is double that of normal adult
   (d) Is two standard deviations mean to normal adult

2. **Formula milk is deficient in:**
   (a) Short chain polyunsaturated fatty acid
   (b) Long chain polyunsaturated fatty acid
   (c) Short chain saturated fatty acid
   (d) Long chain saturated fatty acid

3. **Exclusive breast feeding has following disadvantages *except:***
   (a) Hemolysis because of vit K deficiency
   (b) Intestinal colic
   (c) Golden colour stool
   (d) Prevention of physiological jaundice

4. **When should start breast feeding?**
   (a) 2-3 hours after birth (b) Half hour after birth
   (c) 1-4 hours after birth (d) 4-5 hours after birth

5. **Human mother milk is deficient in:**
   (a) Ca (b) Vitamin D
   (c) Fluoride (d) (b) and (c)

6. **HIV positive mother gives birh, she should:**
   (a) She should not breast feed child at least for 1st 6 months
   (b) She should feed child with bottle
   (c) She should give cow milk to child
   (d) She should continue breast-feeding

7. **Which of the following viruses may be present in the fresh donor milk:**
   (a) CMV (b) Hepatitis B
   (c) Herpes simplex (d) All of the above

8. **Human breast milk having high concentration of:**
   (a) IgM antibodies (b) Lysozymes
   (c) Mast cells (d) IgA antibodies

9. **Accordingly baby friendly hospital which of the following is true?**
   (a) Should not give breast feeding for at least 1 day after child birth
   (b) Only breast feed and no other feed
   (c) For 24 hours baby is kept with mother
   (d) Both (b) and (c)

10. **Infants who can't fed on demand like who are in NICU should fed:**
    (a) Every 6 hourly during day and night
    (b) Every 12 hourly during day and night
    (c) Every 3 hourly during day and night
    (d) Should feed with bottle

11. **Breast milk in a refrigerator is stored for:**
    (a) 4 hours (b) 8 hours
    (c) 12 hours (d) 24 hours

12. **Which of the following is factor for successful breast feeding?**
    (a) Mother should be at big hospital
    (b) Mother should be at her home
    (c) Mother should start breast feeding after 6 days of child birth
    (d) Mother should be happy and relaxed state of mind

13. **Which of the following is coming first in breast feeding process?**
    (a) Rooting reflex (b) Sucking reflex
    (c) Swallowing reflex (d) Satiety reflex

14. **Infant will turn towards the object and open his or her mouth in anticipation of grasping the nipple is called as:**
    (a) Rooting reflex (b) Sucking reflex
    (c) Swallowing reflex (d) All of the above

15. La Leche League is related to:
(a) Providing vaccination to babies
(b) Providing balanced diet to children
(c) Giving assistance with nursing for nursing mothers
(d) None of the above

16. Expression of milk is done for:
(a) To feed baby
(b) It is one of the method of breast feeding
(c) To prevent engorgement of breast
(d) Expression never done

17. Weaning period is:
(a) 1 year of age (b) 3 months of age
(c) 6 months of age (d) 4 months of age

18. Which of the following is contraindication for breast feeding?
(a) Septicemia (b) Active tuberculosis
(c) Psycosis (d) All of the above

19. Food and Drug Administration (FDA) is manufactured by:
(a) United Kingdom (b) USA
(c) France (d) German

20. Underfeeding is suggested by:
(a) Less consumption of milk by infant
(b) Excessive sleeping
(c) Restlessness, crying and not weight gain
(d) Excessive diarrhoea

21. For malnutrition and undernutrition which of the following works?
(a) WHO (b) UNICEF
(c) ASHA (d) None

22. Measurement of undernutrition is done with:
(a) Height for age (b) Weight for age
(c) Weight for height (d) All of the above

23. Non-edematous SCU is known as:
(a) Kwashiorkar (b) Marasmus
(c) Marasmic kwashiorkor (d) All of the above

24. Non - edematous SCU is believed to result due to:
(a) Inadequate intake of energy
(b) Inadequate intake of both energy and protein
(c) Inadequate intake of protein
(d) Inadequate intake of carbohydrates

25. Edema in kwashiorkor is mainly due to:
(a) Decreased secretion of water
(b) Hypoalbuminemia
(c) Hypoproteinemia
(d) Excessive intake of water

26. What is the hallmark of Refeeding Syndrome?
(a) Hypophosphatemia (b) Hyponatremia
(c) Hypokalemia (d) Hyperphoshatemia

27. Which of the following condition do not consists child obesity?
(a) Turner's syndrome (b) Muscular dystrophy
(c) Marasmus (d) Carpenter syndrome

28. Normal weight is considered as per BMI:
(a) 5th-84th percentile (b) 5th-50th percentile
(c) <50th percentile (d) None of the above

29. Kwashiorkor is characterised by all *except:*
(a) Dermatitis (b) Edema
(c) Flag sign (d) Alertness

30. Vitamin A deficiency leads to all of the following *except:*
(a) Nyctalopia (b) Photophobia
(c) Keratomalacia (d) Sterility

31. The normal range of vitamin A is:
(a) 20-60 g/dl (b) 10-40 g/dl
(c) 200-600 g/dl (d) 2-6 g/dl

32. A daily dose of vitamin A is:
(a) 1500 μg (b) 2000 μg
(c) 2500 μg (d) 1000 μg

33. On the radiograph hyper vitaminosis A shows:
(a) Benign lesion (b) Osteolytic lesion
(c) Hyperostosis (d) Hypoostosis

34. Toxicity of vitamin A in children occurs when chronic daily intake is of about:
(a) 6000 μg (b) 1500 μg
(c) 1000 μg (d) 2000 μg

35. Carotenemia is:
(a) Deficiency of vitamin A
(b) Vitamin A toxicity
(c) Yellow discolouration of skin because of excessive intake of carotenoids
(d) All of the above

36. Xeropthalmia is due to:
(a) Vit. A deficiency (b) Vit. D deficiency
(c) Vit. E deficiency (d) Vit. B deficiency

37. First stage of Vitamin A deficiency is:
(a) Cojunctival xerosis (b) Bitots spots
(c) Xeropthalmia (d) Night blindness

38. Which of the following is anti-pellagra vitamin?
(a) Biotin (b) Pantothenic acid
(c) Niacin (d) Cynocobalamine

39. Which of the following vitamin deficiency causes beriberi?
(a) Niacin (b) Cynocobalamine
(c) Thiamine (d) Biotin

40. In which of the following patient urine contains albumin and cast?
(a) Dry beriberi (b) Wet beriberi
(c) Pellagra (d) None of the above

41. Which of the following vitamin deficiency causes impaired nerve conduction?
(a) Biotin (b) Thiamine
(c) Riboflavin (d) Cyanocobalamine

42. Epidemic thiamine deficiency is seen in:
(a) Cow milk fed infants
(b) Cuffalo milk fed infants
(c) Soy based formula fed infants
(d) Coconut based formula fed infants

43. Death due to thiamine deficiency is due to mainly:
(a) Asphyxia (b) Shock
(c) Brain haemorrhages (d) Cardiac involvement

44. Electrocardiogram of thiamine deficiency shows:
(a) Decreased Q-T interval, everted T wave
(b) Increased Q-T interval, inverted T wave
(c) Decreased Q-T interval, inverted T wave
(d) Increased Q-T interval, everted T wave

45. Best indicator of the vitamin thiamine deficiency:
(a) Urinary excretion of thiamine
(b) High level of blood or urinary glyoxylate
(c) Low blood cell transketolase activity
(d) Clinical

46. The daily dose of vitamin thiamine for children and adults are respectively:
(a) 10 mg and 50 mg (b) 100 mg and 500 mg
(c) 25 mg and 500 mg (d) 50 mg and 500 mg

47. Thiamine dependence is described in terms of:
(a) Heart failure and psychic disorders
(b) Megaloblastic anemia and typical maple syrup urine disease
(c) Hoarsesness of voice and meningitis
(d) Asphyxia and heart failure

48. Co-enzyme that provided by thiamine:
(a) Thiamine pyrophosphate
(b) Thiamine decarboxylase
(c) Thiamine hexolase
(d) Thiamine enolase

49. Good source of thiamine include:
(a) Rice, jowar, groundnut
(b) Meat, legumes, cereals
(c) Legumes, rice, spinatch
(d) Spinatch, meat, rice

50. Riboflavin co-enzymes take part in:
(a) HMP shunt
(b) Electron transport chain
(c) TCA cycle
(d) Glycolysis

51. Chelosis is mainly due to deficiency of:
(a) Thiamine (b) Riboflavin
(c) Cynocobalamine (d) Biotin

52. Activity of Erythrocyte Glutathione Reductase (EGR) is functional test of:
(a) Riboflavin deficiency
(b) Biotin deficiency
(c) Cynocobalamine deficiency
(d) Vitamin A deficiency

53. The major source of riboflavin is:
(a) Eggs
(b) Milk and milk products (c) Green vegetables

54. Oral dose for riboflavin deficiency:
(a) 3-10 mg/day (b) 2-5 mg/day
(c) 10-20 mg/day

55. In the diet Niacin is in the form of:
(a) Tryptophan (b) Arachedonic acid
(c) Cholesterol (d) Amino acids

56. Pellagra is due to deficiency of:
(a) Riboflavin (b) Niacin
(c) Biotin (d) Cynocobalamine

57. Classic triad of pellagra is:
(a) Dermatitis, diarrhoea, dementia
(b) Dacryocystitis, diarrhoea, diminution of vision
(c) Dementia, dacryocystitis, diarrhoea
(d) Diminution of vision, diarrhoea, dementia

58. Casal necklace appearance is seen in which condition?
(a) Beriberi
(b) Pellagra
(c) Rickets
(d) Chelosis

59. In pellagra demylination of which column of spinal cord takes place?
(a) Medial and lateral columns
(b) Posterior and lateral columns
(c) Anterior and medial columns
(d) Posterior and medial columns

60. Niacin toxicity is:
(a) Anemia
(b) Cholestatic jaundice
(c) Hepatotoxicity
(d) Both (b) and (c)

61. For conversion of tryptophan to niacin which of the following enzyme is required?
(a) Biotin
(b) Pyridoxine
(c) Cynocobalamine
(d) Vitamin D

62. To treat convulsions due to Vitamin B_6 deficiency which of the following is used?
(a) 100 mg oral dose
(b) 100 mg intramuscular dose
(c) 1000 mg oral dose
(d) 1000 mg intramuscular dose

Answers

1. **(c)** Is double that of normal adult

Expressed per unit of body weight, the EER of the normal infant is approximately twice that of the normal adult. The greater energy requirement of the infant reflects primarily the higher metabolic rate of infants and children and their special needs for growth and development. The inefficient intestinal absorption of the neonate compared with the adult contributes only minimally to the higher energy requirement of infants fed human milk or modern infant formula.

2. **(b)** Long chain polyunsaturated fatty acid

Although infants can convert LA and ALA, respectively, to ARA and DHA, the contents of ARA and, particularly, DHA in the plasma and erythrocyte lipids of formula-fed infants are lower than the contents in breast-fed infants. Autopsy studies show that the low erythrocyte lipid content of DHA, but not ARA, is accompanied by a lower concentration in the brain. These differences are assumed to reflect the presence of LC-PUFA in human milk, but not in formula, suggesting that the synthetic pathway, although intact, does not synthesize enough LC-PUFA. The better visual and, particularly, cognitive development of breast-fed compared with formula-fed infants also has been attributed to the presence of LC-PUFA in human milk, but not in formula.

3. **(b)** Intestinal colic

Macrophages in human milk may synthesize complement, lysozyme, and lactoferrin. In addition, breast milk contains lactoferrin, an iron-binding whey protein that is normally approximately 1/3 saturated with iron and has an inhibitory effect on the growth of *Escherichia coli* in the intestine. Further, the lower pH of the stool of breast-fed infants is thought to contribute to the favorable intestinal flora of infants fed human milk compared with formula (more bifidobacteria and lactobacilli; fewer *Escherichia coli*), and this helps protect against infections caused by some species of *E. coli*. Human milk also contains bile salt-stimulated lipase, which kills *Giardia lamblia* and *Entamoeba histolytica*. Transfer of tuberculin responsiveness by breast milk suggests passive transfer of T-cell immunity.

4. **(b)** Half hour after birth

Feedings should be initiated as soon after birth as possible, depending on the infant's ability to tolerate enteral nutrition. This helps maintain normal metabolism during the transition from fetal to extrauterine life and also promotes bonding between the mother and infant. Most infants can start breast-feeding immediately after birth, almost always within 1–4 hours. Mothers who wish to initiate breast-feeding in the delivery room should be supported in doing so, provided there is no question about the infant's tolerance of enteral feeding. If so, feedings should be withheld until the infant is carefully evaluated. It if appears that feedings must be withheld for some time, parenteral fluids should be administered.

5. **(d)** (b) and (c)

Milk from the mother whose diet is sufficient and properly balanced will supply all the necessary nutrients except fluoride and vitamin D.

6. **(d)** She should continue breast-feeding

Transmission of **HIV** by breast-feeding is well documented. Thus, if safe alternatives are available, breast-feeding by HIV-infected mothers is not recommended. However, in many developing countries, breast-feeding may be crucial for infant survival; the risk of HIV transmission by breast-feeding may be less than the risk of other feeding methods. The World Health Organization (WHO) recommends that breast-feeding be continued, even in areas of high endemic rates of HIV infection, unless safe infant formula is readily available. This reflects the belief that the risk of formula-feeding in many developing countries is significantly greater than the risk of HIV infection with breast-feeding.

7. **(d)** All of the above

Cytomegalovirus (CMV), human T-cell lymphotropic virus type 1, rubella virus, hepatitis B virus, and herpes simplex virus have also been demonstrated in breast milk. Approximately 2/3 of CMV-seronegative breast-fed infants may become infected with CMV. In term infants, this appears to occur without symptoms or sequelae, but the risk of more serious infection in preterm infants may be greater. Thus, the use of fresh donor milk for feeding preterm infants is contraindicated unless the milk is known to be CMV-negative.

8. **(d)** IgA antibodies

Human milk contains bacterial and viral antibodies, including relatively high concentrations of secretory immunoglobulin A, that prevent microorganisms from adhering to the intestinal mucosa.

9. **(d)** Both (b) and (c)

To Encourage Breast-Feeding in the Hospital: UNICEF/WHO Baby-Friendly

Hospital Initiatives

- Provide all pregnant women with information and counseling.
- Document the desire to breast-feed in the medical record.
- Document the method of feeding in the infant's record.
- Place the newborn and mother skin-to-skin, and initiate breast-feeding within 1 hour of birth.
- Continue skin-to-skin contact at other times and encourage rooming in.
- Assess breast-feeding and continue encouragement and teaching on each shift.

Mothers to Learn

- Proper position and latch on
- Nutritive sucking and swallowing
- Milk production and release
- Frequency and feeding cues
- Expression of milk if needed
- Assessment of the infant's nutritional status
- When to contact the clinician

Additional Instructions

- Refer to lactation consultation if any concerns arise.
- Infants should go to the breast at least 8–12 times/24 hours, day and night.
- Avoid time limits on the breasts; offer both breasts at each feeding.
- Do not give sterile water, glucose, or formula unless indicated.
- If supplements are given, use cup feeding, a Haberman feeder, fingers, or syringe feedings.
- Avoid pacifiers in the newborn nursery except during painful procedures.
- Avoid antilactation drugs.

10. **(c)** Every 3 hourly during day and night

Infants who can't be fed on demand should be brought to the mother for feeding approximately every 3 hours during the day and night.

11. **(d)** 24 hours

Extra milk and store it (in a home freezer for up to 1 month or in a refrigerator for up to 24 hours) for use when she is not available.

12. **(d)** Mother should be happy and relaxed state of mind

No factor is more important for successful breast-feeding than the mother's happy, relaxed state of mind. Mothers may worry that their infants are abnormal when they cry, are drowsy, sneeze, or regurgitate milk. They are often upset by any suggestion that their milk may be lacking in quantity or quality, and they may be disturbed by the scanty supply of colostrum, nipple tenderness, and the fullness of the breasts on the 4th or 5th day after delivery. Many mothers do not feel comfortable when trying to nurse in an open ward, or even with another person in the room. Many also may worry about what is going on at home while they are in the hospital or what is going to happen when they return home. An alert physician recognizes and appreciates these worries, particularly if the infant is a first born, and provides tactful reassurance and explanations that minimize worry and enhance the likelihood of successful breast-feeding. The support plan for individual mothers, of course, must include consideration of social and cultural factors.

13. **(a)** Rooting reflex

Several reflexes or behavior patterns that facilitate breast-feeding are present at birth. These include the rooting, sucking, swallowing, and satiety reflexes. The **rooting reflex** is the 1st to come into play.

14. **(a)** Rooting reflex

If the cheek is touched by a smooth object (the mother's breast), the infant will turn toward that object and open his or her mouth in anticipation of grasping the nipple (rooting with the mouth for the nipple).

15. **(c)** Giving assistance with nursing for nursing mothers

The **La Leche League**, which establishes close relationships between successful nursing mothers and mothers needing assistance with nursing, is often helpful in such circumstances.

16. **(c)** To prevent engorgement of breast

Expression of breast milk is useful to relieve engorgement of the breasts.

17. **(c)** 6 months of age

Between 6 and 12 months of age, after they become accustomed to solid foods and liquids by bottle and/or cup, most infants decrease the volume and frequency of breast-feeding. As the infant demands less milk, the mother's supply gradually diminishes without causing discomfort from engorgement. Weaning can be initiated when mutually desired by the mother and infant by substituting formula by bottle or cup for part and, subsequently, all of a breast-feeding. Breast-feeding is eventually replaced with formula-feeding, at which time the infant is weaned completely. Occasionally, an infant takes a cup as readily as a bottle. If so, the intermediate transfer from breast to bottle before transferring from bottle to cup can be avoided. These changes should be made gradually and should be a pleasant experience, not a conflict, for both the mother and the infant.

18. **(d)** All of the above

There also are few maternal contraindications to breast-feeding. Markedly inverted nipples may be troublesome, as may fissuring or cracking of the nipples, but the latter can usually be avoided by preventing engorgement. **Mastitis** usually can be alleviated by continued and frequent nursing on the affected breast to keep it from becoming engorged, but local heat applications and antibiotics may occasionally be necessary. Acute maternal infection may contraindicate breast-feeding if the infant does not have the same infection; otherwise, there is no need to stop nursing unless the condition of either the mother or the infant necessitates it. When the infant is unaffected, the breast may be emptied and the milk given to the infant by bottle or cup. Mothers with septicemia, active tuberculosis, typhoid fever, breast cancer, or malaria should not breast-feed. Substance abuse and severe neuroses or psychoses also are contraindications to breast-feeding. Infants with galactosemia should not be breast-fed, but should receive a non-lactose-containing formula.

19. **(b)** USA

The nutrient content of infant formulas marketed in the USA is regulated by the Food and Drug Administration (FDA) according to the Infant Formula Act, and most industrialized as well as many developing countries have similar regulations.

20. **(c)** Restlessness, crying and not weight gain

Underfeeding is suggested by restlessness and crying as well as by failure to gain weight adequately.

21. **(b)** UNICEF

In response to this situation, the United Nations International Children's Emergency Fund (UNICEF) has developed and is promoting an inclusive conceptual framework for organizing scientific knowledge and experience concerning undernutrition (or malnutrition).

22. **(d)** All of the above

Despite the need for additional approaches, a number of anthropometric indices have been used successfully for many years to estimate the prevalence of undernutrition among preschool-aged children. These include height-for-age, weight-for-age, and weight-for-height.

23. **(b)** Marasmus

Severe childhood undernutrition (SCU), whether primary or secondary, is a spectrum ranging from mild undernutrition resulting in some decrease in length-for-age and/or weight-for-age through severe forms of undernutrition resulting in more marked deficits in weight-for-age and length-for-age as well as wasting (a low weight-for-length measure). Historically, the most severe forms of SCU, **marasmus** (non-edematous SCU with severe wasting) and **kwashiorkor** (edematous SCU), were considered distinct disorders.

24. **(b)** Inadequate intake of both energy and protein

Non-edematous SCU was believed to result primarily from inadequate energy intake or inadequate intakes of both energy and protein, whereas edematous SCU was believed to result primarily from inadequate protein intake.

25. **(b)** Hypoalbuminemia

Why edematous SCU develops in some children and non-edematous SCU develops in others is unknown. Although no specific factor has been identified, a number have been suggested. One concerns the variability among infants in nutrient requirements and in body composition at the time the dietary deficit is incurred. It also has been proposed that giving excess carbohydrate to a child with non-edematous SCU reverses the adaptive responses to low protein intake, resulting in mobilization of body protein stores. Eventually, albumin synthesis decreases, resulting in hypoalbuminemia with edema. Fatty liver also develops secondary, perhaps, to lipogenesis from the excess carbohydrate intake and reduced apolipoprotein synthesis. Other causes of edematous SCU are aflatoxin poisoning as well as diarrhea, impaired renal function and decreased Na^+ K^+ ATPase activity. Finally, free radical damage has been proposed as an important factor in the development of edematous SCU. This proposal is supported by low plasma concentrations of methionine, a dietary precursor of cysteine, which is needed for synthesis of the major antioxidant factor, glutathione. This possibility also is supported by lower rates of glutathione synthesis in children with edematous compared with non-edematous SCU.

26. **(a)** Hypophosphatemia

Refeeding syndrome may complicate the acute nutritional rehabilitation of children who are undernourished from any cause. The hallmark of refeeding syndrome is the development of severe hypophosphatemia after the cellular uptake of phosphate during the 1st week of starting to refeed. Serum phosphate levels of ≤ 0.5 mmol/L can produce weakness, rhabdomyolysis, neutrophil dysfunction, cardiorespiratory failure, arrhythmias, seizures, altered level of consciousness, or sudden death.

27. **(c)** Marasmus

Diseases Associated with Childhood Obesity[*]

Syndrome	Manifestation
Alström syndrome	Hypogonadism, retinal degeneration, deafness, diabetes mellitus
Bardet-Biedl syndrome	Retinal degeneration, syndactyly, polydactyly, hypogonadism, mental retardation, autosomal recessive
Carpenter syndrome	Polydactyly, syndactyly, cranial synostosis, mental retardation
Cohen syndrome	Midchildhood-onset obesity, short stature, prominent maxillary incisors, hypotonia, mental retardation, microcephaly, decreased visual activity
Cushing syndrome	Adrenal hyperplasia or pituitary tumor
Deletion 9q 34	Early-onset obesity, mental retardation, brachycephaly, synophrys, prognathism, behavior and sleep disturbances
ENPP1 gene mutations	Insulin resistance, childhood obesity, chromosome 6q
Fröhlich syndrome	Hypothalamic tumor
Hyperinsulinism	Nesidioblastosis, pancreatic adenoma, hypoglycemia, Mauriac syndrome (poor diabetic control)
Leptin or leptin receptor gene mutation	Early-onset severe obesity, infertility (hypogonadotropic hypogonadism); uncommon;leptin deficiency treatable with recombinant leptin
Melanocortin 4 receptor gene mutation	Early-onset severe obesity, increased linear growth, hyperphagia, hyperinsulinemia; homozygous worse than heterozygous; common genetic cause of obesity
Muscular dystrophy	Late-onset obesity due in part to inactivity
Myelodysplasia	Spina bifida due in part to inactivity
Prader-Willi syndrome	Neonatal hypotonia, normal growth immediately after birth, small hands and feet, mental retardation, hypogonadism; some have partial deletion of chromosome 15 and loss of paternally expressed genes; hyperphagia leading to severe childhood obesity; ghrelin paradoxically elevated
Pro-opiomelanocortin deficiency	Obesity, red hair, adrenal insufficiency, hyperproinsulinemia
Pseudohypopara-thyroidism	Variable hypocalcemia, cutaneous calcifications
Turner syndrome	Ovarian dysgenesis, lymphedema, web neck, XO chromosome

28. **(a)** 5th-84th percentile

BMI percentile for age	Weight status
<5th percentile	Underweight
5th–84th percentile	Normal weight
85th–94th percentile	At risk for overweight
≥ 95th percentile	Overweight

29. **(d)** Alertness

Edematous SCU (kwashiorkor) may initially present as vague manifestations that include lethargy, apathy, and/or irritability. When advanced, there is lack of growth, lack of stamina, loss of muscle tissue, increased susceptibility to infections, vomiting, diarrhea, anorexia, flabby subcutaneous tissues, and edema. The edema usually develops early and may mask the failure to gain weight. It is often present in internal organs before it is recognized in the face and limbs. Liver enlargement may occur early or late in the course of disease. Dermatitis is common, with darkening of the skin in irritated areas, but in contrast to pellagra, not in areas exposed to sunlight. Depigmentation may occur after desquamation in these areas, or it may be generalized. The hair is sparse and thin, and in dark-haired children, it may become streaky red or gray. Eventually, there is stupor, coma and death.

30. **(c)** Keratomalacia

(See Table on the next page)

31. **(a)** 20-60 g/dl

The range of normal vitamin A levels is 20–60 g/dL; a level <20 μg/dL occurs in deficiency.

32. **(a)** 1500 μg

The safety and efficacy of vitamin A supplementation depend on the individual's state of health and the regimens of other treatments. A daily supplement of 1,500 μg of vitamin A is sufficient for treating latent vitamin A deficiency.

33. **(c)** Hyperostosis

Chronic hypervitaminosis A results from excessive ingestion of vitamin A for several weeks or months. Toxicity can be induced in adults and children with chronic daily intakes of 15,000 μg and 6,000 μg, respectively. Symptoms subside rapidly on withdrawal of the vitamin. Signs of subacute or chronic toxicity may include headache; vomiting; anorexia; dry, itchy desquamating skin; seborrheic cutaneous lesions; fissuring at the corners of the mouth; alopecia and/or

Names and synonyms	Characteristics	Biochemical action	Effects of deficiency	Effects of excess	Sources
Vitamin A					
Retinol (vitamin A_1): 1 μg retinol = 3.3 IU by vitamin A = 1 RAE Provitamins A: the plant pigments α-, β-, and γ-carotenes and cryptoxanthin have partial retinol activity: 12 μg β-carotene, or 24 μg of other provitamin A carotenoids = 1 μg retinol	Fat-soluble;heat-stable; destroyed oxidation, drying; bile necessary for absorption; stored in liver; protected by vitamin E	In vision, as retinal, for synthesis of the visual pigments rhodopsin and iodopsin; in growth, reproduction, embryonic and fetal development, bone growth, immune and epithelial functions, via retinoic acid as a ligand for specific nuclear transcription factors, regulating genes involved in many fundamental cellular processes	Nyctalopia;photophobia, xerophthalmia, Bitot spots, conjunctivitis, keratomalacia leading to blindness; faulty epiphyseal bone formation; defective tooth enamel; keratinization of mucous membranes and skin; retarded growth; impaired resistance to infection, anemia, reproductive failure, fetal abnormalities	Anorexia, slow growth, drying and cracking of skin, enlargement of liver and spleen, swelling and pain of long bones, bone fragility, increased intracranial pressure, alopecia, carotenemia; fetal abnormalities	Liver, fish liver oils, dairy products, except skim milk; egg yolk, fortified margarines and fortified skim milk; carotenoids from plants: green vegetables, yellow fruits and vegetables

coarsening of the hair; bone abnormalities; swelling of the bones; enlargement of the liver and spleen; diplopia; increased intracranial pressure; irritability; stupor; limited motion; and dryness of the mucous membranes. In addition, desquamation of the palms and the soles of the feet is common. Radiographs show **hyperostosis** affecting several long bones, especially in the middle of the shafts. Serum levels of vitamin A are elevated. Hypercalcemia and/or liver cirrhosis may be present. Hypervitaminosis A is distinct from cortical hyperostosis.

34. (a) 6000 μg

Toxicity can be induced in adults and children with chronic daily intakes of 15,000 μg and 6,000 μg, respectively.

35. (c) Yellow discolouration of skin because of excessive intake of carotenoids

Excessive intake of carotenoids is not associated with toxicity, but may cause yellow coloration of the skin that disappears when intake is reduced; this disorder (carotenemia) is especially likely to occur in children with liver disease, diabetes mellitus, or hypothyroidism, and in those who do not have enzymes that metabolize carotenoids.

36. (a) Vit. A deficiency

The cornea protects the eye from the environment and is also important in light refraction. In early vitamin A deficiency, the cornea keratinizes, becomes opaque, is susceptible to infection, and forms dry, scaly layers of cells **(xerophthalmia).**

37. (c) Xeropthalmia

The cornea protects the eye from the environment and is also important in light refraction. In early vitamin A deficiency, the cornea keratinizes, becomes opaque, is susceptible to infection, and forms dry, scaly layers of cells **(xerophthalmia).** In later stages, infection occurs, lymphocytes infiltrate, and the cornea becomes wrinkled; it degenerates irreversibly (keratomalacia), resulting in blindness. The conjunctiva keratinizes and develops plaques (**Bitot spots**), it becomes dry **(conjunctival xerosis),** and the lacrimal glands keratinize.

38. (c) Niacin

Niacin: Nicotinamide; nicotinic acid (antipellagra vitamin).

39. (c) Thiamine

A severe deficiency of thiamine leads to the deficiency disease **beriberi.**

40. (b) Wet beriberi

A severe deficiency of thiamine leads to the deficiency disease **beriberi.** Two forms exist, wet beriberi and dry beriberi. The child with wet beriberi is undernourished, pale, and edematous; has dyspnea, vomiting, and tachycardia; and has waxy skin. The urine often contains albumin and casts. The child with dry beriberi appears plump, but is pale, flabby, and listless, with dyspnea, tachycardia and hepatomegaly.

41. (b) Thiamine

Thiamine also is required for the synthesis of acetylcholine, and deficiency results in impaired nerve conduction.

42. (c) Soy based formula fed infants

An epidemic of life-threatening thiamine deficiency was seen in infants fed a defective soy-based formula that had undetectable thiamine levels.

43. **(d)** Cardiac involvement

Death from thiamine deficiency usually is secondary to cardiac involvement. The initial signs are slight cyanosis and dyspnea, but tachycardia, enlargement of the liver, loss of consciousness, and convulsions may develop rapidly. The heart, especially the right side, is enlarged. The electrocardiogram shows an increased Q-T interval, inverted T waves, and low voltage. These changes as well as the cardiomegaly rapidly revert to normal with treatment, but without prompt treatment, cardiac failure can develop rapidly and result in death. In fatal cases of beriberi, lesions are located principally in the heart, peripheral nerves, subcutaneous tissue, and serous cavities. The heart is dilated, and fatty degeneration of the myocardium is common. Generalized edema or edema of the legs, serous effusions, and venous engorgement are often present. Degeneration of myelin and axon cylinders of the peripheral nerves, with wallerian degeneration beginning in the distal locations, also is common, particularly in the lower extremities. Lesions in the brain include vascular dilation and hemorrhage.

44. **(b)** Increased Q-T interval, inverted T wave

Death from thiamine deficiency usually is secondary to cardiac involvement. The initial signs are slight cyanosis and dyspnea, but tachycardia, enlargement of the liver, loss of consciousness, and convulsions may develop rapidly. The heart, especially the right side, is enlarged. The electrocardiogram shows an increased Q-T interval, inverted T waves and low voltage.

45. **(c)** Low blood cell transketolase activity

The early symptoms of thiamine deficiency are nonspecific and of limited value in establishing a diagnosis. Low red blood cell transketolase activity is the best indicator of deficiency of thiamine in body tissues. Urinary excretion of thiamine or its metabolites, thiazole or pyrimidine, after an oral loading dose of thiamine may be measured to help identify the deficiency state. High blood or urinary glyoxylate levels also may be used as diagnostic indicators. Clinical response to administration of thiamine is the best test for thiamine deficiency, but does not necessarily rule out the coexistence of other B vitamin deficiencies.

46. **(a)** 10 mg and 50 mg

If beriberi develops in a breast-fed infant, both the mother and the child should be treated with thiamine. The daily dose for children and adults, respectively, is 10 mg and 50 mg.

47. **(b)** Megaloblastic anemia and typical maple syrup urine disease

Thiamine dependence has been described in a child with megaloblastic anemia and in an infant with otherwise typical maple syrup urine disease.

48. **(a)** Thiamine pyrophosphate

Thiamine (vitamin B_1) provides the functional group for the coenzyme thiamine pyrophosphate, which is involved in decarboxylation of pyruvate and α-ketoglutarate and, thus, is important in the release of energy from carbohydrates. It also participates in the hexose monophosphate shunt.

49. **(b)** Meat, legumes, cereals

Good sources of thiamine include meat (especially lean pork), legumes and cereals.

50. **(b)** Electron transport chain

Riboflavin is part of the structure of the coenzymes flavin adenine dinucleotide (FAD) and flavin mononucleotide, which provide the functional groups for several enzymes important in electron transport.

51. **(b)** Riboflavin

Signs and/or symptoms of riboflavin deficiency include cheilosis (perlèche).

52. **(a)** Riboflavin deficiency

The signs and symptoms of riboflavin deficiency are too nonspecific to make a definitive diagnosis. A functional test of riboflavin status is done by measuring the activity of erythrocyte glutathione reductase (EGR), with and without the addition of FAD.

53. **(b)** Milk and milk products

The major sources of riboflavin are milk and milk drinks, followed by enriched and fortified cereals and bread products. Other sources of riboflavin are eggs, legumes, meat, dark green vegetables, organ meats, and brewer's yeast..legumes.

54. **(a)** 3-10 mg/day

Treatment includes oral administration of 3–10 mg/day of riboflavin. If no response occurs within a few days, intramuscular injections of 2 mg of riboflavin in saline may be given as often as 3 times/day.

55. **(a)** Tryptophan

Dietary tryptophan can be converted to niacin, but the amount is insufficient to meet the total needs for the vitamin. Major food sources of niacin in the diet are meat, fish and poultry. Enriched and whole-grain bread and bread products as well as fortified cereal products and legumes.

56. **(b)** Niacin

Pellagra, the deficiency disease caused by a lack of niacin, affects all tissues of the body. It occurs chiefly in countries where corn (maize), a poor source of tryptophan, is the major foodstuff.

57. **(a)** Dermatitis, diarrhoea, dementia

The early symptoms of pellagra are vague: anorexia, lassitude, weakness, burning sensations, numbness, and dizziness. After a long period of deficiency, the classic triad of dermatitis, diarrhea, and dementia appears. Manifestations in children with parasites or chronic disorders may be especially severe.

58. **(b)** Pellagra

Dermatitis, the most characteristic manifestation of pellagra, may develop suddenly or insidiously and may be elicited by irritants, including intense sunlight. The lesions first appear as symmetric areas of erythema on exposed surfaces, resembling sunburn. Thus, in mild cases, the dermatitis may not be recognized. The lesions are usually sharply demarcated from the healthy skin around them, and their distribution may change frequently. The lesions on the hands often have the appearance of a glove. Similar demarcations may also occur on the foot and leg (pellagrous boot) or around the neck (Casal necklace). In some cases, vesicles and bullae develop (wet type). In others, there may be suppuration beneath the scaly, crusted epidermis, and in still others, the swelling may disappear after a short time, followed by desquamation. The healed parts of the skin may remain pigmented. The cutaneous lesions may be preceded by or accompanied by stomatitis, glossitis, vomiting, and/or diarrhea. Swelling and redness of the tip of the tongue and its lateral margins is often followed by intense redness, even ulceration, of the entire tongue and the papillae. Nervous symptoms include depression, disorientation, insomnia and delirium.

59. **(b)** Posterior and lateral columns

The walls of the colon are thickened and inflamed, with patches of pseudomembrane and usually mucosal atrophy. Changes in the nervous system occur relatively late in the disease. These include patchy areas of demyelination and degeneration of ganglion cells; demyelination of both the posterior and the lateral columns may be seen in the spinal cord.

60. **(d)** Both (b) and (c)

These adverse effects are not produced by niacinamide. Large doses of niacin also may have nonspecific gastrointestinal effects and may cause cholestatic jaundice or hepatotoxicity. Tolerable upper intake levels for children are approximately double the recommended dietary allowance.

61. **(b)** Pyridoxine

Other roles of vitamin B_6 include participation in the metabolism of glycogen, conversion of tryptophan to niacin, synthesis of cysteine from methionine, active transport of amino acids across cell membranes, chelation of metals, and synthesis of arachidonic and docosahexaenoic acids from linoleic and linolenic acids, respectively. If vitamin B_6 is lacking, glycine metabolism may lead to oxaluria. The major excretory product in the urine is 4-pyridoxic acid.

62. **(b)** 100 mg intramuscular dose

Intramuscular administration of 100 mg of pyridoxine is used to treat convulsions due to vitamin B_6 deficiency. One dose should be sufficient if adequate dietary intake follows. For pyridoxine-dependent children, daily doses of 2–10 mg intramuscularly or 10–100 mg orally may be necessary.

Chapter 8

Cardiovascular System (1)

1. **In the early presomite embryo, which is the 1st identifiable cardiac precursor?**
   (a) Cardiac jelly
   (b) Atrium
   (c) Mesoderm
   (d) Angiogenetic cell clusters

2. **In the early presomite embryo, at what intrauterine age the 1st identifiable cardiac precursor is seen?**
   (a) 18 days (b) 25 days
   (c) 35 days (d) 44 days

3. **At what intrauterine age the paired tubes fuse in the midline on the ventral surface of the embryo to form the primitive heart tube?**
   (a) 18 days (b) 22 days
   (c) 35 days (d) 44 days

4. **At what early age the embryonic heart begins to contract and exhibit phases of the cardiac cycle?**
   (a) 20-22 days (b) 6-8 days
   (c) 10-12 days (d) 50-52 days

5. **At what intrauterine age the septation of the heart begins?**
   (a) Day 14 (b) Day 20
   (c) Day 8 (d) Day 26

6. **What is PO_2 value of umbilical vein?**
   (a) 15-20 mmHg (b) 20-25 mmHg
   (c) 30-35 mmHg (d) 40-45 mmHg

7. **In foetal life the combined output of both the left and right ventricles is:**
   (a) 150 mL/kg/min (b) 200 mL/kg/min
   (c) 350 mL/kg/min (d) 450 mL/kg/min

8. **What is average central aortic pressure in a term neonate?**
   (a) 75/50 mmHg (b) 90/60 mmHg
   (c) 100/70 mmHg (d) 50/30 mmHg

9. **What is normal newborn cardiac output?**
   (a) 125 mL/kg/min (b) 175 mL/kg/min
   (c) 350 mL/kg/min (d) 450 mL/kg/min

10. **Cardiac defect associated with Down syndrome:**
    (a) Endocardial cushion defect
    (b) VSD
    (c) ASD
    (d) Any of the above

11. **Radial-femoral delay is commonly observed in:**
    (a) Coarctation of the aorta
    (b) Deep venous thrombosis
    (c) Preductal stenosis
    (d) All

12. **The 1st Korotkoff's sounds indicate:**
    (a) Systolic pressure (b) Diastolic pressure
    (c) Both (d) None

13. **What is difference of pressure recorded in the legs with the cuff technique and that in the arms?**
    (a) About 10 mmHg (b) 15 mmHg
    (c) 22 mmHg (d) 30 mmHg

14. **A silent precordium with a barely detectable apical impulse suggests:**
    (a) Pericardial effusion
    (b) Severe cardiomyopathy
    (c) Normal in obese patient
    (d) All of the above

15. **Right-sided apical impulses is seen in:**
    (a) Dextrocardia
    (b) Tension pneumothorax
    (c) Left-sided thoracic space-occupying lesions
    (d) All of the above

16. **Wide splitting 2nd heart sound is observed in:**
    (a) Atrial septal defect
    (b) Pulmonary stenosis

(c) Total anomalous pulmonary venous return
(d) All of the above

17. Narrow splitting of 2nd sound is observed in:
(a) Pulmonary stenosis
(b) Pulmonary hypertension
(c) Mitral regurgitation
(d) All of the above

18. A single 2nd sound occurs in:
(a) Aortic atresia
(b) Truncus arteriosus
(c) Transposition of the great arteries
(d) All of the above

19. Pansystolic murmur is observed in:
(a) Ventricular septal defect
(b) Mitral valve insufficiency
(c) Tricuspid valve insufficiency
(d) All of the above

20. A continuous murmur indicates:
(a) Patent ductus arteriosus
(b) VSD
(c) ASD
(d) MR

21. Holt-Oram syndrome is associated with:
(a) Absent radii
(b) 1st degree heart block
(c) ASD
(d) All of the above

22. Feature of ASD is:
(a) Right ventricular systolic
(b) Loud 1st heart sound
(c) Wide and fixed split
(d) All of the above

23. Most common congenital heart disease in children is:
(a) ASD (b) PDA
(c) TA (d) VSD

24. Williams syndrome is associated with:
(a) Supravalvular aortic stenosis
(b) Idiopathic hypercalcemia of infancy
(c) Elfin facies
(d) All of the above

25. PHACE syndrome is associated with:
(a) Posterior brain fossa anomalies
(b) Facial hemangiomas
(c) Aortic coarctation
(d) All of the above

26. CATCH 22 is associated with:
(a) Cardiac defects (b) Thymic hypoplasia
(c) Hypocalcemia (d) All of the above

27. Tetralogy of Fallot has component of:
(a) Pulmonary stenosis
(b) Ventricular septal defect
(c) Right ventricular hypertrophy
(d) All of the above

28. Osler-Weber-Rendu syndrome is characterized by:
(a) Hereditary hemorrhagic telangiectasia type I
(b) Angiomas of the nasal and buccal mucous membranes
(c) Angiomas of liver
(d) All of the above

29. Eisenmenger syndrome occur frequently with:
(a) Atrial septal defect
(b) Atrioventricular septal defect
(c) Patent ductus arteriosus
(d) All of the above

30. Cardiac feature of hyperthyroidism is:
(a) Tachycardia (b) A wide pulse pressure
(c) Cardiac enlargement (d) All of the above

31. Cardiac feature of hypothyroidism:
(a) Bradycardia
(b) Low voltage the P and T waves
(c) Left axis deviation
(d) All of the above

32. How much pericardial fluid is present in a healthy child?
(a) 10-15 Ml (b) 15-20 Ml
(c) 20-25 Ml (d) Above 30 Ml

33. Aneurysms of the coronary or systemic arteries is commonly seen in:
(a) Kawasaki disease
(b) Coarctation of the aorta
(c) Marfan syndrome
(d) All of the above

Answers

1. **(d)** Angiogenetic cell clusters
2. **(a)** 18 days
3. **(b)** 22 days
4. **(a)** 20–22 days
5. **(d)** Day 26
6. **(c)** 30–35 mmHg
7. **(d)** 450 mL/kg/min
8. **(a)** 75/50 mmHg
9. **(c)** 450 mL/kg/min
10. **(a)** Endocardial cushion defect
11. **(a)** Coarctation of the aorta
12. **(a)** Systolic pressure
13. **(a)** About 10 mmHg
14. **(d)** All of the above
15. **(d)** All of the above
16. **(d)** All of the above
17. **(b)** Pulmonary hypertension
18. **(d)** All of the above
19. **(d)** All of the above
20. **(a)** Patent ductus arteriosus
21. **(d)** All of the above
22. **(c)** Wide and fixed split
23. **(d)** VSD
24. **(d)** All of the above
25. **(d)** All of the above
26. **(d)** All of the above
27. **(d)** All of the above
28. **(d)** All of the above
29. **(d)** All of the above
30. **(d)** All of the above
31. **(d)** All of the above
32. **(a)** 10–15 Ml
33. **(d)** All of the above

Chapter 9

Cardiovascular System (2)

1. **Condition in which pulmonary blood flow is increased is in all *except:***
   (a) Single ventricle
   (b) Truncus arteriosus
   (c) Total anomalous pulmonary venous return without obstruction
   (d) Total anomalous pulmonary venous return with obstruction

2. **Holt-Oram syndrome consists of the following *except:***
   (a) Hypoplastic or absent radii
   (b) VSD
   (c) ASD
   (d) 1st degree heart block

3. **Which is the most common cardiac malformation?**
   (a) VSD (b) PDA
   (c) Tetralogy of Fallot (d) Tricuspid atresia

4. **Restrictive VSD are characterized by the following size:**
   (a) >1.0 cm^2 (b) <0.5 cm^2
   (c) >2.5 cm^2 (d) >3.5cm^2

5. **Indications for surgical closure of a VSD include all *except:***
   (a) Clinical symptoms and failure to thrive cannot be controlled medically
   (b) Clinical symptoms and failure to thrive cannot be controlled medically
   (c) Patients with supracristal VSD of any size
   (d) Severe pulmonary vascular disease

6. **All are true about PDA *except:***
   (a) The aortic end of the ductus is just proximal to the origin of the left subclavian artery
   (b) The ductus enters the pulmonary artery at its bifurcation
   (c) Female patients with PDA outnumber males 2 : 1
   (d) PDA is also associated with maternal rubella infection during early pregnancy

7. **True about an aorticopulmonary window defect are all *except:***
   (a) The presence of pulmonary and aortic valves with an ventricular septal defect
   (b) The cardiac murmur is systolic with a mid-diastolic rumble
   (c) Window defect is surgically corrected during infancy with cardiopulmonary bypass
   (d) The window defect can best be delineated with color flow Doppler

8. **True about Noonan syndrome are all *except:***
   (a) Pulmonary stenosis is the most common cardiac abnormality
   (b) Mutation in the gene PTPN11
   (c) PS, ASD, hypertrophic cardiomyopathy
   (d) Chromosomal location 3p21-p24

9. **True about arteriovenous fistulas are all *except:***
   (a) Common sites are liver, in the lung, in the extremities
   (b) Associated with tachycardia and increased stroke volume
   (c) Be a manifestation of hereditary hemorrhagic telangiectasia (Osler-Weber-Rendu disease)
   (d) Surgical treatment is indicated when lesion is extensive and diffuse

10. **Conditions associated with continuous murmur and a wide pulse pressure are all *except:***
   (a) PDA
   (b) A sinus of valsalva aneurysm that has ruptured into the right side of the heart
   (c) Coronary arteriovenous fistulas
   (d) Pulmonary branch stenosis

11. All are true about coronary-arteriovenous fistula *except:*
(a) Also known as coronary-cameral fistula
(b) Machinery-like murmur
(c) Small fistulas need to be treated immediately
(d) Coronary artery may be dilated or aneurysmal

12. All are true about ruptured sinus of valsalva aneurysm *except:*
(a) Congenital or acquired disease
(b) Onset is usually slow and progressive
(c) Symptoms of acute heart failure
(d) Often associated with infective endocarditis of the aortic valve

13. Partial anomalous pulmonary venous return usually involves which lung?
(a) Right (b) Left
(c) Both the lungs (d) No such corelation

14. PHACE syndrome includes all *except:*
(a) Posterior brain fossa anomalies
(b) Eye anomalies
(c) Facial hemangiomas
(d) Renal anomalies

15. CATCH 22 includes all *except:*
(a) Cardiac defects (b) Thyroid enlargement
(c) Thymic hypoplasia (d) Hypocalcemia

16. DiGeorge syndrome includes all *except:*
(a) Hypocalcemia (b) Thymic hypoplasia
(c) Hypercalcemia (d) Mild facial anomalies

17. Symptoms of congenital mitral stenosis usually manifests around:
(a) Within 3 years
(b) Within 4 years
(c) Within the 1st 2 years of life
(d) Within 5 years

18. Congenital mitral insufficiency may be associated with the following anomalies *except:*
(a) Patent ductus arteriosus
(b) Coarctation of the aorta
(c) DiGeorge syndrome
(d) Ventricular septal defect

19. All are true about mitral valve prolapse *except:*
(a) Usually sporadic
(b) Is more common in girls
(c) Common in patients with Marfan syndrome
(d) Inherited as autosomal recessive

20. Tetralogy of Fallot does not include:
(a) Ventricular septal defect (VSD)
(b) Right ventricular hypertrophy
(c) Pulmonary stenosis
(d) Aortic stenosis

21. Not true about paroxysmal hypercyanotic attacks is:
(a) Problem during the 1st 2 years of life
(b) Most frequently in the morning
(c) Infant becomes hyperpneic and restless
(d) Increase in intensity of the systolic murmur is usual as flow across the right ventricular outflow tract diminishes

22. A 2-year-old boy presented with c/o turning blue. O/E central cyanosis, clubbing, was present there was no pallor or edema or breathing difficulties — There was parasternal heave, and systolic thrill, liver was not enlarged, what is the probable diagnosis?
(a) Tetralogy of Fallot
(b) Aortic stenosis
(c) Eisenmenger syndrome
(d) Ventricular septal defect (VSD)

23. Preterm infant is given _____ for closure of PDA.
(a) Indomethacin (b) Steroids
(c) Oxygen (d) Aspirin

24. TGA is more common in ____.
(a) Males (b) Females
(c) Both (d) No such co-relation

25. The pulmonary arteries may arise together from the posterior left side of the persistent truncus arteriosus and then divide into left and right pulmonary arteries this is _____ type.
(a) I (b) II
(c) III (d) IV

26. EGG on side appearance is seen in:
(a) Tetralogy of Fallot
(b) Aortic stenosis
(c) Eisenmenger syndrome
(d) TGA

27. The surgical treatment of choice for neonates with d-TGA and an intact ventricular septum is:
(a) (Jantene) procedure
(b) Aortic pulmonary window
(c) Rashkind's operation
(d) Taussig Blalock procedure

28. **Right aortic arch is associated with all *except:***
(a) The aorta curves to the right
(b) It is found in 20% of cases of tetralogy of Fallot
(c) Trachea is deviated to the left of the midline
(d) Trachea is deviated to the right of the midline

29. **The pathologic changes of Eisenmenger syndrome of medial hypertrophy and intimal hyperplasia is classified under ____ grade.**
(a) I (b) III
(c) II (d) IV

30. **Eisenmenger syndrome is common in patients with:**
(a) VSD (b) ASD
(c) PDA (d) Cushion defect

31. **According to Vaughan Williams classification system repolarization blockers are under class:**
(a) Class II (b) Class IV
(c) Class III (d) Class I

32. **Sinus bradycardia in neonates:**
(a) <90 beats/min (b) <60 beats/min
(c) <40 beats/min (d) <50 beats/min

33. **All are true about PVCs *except:***
(a) May arise in any region of the ventricles
(b) Preceded by a P wave
(c) Characterized by premature, widened, bizarre QRS complexes
(d) Presence of fusion beats

34. **PVCs that could require suppressive therapy are all *except:***
(a) Increased ventricular ectopic activity with exercise
(b) Two or more ventricular premature beats in a row
(c) Unifocal origin
(d) R on T phenomenon

35. **Malignant PVCs are usually secondary to:**
(a) Shock
(b) Drug toxicity
(c) Electrolyte imbalance
(d) Intraventricular catheter

36. **Leading causative agents for endocarditis in pediatric patients is:**
(a) Staphylococcus aureus
(b) Pseudomonas aeruginosa
(c) Coagulase-negative staphylococci
(d) Cardiobacterium

37. **Endocarditis more common in patients with no underlying heart disease:**
(a) Staphylococcus
(b) Group D enterococci
(c) Viridans group streptococci
(d) Serratia marcescens

38. **Endocarditis more common in patients after dental procedures:**
(a) Staphylococcus
(b) Group D enterococci
(c) Viridans group streptococci
(d) Serratia marcens

39. **Endocarditis more common in patients after lower bowel or genitourinary manipulation:**
(a) Staphylococcus
(b) Group D enterococci
(c) Viridans group streptococci
(d) Serratia marcens

40. **Endocarditis seen more frequently in intravenous drug users:**
(a) Staphylococcus
(b) Group D enterococci
(c) Viridans group streptococci
(d) Serratia marcens

41. **Endocarditis common in the presence of an indwelling central venous catheter is:**
(a) Pseudomonas aeruginosa
(b) Group D enterococci
(c) Viridans group streptococci
(d) Coagulase-negative staphylococci

42. **The Duke criteria include all *except:***
(a) Glomerulonephritis
(b) Positive blood cultures
(c) Evidence of endocarditis on echocardiography
(d) Fever
(e) None of the above

43. **Infective endocarditis is not seen in:**
(a) ASD (b) VSD
(c) TOF (d) MR

44. **In infective endocarditis tender, pea-sized intradermal nodules in the pads of the fingers and toes are known as:**
(a) Osler nodes (b) Janeway lesions
(c) Splinter hemorrhages (d) Roth spots

45. In infective endocarditis painless small erythematous or hemorrhagic lesions on the palms and soles are known as:

(a) Osler nodes
(b) Janeway lesions
(c) Splinter hemorrhages
(d) Roth spots

46. In infective endocarditis, linear lesions beneath the nails are known as:

(a) Osler nodes (b) Janeway lesions
(c) Splinter hemorrhages (d) Roth spots

47. The lesions representing vasculitis produced by circulating antigen-antibody complexes are all *except:*

(a) Osler nodes (b) Janeway lesions
(c) Splinter hemorrhages (d) None

48. In infants and children, severe anemia may be associated with all *except:*

(a) Heart rate is rapid
(b) Pulse pressure is widened
(c) A systolic flow murmur at the apex
(d) Elevated ST segments

49. Hypersensitivity myocarditis is characterized by all *except:*

(a) Fever
(b) Bradycardia
(c) Eosinophilia
(d) Arrhythmias

50. Most common cause of myocarditis is:

(a) Viral (b) Bacterial
(c) Fungal (d) Protozoal

Answers

1. **(d)** Total anomalous pulmonary venous return with obstruction

(Kliegman: Nelson Book of Pediatrics, 18th ed.)

Pulmonary blood flow is decreased (Tetralogy of Fallot, pulmonary atresia with an intact septum, tricuspid atresia, total anomalous pulmonary venous return with obstruction) or increased (transposition of the great vessels, single ventricle, truncus arteriosus, total anomalous pulmonary venous return without obstruction). The chest radiograph is a valuable tool for initial differentiation between these two categories.

2. **(b)** VSD

(Kliegman: Nelson Book of Pediatrics, 18th ed.)

Holt-Oram syndrome (hypoplastic or absent radii, 1st-degree heart block, ASD). Secundum ASDs are associated with the autosomal dominant Holt-Oram syndrome. The gene responsible for this syndrome, situated in the region 12q21-q22 of chromosome 12, is TBX5, a member of the T-box transcriptional family.

3. **(a)** VSD

(Kliegman: Nelson Book of Pediatrics, 18th ed.)

Relative Frequency of Major Congenital Heart Lesions

Lesion	% of all lesions
Ventricular septal defect	35-30
Atrial septal defect (secundum)	6-8
Patent ductus arteriosus	6-8
Coarctation of aorta	5-7
Tetralogy of Fallot	5-7
Pulmonary valve stenosis	5-7
Aortic valve stenosis	4-7
d-Transposition of great arteries	3-5
Hypoplastic left ventricle	1-3
Hypoplastic right ventricle	1-3
Truncus arteriosus	1-2
Total anomalous pulmonary venous return	1-2
Tricuspid atresia	1-2
Single ventricle	1-2
Double-outlet right ventricle	1-2
Others	5-10

4. Restrictive VSD are characterized by the following size

(Kliegman: Nelson Book of Pediatrics, 18th ed.)

When a small communication is present (usually <0.5 cm^2), the VSD is called restrictive and right ventricular pressure is normal. The higher pressure in the left ventricle drives the shunt left to right; the size of the defect limits the magnitude of the shunt. In large non-restrictive VSDs (usually >1.0 cm^2).

5. **(d)** Severe pulmonary vascular disease

(Kliegman: Nelson Book of Pediatrics, 18th ed.)

Indications for surgical closure of a VSD include patients at any age with large defects in whom clinical symptoms and failure to thrive cannot be controlled medically; infants between 6 and 12 months of age with large defects associated with pulmonary hypertension, even if the symptoms are controlled by medication; and patients older than 24 months with a Qp : Qs ratio greater than 2 : 1. Patients with supracristal VSD of any size are usually referred for surgery because of the high risk for aortic valve regurgitation. Severe pulmonary vascular disease is a contraindication to closure of a VSD.

6. **(a)** The aortic end of the ductus is just proximal to the origin of the left subclavian artery

(Kliegman: Nelson Book of Pediatrics, 18th ed.)

Functional closure of the ductus normally occurs soon after birth, but if the ductus remains patent when pulmonary vascular resistance falls, aortic blood is shunted into the pulmonary artery. The aortic end of the ductus is just distal to the origin of the left subclavian artery, and the ductus enters the pulmonary artery at its bifurcation. Female patients with PDA outnumber males 2: 1. PDA is also associated with maternal rubella infection during early pregnancy. It is a common problem in premature infants, where it can cause severe hemodynamic derangements and several major sequelae.

7. **(a)** The presence of pulmonary and aortic valves with an ventricular septal defect

(Kliegman: Nelson Book of Pediatrics, 18th ed.)

An aorticopulmonary window defect consists of a communication between the ascending aorta and the main pulmonary artery. The presence of pulmonary and aortic valves and an intact ventricular septum distinguishes this anomaly from truncus arteriosus. Symptoms of heart failure appear during early infancy; occasionally, minimal cyanosis is present. The defect is usually large, and the cardiac murmur is systolic with a mid-diastolic rumble as a result of the increased blood flow across the mitral valve. In the rare instance when the communication is somewhat smaller and pulmonary hypertension is absent, the findings on examination can mimic those of a PDA (wide pulse pressure and a continuous murmur at the upper sternal borders). The electrocardiogram shows either left ventricular or biventricular hypertrophy. Radiographic studies demonstrate cardiac enlargement and prominence of the pulmonary artery and intrapulmonary vasculature. The echocardiogram shows enlarged left-sided heart chambers; the window defect can best be delineated with color flow Doppler. Magnetic resonance angiography (MRA) can also be utilized to visualize the defect. Cardiac catheterization reveals a left-to-right shunt at the level of the pulmonary artery, as well as hyperkinetic pulmonary hypertension, because the defect is almost always large. Selective aortography with injection of contrast medium into the ascending aorta demonstrates the lesion, and manipulation of the catheter from the main pulmonary artery directly to the ascending aorta is also diagnostic.

An aorticopulmonary window defect is surgically corrected during infancy with cardiopulmonary bypass. If surgery is not carried out in infancy, survivors carry the risk of progressive pulmonary vascular obstructive disease, similar to that of other patients who have large intracardiac or great vessel communications.

8. **(d)** Chromosomal location 3p21-p24

(Kliegman: Nelson Book of Pediatrics, 18th ed.)

Pulmonary stenosis as a result of valve dysplasia is the most common cardiac abnormality in Noonan syndrome, and is associated in about 50% of cases with a mutation in the gene PTPN11, encoding the protein tyrosine phosphotase SHP-2 on chromosome 12. The mechanism for pulmonic stenosis is unknown, although maldevelopment of the distal portion of the bulbus cordis and the sequelae of fetal endocarditis.

9. **(d)** Surgical treatment is indicated when lesion is extensive and diffuse

(Kliegman: Nelson Book of Pediatrics, 18th ed.)

Arteriovenous Fistulas: The most common sites in infants and children are within the cranium, in the liver, in the lung, in the extremities, and in vessels in or near the thoracic wall. Clinical symptoms occur only in association with large arteriovenous communications when arterial blood flows into a low-pressure venous system; local venous pressure is increased, and arterial flow distal to the fistula is decreased. Systemic arterial resistance falls because of the runoff of blood through the fistula. Compensatory mechanisms include tachycardia and increased stroke volume so that cardiac output rises. Total blood volume is also increased. In large fistulas, left ventricular dilatation, a widened pulse pressure, and heart failure occur.

Medical management of heart failure is initially helpful in neonates with these conditions; with time, the size of the shunt may diminish and symptoms spontaneously regress. Hemangiomas of the liver often eventually disappear completely. Large liver hemangiomas have been treated with steroids, ε-aminocaproic acid, interferon, local compression, embolization, or local irradiation; the beneficial effects of these management options are not firmly established because individual patients display marked variation in clinical course without treatment. Catheter embolization is becoming the treatment of choice for many patients with a symptomatic arteriovenous fistula. Embolic agents that have been used include detachable balloons, steel (Gianturco) coils, and liquid tissue adhesives (cyanoacrylate). Often, multiple procedures are necessary before flow is significantly reduced. Surgical removal of a large fistula may be attempted in patients with severe cardiac failure and lack of improvement with medical treatment. Surgical treatment may be contraindicated or unsuccessful when the lesion is extensive and diffuse or is located in a position where adjoining tissue may be injured during the surgery or related procedures.

10. **(d)** Pulmonary branch stenosis

(Kliegman: Nelson Book of Pediatrics, 18th ed.)

An aorticopulmonary window defect may rarely be clinically indistinguishable from a patent ductus, although, in most cases, the murmur is only systolic and is loudest at the right rather than the left upper sternal border. A sinus of Valsalva aneurysm that has ruptured into the right side of the heart or pulmonary artery, coronary arteriovenous fistulas, and an aberrant left coronary artery with massive collaterals from the right coronary display dynamics similar to that of a PDA with a continuous murmur and a wide pulse pressure. Pulmonary branch stenosis can be associated with systolic and diastolic murmurs, but the pulse pressure will be normal.

11. **(c)** Small fistulas need to be treated immediately

(Kliegman: Nelson Book of Pediatrics, 18th ed.)

Coronary-Arteriovenous Fistula (Coronary-Cameral Fistula): A congenital fistula may exist between a coronary artery and an atrium, ventricle (especially the right), or pulmonary artery. Sometimes, multiple fistulas exist. Regardless of the recipient chamber, the clinical signs are similar to those of PDA, although the machinery-like murmur may be more diffuse. If the flow is substantial, the involved coronary artery may be dilated or aneurysmal. The anatomic abnormality is usually demonstrable by color flow Doppler echocardiography and, during catheterization, by injection of contrast medium into the ascending aorta. Small fistulas may be hemodynamically insignificant and may even close spontaneously. If the shunt is large, treatment consists of either transcatheter coil embolization or, for lesions not amenable to catheter intervention, surgical closure of the fistula.

12. **(b)** Onset is usually slow and progressive

(Kliegman: Nelson Book of Pediatrics, 18th ed.)

Ruptured Sinus of Valsalva Aneurysm : When one of the sinuses of Valsalva of the aorta is weakened by congenital or acquired disease, an aneurysm may form and eventually rupture, usually into the right atrium or ventricle. This condition is extremely rare in childhood. The onset is usually sudden. The diagnosis should be suspected in a patient in whom symptoms of acute heart failure develop in association with a new loud to-and-fro murmur. Color Doppler echocardiography and cardiac catheterization demonstrate the left-to-right shunt at the atrial or ventricular level. Urgent surgical repair is generally required. This condition is often associated with infective endocarditis of the aortic valve.

13. **(a)** Right

(Kliegman: Nelson Book of Pediatrics, 18th ed.)

Partial anomalous pulmonary venous return usually involves some or all of the veins from only one lung, more often the right one.

14. **(d)** Renal anomalies

(Kliegman: Nelson Book of Pediatrics, 18th ed.)

PHACE syndrome (posterior brain fossa anomalies), facial hemangiomas, arterial anomalies, cardiac anomalies and aortic coarctation, eye anomalies.

15. **(b)** Thyroid enlargment

(Kliegman: Nelson Book of Pediatrics, 18th ed.)

CATCH 22 (cardiac defects, abnormal facies, thymic hypoplasia, cleft palate, hypocalcemia).

16. **(c)** Hypercalcemia

(Kliegman: Nelson Book of Pediatrics, 18th ed.)

DiGeorge syndrome (hypocalcemia, thymic hypoplasia, mild facial anomalies).

17. **(c)** Within the 1st 2 years of life

(Kliegman: Nelson Book of Pediatrics, 18th ed.)

Congenital mitral stenosis is a rare anomaly that can be isolated or associated with other defects, the most common being aortic stenosis and coarctation of the aorta (Shone complex). Symptoms usually appear within the 1st 2 years of life.

18. **(c)** DiGeorge syndrome

(Kliegman: Nelson Book of Pediatrics, 18th ed.)

Congenital mitral insufficiency may be isolated but is more often associated with other anomalies, including patent ductus arteriosus. Coarctation of the aorta, ventricular septal defect, corrected transposition of the great vessels, anomalous origin of the left coronary artery from the pulmonary artery, or Marfan syndrome. Mitral insufficiency is common in patients with atrioventricular septal defects. Mitral insufficiency can also be seen in patients with dilated cardiomyopathy secondary to dilatation of the valve ring.

19. **(d)** Inherited as autosomal recessive

(Kliegman: Nelson Book of Pediatrics, 18th ed.)

Mitral valve prolapse results from an abnormal mitral valve mechanism that causes billowing of one or both mitral leaflets, especially the posterior cusp, into the left atrium toward the end of systole. The abnormality is predominantly congenital but may not be recognized until adolescence or adulthood. Mitral valve prolapse is usually sporadic, is more common in girls, and may be inherited as an autosomal dominant trait with variable expression. It is common in patients with Marfan syndrome, straight back syndrome, pectus excavatum, scoliosis, Ehlers-Danlos syndrome, osteogenesis imperfecta, and pseudoxanthoma elasticum.

20. **(d)** Aortic stenosis

(Kliegman: Nelson Book of Pediatrics, 18th ed.)

Tetralogy of Fallot is one of the conotruncal family of heart lesions in which the primary defect is an anterior deviation of the infundibular septum (the muscular septum that separates the aortic and pulmonary outflows). The consequences of this deviation are (1) obstruction to right ventricular outflow (pulmonary stenosis), (2) ventricular septal defect (VSD), (3) dextroposition of the aorta with override of the ventricular septum, and (4) right ventricular hypertrophy.

21. **(d)** Increase in intensity of the systolic murmur is usual as flow across the right ventricular outflow tract diminishes

(Kliegman: Nelson Book of Pediatrics, 18th ed.)

Paroxysmal hypercyanotic attacks (hypoxic, "blue", or "tet" spells) are a particular problem during the 1st 2 years of life. The infant becomes hyperpneic and restless, cyanosis increases, gasping respirations ensue, and syncope may follow. The spells occur most frequently in the morning on initially awakening or after episodes of vigorous crying. Temporary disappearance or a decrease in intensity of the systolic murmur is usual as flow across the right ventricular outflow tract diminishes.

22. **(a)** Tetralogy of Fallot

(Kliegman: Nelson Book of Pediatrics, 18th ed.)

23. **(a)** Indomethacin

(Kliegman: Nelson Book of Pediatrics, 18th ed.)

24. **(a)** Males

(Kliegman: Nelson Book of Pediatrics, 18th ed.)

TGA is more common in infants of diabetic mothers and in males (3 : 1).

25. **(a)** I

(Kliegman: Nelson Book of Pediatrics, 18th ed.)

In truncus arteriosus: The pulmonary arteries may arise together from the posterior left side of the persistent truncus arteriosus and then divide into left and right pulmonary arteries (type I truncus arteriosus). In types II and III truncus arteriosus, no main pulmonary artery is present, and the right and left pulmonary arteries arise from separate orifices in the posterior (type II) or lateral (type III) aspects of the truncus arteriosus. Type IV truncus has no identifiable connection between the heart and pulmonary arteries, and pulmonary blood flow is derived from major aortopulmonary collateral arteries arising from the transverse or descending aorta; this form has also been called pseudotruncus but is essentially a form of pulmonary atresia with a VSD.

26. **(d)** TGA

(Kliegman: Nelson Book of Pediatrics, 18th ed.)

Transposition of the Great Arteries: The electrocardiogram shows the normal neonatal right-sided dominant pattern. Roentgenograms of the chest may show mild cardiomegaly, a narrow mediastinum (hence an egg-shaped heart), and normal to increased pulmonary blood flow.

27. **(a)** (Jantene) procedure

(Kliegman: Nelson Book of Pediatrics, 18th ed.)

The arterial switch (Jantene) procedure is the surgical treatment of choice for neonates with d-TGA and an intact ventricular septum and is usually performed within the 1st 2 weeks of life. The reason for this urgency is that as pulmonary vascular resistance declines after birth, pressure in the left ventricle (connected to the pulmonary vascular bed) also declines.

28. **(d)** Trachea is deviated to the right of the midline

(Kliegman: Nelson Book of Pediatrics, 18th ed.)

In this abnormality, the aorta curves to the right and, if it descends on the right side of the vertebral column, is usually associated with other cardiac malformations. It is found in 20% of cases of tetralogy of Fallot and is also common in truncus arteriosus. A right aortic arch without other cardiac anomalies is not associated with symptoms. It can often be visualized on the chest roentgenogram. The trachea is deviated to the left of the midline rather than to the right, as in the presence of a normal left arch. On a barium esophagogram, the esophagus is indented on its right border at the level of the aortic arch.

29. **(c)** II

(Kliegman: Nelson Book of Pediatrics, 18th ed.)

The pathologic changes of Eisenmenger syndrome occur in the small pulmonary arterioles and muscular arteries (<300 mm) and are graded on the basis of histologic characteristics (Heath-Edwards classification): Grade I changes involve medial hypertrophy alone, grade II consists of medial hypertrophy and intimal hyperplasia, grade III involves near obliteration of the vessel lumen, grade IV includes arterial dilatation, and grades V and VI include plexiform lesions, angiomatoid formation, and fibrinoid necrosis. Grades IV-VI indicate irreversible pulmonary vascular obstructive disease.

30. **(a)** VSD

(Kliegman: Nelson Book of Pediatrics, 18th ed.)

The term Eisenmenger syndrome refers to patients with a ventricular septal defect in which blood is shunted partially or totally from right to left as a result of the development of pulmonary vascular disease.

31. **(c)** Class III

(Kliegman: Nelson Book of Pediatrics, 18th ed.)

Antiarrhythmic drugs are commonly categorized using the Vaughan Williams classification system. This system comprises four classes: Class I is the sodium channel blockers, class II the β-blockers, class III is the repolarization blockers, and class IV the calcium channel blockers.

32. **(a)** <90 beats/min

(Kliegman: Nelson Book of Pediatrics, 18th ed.)

Sinus bradycardia is due to slow discharge of impulses from the sinus node. A sinus rate <90 beats/min in neonates and <60 beats/min thereafter is considered to be sinus bradycardia.

33. **(b)** Preceded by a P wave

(Kliegman: Nelson Book of Pediatrics, 18th ed.)

PVCs may arise in any region of the ventricles. They are characterized by premature, widened, bizarre QRS complexes that are not preceded by a P wave. When all premature beats have identical contours, they are classified as unifocal in origin. When PVCs vary in contour, they are designated as multifocal. Ventricular extrasystoles are often, but not always followed by a compensatory pause. The presence of fusion beats, that is, complexes with morphologic features that are intermediate between those of normal sinus beats and those of PVCs, is a clue to the ventricular origin of the extrasystole.

34. **(c)** Unifocal origin

(Kliegman: Nelson Book of Pediatrics, 18th ed.)

PVCs that could require suppressive therapy: (1) two or more ventricular premature beats in a row, (2) multifocal origin, (3) increased ventricular ectopic activity with exercise, (4) R on T phenomenon (premature ventricular depolarization occurs on the T wave of the preceding beat), and (5) presence of underlying heart disease.

35. **(a)** Shock

(Kliegman: Nelson Book of Pediatrics, 18th ed.)

Malignant PVCs are usually secondary to another medical problem (electrolyte imbalance, hypoxia, drug toxicity, cardiac injury, or an intraventricular catheter).

36. **(a)** Staphylococcus aureus

(Kliegman: Nelson Book of Pediatrics, 18th ed.)

Viridans-type streptococci (α-hemolytic streptococci) and Staphylococcus aureus are the leading causative agents for endocarditis in pediatric patients.

37. **(a)** Staphylococcus

(Kliegman: Nelson Book of Pediatrics, 18th ed.)

Staphylococcal endocarditis is more common in patients with no underlying heart disease.

38 . **(c)** Viridans group streptococci

(Kliegman: Nelson Book of Pediatrics, 18th ed.)

Viridans group streptococcal infection is more common after dental procedures.

39. **(b)** Group D enterococci

(Kliegman: Nelson Book of Pediatrics, 18th ed.)

Group D enterococci are seen more often after lower bowel or genitourinary manipulation.

40. **(d)** Serratia marcens

(Kliegman: Nelson Book of Pediatrics, 18th ed.)

Pseudomonas aeruginosa or Serratia marcescens is seen more frequently in intravenous drug users and fungal organisms are encountered after open heart surgery.

41. **(d)** Coagulase-negative staphylococci

(Kliegman: Nelson Book of Pediatrics, 18th ed.)

Coagulase-negative staphylococci are common in the presence of an indwelling central venous catheter.

42. **(e)** None of the above

(Kliegman: Nelson Book of Pediatrics, 18th ed.)

The Duke criteria help in the diagnosis of endocarditis. Major criteria include (1) positive blood cultures (two separate cultures for a usual pathogen, two or more for less typical pathogens) and (2) evidence of endocarditis on echocardiography (intracardiac mass on a valve or other site, regurgitant flow near a prosthesis, abscess, partial dehiscence of prosthetic valves, or new valve regurgitant flow). Minor criteria include predisposing conditions, fever, embolic-vascular signs, immune complex phenomena (glomerulonephritis, arthritis, rheumatoid factor, Osler nodes, Roth spots), a single positive blood culture or serologic evidence of infection, and echocardiographic signs not meeting the major criteria. Two major criteria, one major and three minor, or five minor criteria suggest definite endocarditis.

43. (**a**) ASD

(Kliegman: Nelson Book of Pediatrics, 18th ed.)

Patients with congenital heart lesions in which blood is ejected at high velocity through a hole or stenotic orifice are most susceptible to endocarditis. Children with ventricular septal defects (VSDs), left-sided valvular disease such as aortic stenosis, tetralogy of Fallot, and systemic-pulmonary arterial communications (patent ductus arteriosus or Blalock-Taussig shunts) are at highest risk. In older patients, congenital bicuspid aortic valves and mitral valve prolapse with regurgitation pose additional risks for endocarditis. Children who have undergone valve replacement or valved conduit repair are also at high risk.

44. (**a**) Osler nodes

(Kliegman: Nelson Book of Pediatrics, 18th ed.)

Osler nodes (tender, pea-sized intradermal nodules in the pads of the fingers and toes).

45. (**b**) Janeway lesions

(Kliegman: Nelson Book of Pediatrics, 18th ed.)

Janeway lesions (painless small erythematous or hemorrhagic lesions on the palms and soles).

46. (**c**) Splinter hemorrhages

(Kliegman: Nelson Book of Pediatrics, 18th ed.)

Splinter hemorrhages (linear lesions beneath the nails). These lesions may represent vasculitis produced by circulating antigen-antibody complexes.

47. (**d**) None

(Kliegman: Nelson Book of Pediatrics, 18th ed.)

Osler nodes (tender, pea-sized intradermal nodules in the pads of the fingers and toes), Janeway lesions (painless small erythematous or hemorrhagic lesions on the palms and soles), and splinter hemorrhages (linear lesions beneath the nails). These lesions may represent vasculitis produced by circulating antigen-antibody complexes.

48. (**d**) Elevated ST segments

(Kliegman: Nelson Book of Pediatrics, 18th ed.)

In infants and children, severe anemia may be associated with cardiac involvement. Although cardiac output increases when the hemoglobin content is less than about 7 g/dL, significant cardiac enlargement occurs with an extreme reduction in hemoglobin ($\leq$3-4 g). The heart rate is rapid, pulse pressure is widened, and venous pressure is increased. A systolic flow murmur at the apex or along the left sternal border is usual; diastolic murmurs may occur in the same areas, and a gallop rhythm is also common. Electrocardiographic changes include depressed ST segments and flat T waves.

49. (**b**) Bradycardia

(Kliegman: Nelson Book of Pediatrics, 18th ed.)

Hypersensitivity myocarditis (characterized by fever, rash, tachycardia, eosinophilia, drug allergy and arrhythmias).

50. (**a**) Viral

(Kliegman: Nelson Book of Pediatrics, 18th ed.)

Myocarditis refers to inflammation, necrosis, or myocytolysis and may be caused by many infectious, connective tissue, granulomatous, toxic, or idiopathic processes affecting the myocardium with or without associated systemic manifestations of the disease process or involvement of the endocardium or pericardium. Coronary pathology is uniformly absent. The most common manifestation is heart failure, although arrhythmias and sudden death may be the 1st detectable signs. Viral infections are the most common cause.

Chapter 10

Respiratory System (1)

1. **Most common cause of stridor shortly after birth:**
   (a) Laryngeal papilloma (b) Laryngeal web
   (c) Laryngomalacia (d) Vocal cord palsy

2. **Most common presentation of laryngeal web is:**
   (a) Complete laryngeal web
   (b) Laryngeal web in supraglottic area
   (c) Glottic with subglottic extension
   (d) In posterior interarytenoid area

3. **Most common cause of open (incompete) vascular ring is:**
   (a) Aberrant right subclavian artery
   (b) Aberrant right subclavian artery
   (c) Right aortic arch
   (d) Anomalous origin of left subclavian artery

4. **The most common pathogens associated with syndromes:**
   (a) Rhinoviruses
   (b) Respiratory syncytial viruses
   (c) Influenza viruses
   (d) Adenoviruses

5. **1st symptom noted in common cold is:**
   (a) Sore or "scratchy" throat
   (b) Nasal obstruction
   (c) Rhinorrhea
   (d) Fever

6. **Persistent rhinorrhea with onset in the 1st 3 months of life is seen in:**
   (a) Sinusitis (b) Pertussis
   (c) Allergic rhinitis (d) Congenital syphilis

7. **The most common complication of a common cold is:**
   (a) Otitis media (b) Sinusitis
   (c) Exacerbation of asthma (d) Croup

8. **Acute onset of cough, stridor, dyspnea in child is mostly due to:**
   (a) Foreign body (b) Acute asthma
   (c) Primary complex (d) Aspiration pneumonia

9. **In bronchiolitis following is not seen:**
   (a) Caused by R.S.V
   (b) Wheeze present
   (c) Chest X-ray shows hyperinflation bilaterally
   (d) Symptomatic treatment given
   (e) Seen in children 5 months to 3 years

10. **An 8 months old baby coming with history of increasing difficulty in breathing of 2 days duration and on examination baby is febrile, bilateral wheeze and CXR shows bilateral hyperinflation of lung with normal WBC count, the diagnosis is:**
    (a) Bronchiolitis (b) Chronic bronchitis
    (c) Asthma (d) Pneumonia

11. **A child with recent onset of URTI after 2 days presents with acute onset of breathlessness, cough and fever. All of the following can be given *except*:**
    (a) Antipyretic (b) Morphine
    (c) O_2 inhalation (d) Ribavirin

12. **Which of the following is not seen in Swyer-James syndrome?**
    (a) Hemoptysis
    (b) Hyper resonance and a small lung with the mediastinum shifted toward the more abnormal lung
    (c) CT scanning or bronchography may demonstrate bronchiectasis
    (d) Also known as Macleod syndrome
    (e) The pulmonary artery on the affected side is hyperplastic

13. **In case of naphthalene poisoning lung changes seen in:**
    (a) 2-8 hours (b) 10-12 hours
    (c) 2-3 days (d) 1 week

14. Most common micro-organism causing pneumonia in neonates:
(a) Group B streptococci
(b) Streptococcus pneumonia
(c) Haemophilus influenzae type B
(d) Moraxella catarrhalis

15. Most common micro-organism causing pneumonia in infants:
(a) Group B streptococci
(b) Mycoplasma pneumoniae[*]
(c) Chlamydia trachomatis
(d) Moraxella catarrhalis

16. Most common micro-organism causing croup:
(a) Respiratory synctial virus
(b) Parainfluenza types 1-3
(c) Adenovirus
(d) Rhinovirus

17. Focal lobar pneumonia is characteristic of which micro-organism?
(a) S. pneumonia
(b) Group A streptococcus
(c) S. aureus
(d) Chlamydia trachomatis

18. Pneumatocele is caused by:
(a) Staphylococcus (b) Streptococcus
(c) E. coli (d) P. carnii

19. An infant developed cough, fever, tachypnoea, wheeze. The X-ray shows bronchopneumonia. All of the following viruses can be causative agent *except:*
(a) Parainfluenza (b) Influenza virus A
(c) R.S.V. (d) Cytomegalovirus

20. Which of the following is not a criteria for hospitalization of children?
(a) Age >6 months
(b) Severe respiratory distress
(c) Dehydration (d) Vomiting
(e) No response to appropriate oral antibiotic therapy

21. In a 6-month-old infant with rapid respirations, intercostals retraction and fever. On auscultation crackles and wheeze is heard. Anteroposterior (AP) radiograph of the chest shows hyperexpansion of the lungs, the diagnosis is:
(a) Pneumonia (b) Bronchiolitis
(c) Pneumothorax (d) Pleural effusion

22. Which of the following sign is not seen in respiratory distress?
(a) Grunting (b) Nasal flaring
(c) Tachycardia (d) Bradycardia

23. Confluence lobar pneumonia is typically seen in:
(a) Pneumococcal pneumonia
(b) Staphylococcal pneumonia
(c) Viral pneumonia
(d) Klebsiella pneumonia

24. Growth of respiratory viruses in tissue culture usually requires:
(a) 10-12 hours (b) 1-2 days
(c) 5-10 days (d) 2 weeks

25. Which of the following is not used for definitive diagnosis of a bacterial infection in young children?
(a) Isolation of an organism from the blood
(b) Isolation of an organism from the pleural fluid
(c) Isolation of an organism lung
(d) Culture of sputum

26. For school-aged children treatment of choice for atypical pneumonia:
(a) Azithromycin (b) Amoxicillin
(c) Levofloxacin (d) Cefuroxime axetil

27. For mildly ill children who do not require hospitalization treatment of choice is:
(a) Azithromycin (b) Amoxicillin
(c) Gatifloxacin (d) Cefuroxime axetil

28. Patients with uncomplicated community-acquired bacterial pneumonia respond to therapy with improvement in clinical symptoms (fever, cough, tachypnea, chest pain) within:
(a) 24-48 hours (b) 48-96 hours
(c) 7-8 days (d) 10-15 days

29. Most common cause of clinically significant bronchiectasis:
(a) Cystic fibrosis
(b) Right middle lobe syndrome
(c) Yellow nail syndrome
(d) Tuberculosis

30. Gold standard investigation for bronchiectasis:
(a) Thin-section HRCT (b) MRI
(c) X-ray (d) Bronchogram

Answers

1. **(a)** Laryngomalacia

(Nelson Textbook of Pediatrics, 18th ed.)

Of congenital laryngeal anomalies in children with stridor, 60% are caused by laryngomalacia, the most common congenital laryngeal anomaly and the most frequent cause of stridor in infants and children. Typically, stridor is inspiratory, low pitched, and exacerbated by any exertion (crying, agitation, feeding), supine position, and viral infections of the upper airway. Stridor results from the collapse of supraglottic structures inward during inspiration. Symptoms usually appear in the first 2 weeks of life and increase in severity for up to 6 months although gradual improvement can begin at any time. Laryngopharyngeal reflux is commonly associated with laryngomalacia.

2. **(c)** Glottic with subglottic extension

(Nelson Textbook of Pediatrics, 18th ed.)

Most congenital laryngeal webs are glottic with subglottic extension and associated subglottic stenosis.The cry may be high pitched. Airway obstruction is not always present and may be related to the subglottic stenosis. Thick webs may be suspected in lateral radiographs of the airway. Diagnosis is made by direct laryngoscopy. Treatment may require only incision or dilation. Webs with associated subglottic stenosis are likely to require cartilage augmentation of the cricoid (laryngotracheal reconstruction).

3. **(a)** Aberrant right subclavian artery

(Nelson Textbook of Pediatrics, 18th ed.)

The most common open (incomplete) vascular ring is the aberrant right subclavian artery. The term vascular ring is used to describe vascular anomalies that result from abnormal development of the aortic arch complex. The double aortic arch is the most common complete vascular ring, encircling both the trachea and esophagus, compressing both. With rare exception, these patients are symptomatic by 3 months of age. Respiratory symptoms predominate, but dysphagia may be present. The diagnosis is established by barium esophagram, which shows a posterior indentation of the esophagus by the vascular ring.

4. **(b)** Respiratory syncytial viruses

(Nelson Textbook of Pediatrics, 18th ed.)

Pathogens associated with the common cold

Association	Pathogen	Relative Frequency[*]
Agents primarily associated with colds	Rhinoviruses	Frequent
	Coronaviruses	Occasional
Agents primarily associated with other clinical syndromes that also cause common cold symptoms	Respiratory syncytial viruses	Occasional
	Human metapneumovirus	Occasional
	Influenza viruses	Uncommon
	Parainfluenza viruses	Uncommon
	Adenoviruses	Uncommon
	Enteroviruses	Uncommon
	Bocavirus	Uncommon

5. **(a)** Sore or "scratchy" throat

(Nelson Textbook of Pediatrics, 18th ed.)

The onset of common cold symptoms typically occurs 1-3 days after viral infection. The 1st symptom noted is frequently sore or "scratchy" throat, followed closely by nasal obstruction and rhinorrhea. The sore throat usually resolves quickly and, by the 2nd and 3rd day of illness, nasal symptoms predominate. Cough is associated with ≈30% of colds and usually begins after the onset of nasal symptoms. Influenza viruses, RSV, and adenoviruses are more likely than rhinoviruses or coronaviruses to be associated with fever and other constitutional symptoms.

6. **(d)** Congenital syphilis

(Nelson Textbook of Pediatrics, 18th ed.)

Conditions that can mimic the common cold

Condition	Differentiating Features
Allergic rhinitis	Prominent itching and sneezing
	Nasal eosinophils
Foreign body	Unilateral, foul-smelling secretions
	Bloody nasal secretions
Sinusitis	Presence of fever, headache or facial pain, or periorbital edema or persistence of rhinorrhea or cough for >14 days
Streptococcosis	Nasal discharge that excoriates the nares
Pertussis	Onset of persistent or severe cough
Congenital syphilis	Persistent rhinorrhea with onset in the 1st 3 months of life

7. **(a)** Otitis media

(Nelson Textbook of Pediatrics, 18th ed.)

The most common complication of a cold is **otitis media,** which is reported in 5-30% of children who have a cold, with the higher incidence occurring in children cared for in a group daycare setting. **Sinusitis** is another complication of the common cold. 0.5-2% of viral upper respiratory tract infections in adults, and 5-13% in children, are complicated by acute bacterial sinusitis.

Exacerbation of asthma is a relatively uncommon but potentially serious complication of colds.

8. **(a)** Foreign body

(Nelson Textbook of Pediatrics, 18th ed.)

Coughing, choking, gagging, and possibly airway obstruction occur immediately when the foreign body is aspirated.

Three stages of symptoms may result from aspiration of an object into the airway:

1. **Initial event:** Violent paroxysms of coughing, choking, gagging, and possibly airway obstruction occur immediately when the foreign body is aspirated.
2. **Asymptomatic interval:** The foreign body becomes lodged, reflexes fatigue, and the immediate irritating symptoms subside. This stage is most treacherous and accounts for a large percentage of delayed diagnoses and overlooked foreign bodies. It is during this 2nd stage that the physician may minimize the possibility of a foreign body accident, being reassured by the absence of symptoms that no foreign body is present.
3. **Complications:** Obstruction, erosion, or infection develops to direct attention again to the presence of a foreign body. In this 3rd stage, complications include fever, cough, hemoptysis, pneumonia and atelectasis.
   - Most airway foreign bodies lodge in a bronchus (right bronchus in ≈58% of cases); laryngeal or tracheal locations occur in ≈10% of cases.
   - One third of aspirated objects are nuts, particularly peanuts.
   - Infants and toddlers use their mouths to explore their surroundings.

9. **(e)** Seen in children 5 months to 3 years

(Nelson Textbook of Pediatrics, 18th ed.)

- **Acute bronchiolitis** is predominantly a viral disease. Respiratory syncytial virus (RSV) is responsible for >50% of cases). Other agents include parainfluenza, adenovirus, Mycoplasma, and, occasionally, other viruses. Human metapneumovirus is an important primary cause of viral respiratory infection or it can occur as a co-infection with RSV.
- Wheezing produces an expiratory whistling sound that can be polyphonic or monophonic in nature. Prolonged expiratory time may be present. Biphasic wheezing can occur if there is a central, large airway obstruction. The lack of audible wheezing is not reassuring if the infant shows other signs of respiratory distress because complete obstruction to airflow can eliminate the turbulence, which causes the sound to resonate.
- In **acute bronchiolitis,** chest radiography reveals hyperinflated lungs with patchy atelectasis.

10. **(a)** Bronchiolitis

(Nelson Textbook of Pediatrics, 18th ed.)

- Wheezing produces an expiratory whistling sound that can be polyphonic or monophonic in nature.
- **Acute bronchiolitis** is usually preceded by exposure to an older contact with a minor respiratory syndrome within the previous week. The infant 1st develops a mild upper respiratory tract infection with sneezing and clear rhinorrhea. This may be accompanied by diminished appetite and fever of 38.5-39°C (101-102°F), although the temperature may range from subnormal to markedly elevated.
- In acute bronchiolitis, chest radiography reveals hyperinflated lungs with patchy atelectasis. The white blood cell and differential counts are usually normal.

11. **(b)** Morphine

(Nelson Textbook of Pediatrics, 18th ed.)

- Treatment of an infant with wheezing depends on the underlying etiology. Response to bronchodilators is unpredictable, regardless of cause, but suggests a component of bronchial hyperreactivity. It is appropriate to administer albuterol aerosol and objectively observe the response.
- Infants with **acute bronchiolitis** who are experiencing respiratory distress should be hospitalized; the mainstay of treatment is supportive. If hypoxemic, the child should receive cool humidified oxygen. Sedatives are to be avoided because they may depress respiratory drive.

- Corticosteroids are not recommended in previously healthy infants with RSV. Ribavirin, an antiviral agent administered by aerosol, has been used for infants with congenital heart disease or chronic lung disease.

12. **(b)** The pulmonary artery on the affected side is hyperplastic

(Nelson Textbook of Pediatrics, 18th ed.)

Patients with unilateral hyperlucent lung may present with **clinical manifestations** of pneumonia, but some patients are discovered only when a chest radiograph is obtained for an unrelated reason. A few patients have hemoptysis. Physical findings may include hyperresonance and a small lung with the mediastinum shifted toward the more abnormal lung. This condition has been labeled **Swyer-James** or **Macleod syndrome**. Some patients show a mediastinal shift away from the lesion with exhalation. CT scanning or bronchography may demonstrate bronchiectasis. In some patients, previous chest radiographs have been normal or have shown only an acute pneumonia, suggesting that a hyperlucent lung is an acquired lesion. No specific treatment is known; it may become less symptomatic with time. There is no vascular abnormality.

13. **(a)** 2-8 hours

(Nelson Textbook of Pediatrics, 18th ed.)

Hydrocarbons with lower surface tensions (gasoline, turpentine, naphthalene) have more potential for aspiration toxicity than heavier mineral or fuel oils. Ingestion of >30 mL (approximate volume of an adult swallow) of hydrocarbon is associated with an increased risk of severe pneumonitis. Clinical findings of chest retractions, grunting, cough, and fever may occur as soon as 30 minutes after aspiration, or may be delayed for several hours. Lung radiograph changes usually occur within 2-8 hours, peaking in 48-72 hours. Pneumatoceles and pleural effusions may occur.

14. **(a)** Group B streptococci

(Nelson Textbook of Pediatrics, 18th ed.)

Bacterial	
Common	
Streptococcus pneumoniae	
Group B streptococci	Neonates
Group A streptococci	
Mycoplasma pneumoniae[*]	Adolescents; summerfall epidemics
Chlamydia pneumoniae[*]	Adolescents
Chlamydia trachomatis	Infants
Mixed anaerobes	Aspiration pneumonia
Gram-negative enteric	Nosocomial pneumonia

15. **(c)** Chlamydia trachomatis

(Nelson Textbook of Pediatrics, 18th ed.)

Refer above table.

16. **(b)** Parainfluenza types 1-3

(Nelson Textbook of Pediatrics, 18th ed.)

Respiratory synctial virus	Bronchiolitis
Parainfluenza types 1–3	Croup
Influenza A, B	High fever; winter months

17. **(a)** S. pneumonia

(Nelson Textbook of Pediatrics, 18th ed.)

- S. pneumoniae produces local edema that aids in the proliferation of organisms and their spread into adjacent portions of lung, often resulting in the characteristic focal lobar involvement.
- Group A streptococcus infection of the lower respiratory tract results in more diffuse infection with interstitial pneumonia. The pathology includes necrosis of tracheobronchial mucosa; formation of large amounts of exudate, edema, and local hemorrhage, with extension into the interalveolar septa; and involvement of lymphatic vessels and the increased likelihood of pleural involvement.
- S. aureus pneumonia manifests in confluent bronchopneumonia, which is often unilateral and characterized by the presence of extensive areas of hemorrhagic necrosis and irregular areas of cavitation of the lung parenchyma, resulting in pneumatoceles, empyema, or, at times, bronchopulmonary fistulas.

18. **(a)** Staphylococcus

(Nelson Textbook of Pediatrics, 18th ed.)

S. aureus pneumonia manifests in confluent bronchopneumonia, which is often unilateral and characterized by the presence of extensive areas of hemorrhagic necrosis and irregular areas of cavitation of the lung parenchyma, resulting in pneumatoceles, empyema, or, at times, bronchopulmonary fistulas.

19. **(a)** Cytomegalovirus

(Nelson Textbook of Pediatrics, 18th ed.)

Febrile pneumonia	Respiratory syncytial virus, other respiratory viruses (parainfluenza viruses, influenza viruses, adenoviruses), *S. pneumoniae, H. influenzae* (type B, non-typable)
Afebrile pneumonia	*Chlamydia trachomatis, Mycoplasma hominis, Ureaplasma urealyticum,* cytomegalovirus

20. **(a)** Age >6 months

(Nelson Textbook of Pediatrics, 18th ed.)

Factors Suggesting Need for Hospitalization of Children with Pneumonia

- Age <6 months
- Sickle cell anemia with acute chest syndrome
- Multiple lobe involvement
- Immunocompromised state
- Toxic appearance
- Severe respiratory distress
- Requirement for supplemental oxygen
- Dehydration
- Vomiting
- No response to appropriate oral antibiotic therapy
- Noncompliant parents

21. **(a)** Pneumonia

(Nelson Textbook of Pediatrics, 18th ed.)

Viral and bacterial pneumonias are often preceded by several days of symptoms of an upper respiratory tract infection, typically rhinitis and cough. In viral pneumonia, fever is usually present; temperatures are generally lower than in bacterial pneumonia. Tachypnea is the most consistent clinical manifestation of pneumonia. Increased work of breathing accompanied by intercostal, subcostal, and suprasternal retractions, nasal flaring, and use of accessory muscles is common. Severe infection may be accompanied by cyanosis and respiratory fatigue, especially in infants. Auscultation of the chest may reveal crackles and wheezing, but it is often difficult to localize the source of these adventitious sounds in very young children with hyperresonant chests. It is often not possible to distinguish viral pneumonia clinically from disease caused by Mycoplasma and other bacterial pathogens.

22. **(d)** Bradycardia

(Nelson Textbook of Pediatrics, 18th ed.)

Respiratory distress manifested by grunting; nasal flaring; retractions of the supraclavicular, intercostal and subcostal areas; tachypnea; tachycardia; air hunger; and often cyanosis.

23. **(a)** Pneumococcal pneumonia

(Nelson Textbook of Pediatrics, 18th ed.)

Confluent lobar consolidation is typically seen with pneumococcal pneumonia.

24. **(c)** 5-10 days

(Nelson Textbook of Pediatrics, 18th ed.)

Growth of respiratory viruses in tissue culture usually requires 5-10 days.

25. **(d)** Culture of sputum

(Nelson Textbook of Pediatrics, 18th ed.)

The definitive diagnosis of a bacterial infection requires isolation of an organism from the blood, pleural fluid, or lung. Culture of sputum is of little value in the diagnosis of pneumonia in young children. Blood cultures are positive in only 10% of children with pneumococcal pneumonia.

26. **(a)** Azithromycin

(Nelson Textbook of Pediatrics, 18th ed.)

For school-aged children and in those in whom infection with M. pneumoniae or C. pneumoniae (atypical pneumonias) is suggested, a macrolide antibiotic such as azithromycin is an appropriate choice. In adolescents, a respiratory fluoroquinolone (levofloxacin, gatifloxacin, moxifloxacin, gemifloxacin) may be considered for atypical pneumonias.

27. **(b)** Amoxicillin

(Nelson Textbook of Pediatrics, 18th ed.)

For mildly ill children who do not require hospitalization, amoxicillin is recommended. In communities with a high percentage of penicillin-resistant pneumococci, high doses of amoxicillin (80-90 mg/kg/24 hr) should be prescribed.

28. **(b)** 48-96 hours

(Nelson Textbook of Pediatrics, 18th ed.)

Patients with uncomplicated community-acquired bacterial pneumonia respond to therapy with improvement in clinical symptoms (fever, cough, tachypnea, chest pain) within 48-96 hours of initiation of antibiotics. Radiographic evidence of improvement substantially lags behind clinical improvement.

29. **(a)** Cystic fibrosis

(Nelson Textbook of Pediatrics, 18th ed.)

In the developed world, cystic fibrosis is the most common cause of clinically significant bronchiectasis. Other conditions associated with bronchiectasis include ciliary dyskinesia, immune deficiency syndromes and infection, especially pertussis, measles, and tuberculosis. Bronchiectasis can also be congenital, as in Williams-Campbell syndrome, in which there is an absence of annular bronchial cartilage, and Marnier-Kuhn syndrome (congenital tracheobronchomegaly), in which there is a connective tissue disorder. Other disease entities associated with bronchiectasis include right middle lobe syndrome (chronic extrinsic compression of right middle lobe bronchus by hilar lymph nodes) and yellow nail syndrome (pleural effusion, lymphedema, discolored nails).

30. (**a**) Thin-section HRCT

(Nelson Textbook of Pediatrics, 18th ed.)

Thin-section HRCT scanning is the gold standard, because it has excellent sensitivity and specificity. CT provides further information on disease location, presence of mediastinal lesions, and the extent of segmental involvement. The addition of radiolabeled aerosol inhalation to CT scanning can provide further information. The CT findings in patients with bronchiectasis typically include cylindrical ("tram lines", "signet ring appearance"), varicose (bronchi with "beaded contour"), cystic (cysts in "strings and clusters"), or mixed forms. The lower lobes are most commonly affected.

Chapter 11

Respiratory System (2)

1. **What is tidal volume at rest?**
   (a) 12-14 mL/kg body weight
   (b) 10-12 mL/kg body weight
   (c) 8-10 mL/kg body weight
   (d) 6-7 mL/kg body weight

2. **What is a hallmark of extrathoracic airway obstruction?**
   (a) Increased LC
   (b) Decreased FEV1/FVC
   (c) Increased RV
   (d) Decreased FEV1

3. **Expiratory wheezing is characteristic of:**
   (a) Intrathoracic airway obstruction
   (b) Extrathoracic airway obstruction
   (c) Both
   (d) None

4. **Grunting is observed in:**
   (a) Pulmonary edema
   (b) Hyaline membrane disease
   (c) Bronchiolitis
   (d) All of the above

5. **Pickwickian syndrome is characterized by:**
   (a) Marked obesity
   (b) Chronic alveolar hypoventilation
   (c) Right heart failure
   (d) All of the above

6. **Peripheral chemoreceptors are located in:**
   (a) Blood vessels
   (b) Carotid bodies
   (c) Uterus
   (d) Skin

7. **Stretch receptors are located in:**
   (a) Airway smooth muscle
   (b) Blood vessels
   (c) Uterus
   (d) Skin

8. **Percussion is usually dull in:**
   (a) Restrictive lung disease
   (b) Pleural effusion, pneumonia
   (c) Atelectasis
   (d) All of the above

9. **Nonpulmonary disease associated with clubbing is:**
   (a) Cyanotic congenital heart disease
   (b) Thalassemia
   (c) Subacute bacterial endocarditis
   (d) All of the above

10. **Most common pathogens associated with the common cold is:**
    (a) Streptococcus viridans
    (b) Rhinoviruses
    (c) Staphylococcus aureus
    (d) Vibrio

11. **Most common cause of acute bronchiolitis is:**
    (a) H. influeza
    (b) H. ducrei
    (c) Streptococcus viridans
    (d) Respiratory syncytial virus

12. **Drug of choice for acute bronchiolitis:**
    (a) Ribavirin (b) Acyclovir
    (c) Nevirapin (d) Cabavarinz

13. Recurrent pneumonia is defined as _____ or more episodes in a single year.

(a) 2 (b) 3
(c) 4 (d) 5

14. Most common causes of parapneumonic effusions and of empyema is:

(a) S. aureus (b) S. pneumoniae
(c) S. pyogenes (d) All of the above

15. Complication of cystic fibrosis:

(a) Atelectasis (b) Cor pulmonale
(c) Hemoptysis (d) All of the above

16. What is mode of inheritance of cystic fibrosis?

(a) Autosomal dominant
(b) Autosomal recessive trait
(c) X linked dominant
(d) X linked recessive

17. Newborns with CF identified by:

(a) Determination of immunoreactive trypsinogen
(b) Limited DNA testing on blood spots
(c) Sweat analysis
(d) All of the above

Answers

1. **(d)** 6–7 mL/kg body weight
2. **(b)** Inspiratory stridor
3. **(c)** Intrathoracic airway obstruction
4. **(d)** All of the above
5. **(d)** All of the above
6. **(b)** Carotid bodies
7. **(a)** Airway smooth muscle
8. **(d)** All of the above
9. **(d)** All of the above
10. **(b)** Rhinoviruses
11. **(d)** Respiratory syncytial virus
12. **(a)** Ribavirin
13. **(a)** 2
14. **(a)** S. aureus
15. **(d)** All of the above
16. **(b)** Autosomal recessive trait
17. **(d)** All of the above

Chapter 12

Digestive System

1. **A fetus can swallow amniotic fluid as early as ____ weeks of gestation.**
(a) 12 (b) 14
(c) 16 (d) 18

2. **Nutritive sucking in neonates 1st develops at about ____ weeks of gestation.**
(a) 34 (b) 32
(c) 30 (d) 28

3. **At what age infants appear to show preferences for sweet and salty foods?**
(a) 1 month (b) 2 months
(c) 3 months (d) 4 months

4. **At what age infants' interest in solids increases?**
(a) 2 months (b) 3 months
(c) At about 4 months of age (d) 6 months

5. **Complication of gastroesophageal reflux is:**
(a) Failure to thrive
(b) Aspiration pneumonitis
(c) Esophagitis
(d) All of the above

6. **Normally earliest stool passed after birth is:**
(a) 1st 48 hours (b) First 24 hours
(c) 72 hours (d) After a week

7. **True constipation in the neonatal period is secondary to:**
(a) Hirschsprung disease
(b) Intestinal pseudo-obstruction
(c) Hypothyroidism
(d) All of the above

8. **Supernumerary teeth is seen in:**
(a) Osteogenesis imperfecta
(b) Achondroplasia
(c) Down's syndrome
(d) Cleidocranial dysplasia

9. **Fluorosis result from systemic fluoride consumption of more than:**
(a) 0.02 mg/kg/day (b) 0.05 mg/kg/day
(c) 0.07 mg/kg/day (d) 0.09 mg/kg/day

10. **What is the cause of blue to black discoloration of the primary teeth?**
(a) Fluorosis
(b) Neonatal hyperbilirubinemia
(c) Chondrodysplasia
(d) Porphyria

11. **What is cause of red-brown discoloration of the primary teeth?**
(a) Porphyria
(b) Fluorosis
(c) Neonatal hyperbilirubinemia
(d) Chondrodysplasia

12. **What is cause of brownish discoloration of the primary teeth?**
(a) Fluorosis
(b) Neonatal hyperbilirubinemia
(c) Tetracyclines
(d) Chondrodysplasia

13. **Delayed eruption of the primary teeth is seen in:**
(a) Hypopituitarism (b) Hypothyroidism
(c) Rickets (d) All of the above

14. **Early dentition is seen in:**
(a) Hyperthyroidism (b) Hypothyroidism
(c) Rickets (d) All of the above

15. **Natal teeth is associated with:**
(a) Cleft palate
(b) Pierre Robin syndrome
(c) Ellis-van Creveld syndrome
(d) All of the above

16. Surgical closure of a cleft lip is usually performed by:
(a) 3 months (b) 6 months
(c) 9 months (d) 12 months

17. Surgical closure of the cleft palate is usually done before:
(a) 3 months (b) 6 months
(c) 9 months (d) 1 year

18. Pierre Robin syndrome consists of:
(a) Micrognathia (b) High arched palate
(c) Cleft palate (d) All of the above

19. Bohn nodules are seen normally in which place in neonate?
(a) Buccal and lingual aspects of the mandibular ridges
(b) Hard palate of the neonate
(c) These lesions arise from remnants of mucous gland tissue
(d) All of the above

20. What is normal length of the esophagus at birth?
(a) 4-6 cm (b) 8-10 cm
(c) 12-14 cm (d) 16-20 cm

21. Neonatal swallowing can be seen in utero as early as:
(a) 4 weeks (b) 16-20 weeks
(c) 24-28 weeks (d) 28-30 weeks

22. Neonatal sucking and swallowing in utero becomes coordinated at:
(a) 12 weeks (b) 16 weeks
(c) 20 weeks (d) 34 weeks

23. Facial stimulation by a puff of air can induce swallowing and esophageal peristalsis in healthy young infants. This reflex is termed as:
(a) Rooting reflex (b) Santmyer swallow
(c) Swallowing reflex (d) Sucking reflex

24. Esophageal atresia is most frequently associated with:
(a) Vater syndrome (b) Feingold syndrome
(c) Charge syndrome (d) All of the above

25. What are systemic causes of swallowing dysfunction in child?
(a) Cerebral palsy
(b) Arnold Chiari malformations
(c) Syringomyelia
(d) All of the above

26. In utero primitive gut is recognizable by:
(a) 14th week (b) 12th week
(c) 6th week (d) 4th week

27. What is normal small bowel length at birth in a term neonate?
(a) 120 cm (b) 270 cm
(c) 350 cm (d) 450 cm

28. At what age adult length of small bowel (450-550 cm) is achieved?
(a) 2 years (b) 4 years
(c) 6 years (d) 8 years

29. Which is the hallmark of gastric obstruction in children?
(a) Billous vomiting
(b) Abdominal distention
(c) Nonbilious vomiting
(d) All of the above

30. The most common cause of nonbilious vomiting in children is:
(a) Infantile hypertrophic pyloric stenosis
(b) Pyloric atresia
(c) Gastric volvulus
(d) All of the above

31. Hypertrophic pyloric stenosis is commonly associated with:
(a) Type B and O blood groups
(b) Tracheoesophageal fistula
(c) Agenesis of the inferior labial frenulum
(d) All of the above

32. Pyloric stenosis in child is associated with:
(a) Eosinophilic gastroenteritis
(b) Apert syndrome
(c) Zellweger syndrome
(d) All of the above

33. Recommended eradication drug therapies for H. pylori is:
(a) Amoxicillin (b) Clarithromycin
(c) Metronidazole (d) All of the above

34. What is dietary source of the protein gluten?
(a) Wheat (b) Rye
(c) Barley (d) All of the above

35. Celiac disease is common in:
(a) Type 1 diabetes (b) Down syndrome
(c) William syndrome (d) All of the above

36. What is non-intestinal manifestations of celiac disease?
(a) Osteopenia (b) Epilepsy
(c) Depression (d) All of the above

37. Hartnup disease is characterized by:
(a) Ataxia
(b) Intellectual deterioration
(c) Pellagra-like rash
(d) All of the above

38. In blue diaper syndrome which component absorption is defective?
(a) Tryptophan (b) Tyrosine
(c) Glutamine (d) Aliphatic amines

39. Menkes disease is characterized by:
(a) Growth retardation (b) Abnormal hair
(c) Cerebellar degeneration (d) All of the above

40. Menkes disease is characterized by:
(a) Low serum copper
(b) Low serum ceruloplasmin
(c) Increased cellular copper
(d) All of the above

41. To label persistent diarrhea duration of diarrhea should be at least:
(a) 14 days (b) 21 days
(c) 7 days (d) 5 days

42. What is WHO oral rehydration solutions osmolarity (MOSM/L)?
(a) 215 (b) 220
(c) 230 (d) 245

43. What is apple juice osmolarity (MOSM/L)?
(a) 230 (b) 730
(c) 245 (d) 650

44. What is Coca-Cola osmolarity (MOSM/L)?
(a) 730 (b) 650
(c) 525 (d) 240

45. Which is limitation to oral rehydration therapy?
(a) Shock (b) Ileus, intussusception
(c) Carbohydrate (d) All of the above

46. To label chronic diarrhea duration of diarrhea should be more than:
(a) 14 days (b) 21 days
(c) 30 days (d) 7 days

47. Shwachman syndrome is characterized by:
(a) Short stature
(b) Exocrine pancreatic hypoplasia
(c) Normal sweat chloride
(d) All of the above

48. Johannson-Blizzard syndrome is characterized by:
(a) Anal imperforation
(b) Agenesis of the nasal cartilage
(c) Pancreatic insufficiency
(d) All of the above

49. Pearson syndrome is characterized by:
(a) Refractory sideroblastic anemia
(b) Exocrine pancreatic insufficiency
(c) Mitochondrial DNA deletions
(d) All of the above

50. In utero opening of the anal membrane occurs at:
(a) 4 weeks (b) 8 weeks
(c) 12 weeks (d) 16 weeks

51. At what intrauterine life human pancreas develops from evaginations of primitive duodenum ?
(a) 5 weeks (b) 8 weeks
(c) 12 weeks (d) 16 weeks

52. Which condition is commonly associated with an annular pancreas?
(a) History of maternal polyhydramnios
(b) Children present with chronic vomiting
(c) Treatment of choice is duodenojejunostomy
(d) All of the above

53. Annular pancreas is seen in:
(a) Down syndrome (b) Intestinal atresia
(c) Imperforate anus (d) All of the above

54. At what intrauterine life hepatic lobules are identifiable?
(a) 4th week (b) 6th week
(c) 8th week (d) 12th week

55. At what intrauterine life bile secretion is noted?
(a) 12th week (b) 4th week
(c) 6th week (d) 8th week

56. What is normal gallbladder length at birth?
(a) 0.8-1 cm (b) 2-3 cm
(c) 6.5-8 cm (d) 1.5-5.5 cm

57. Zellweger (cerebrohepatorenal) syndrome is characterised by:
(a) Autosomal recessive genetic disorder
(b) Progressive degeneration of the liver
(c) Psychomotor retardation
(d) All of the above

58. Alagille syndrome has facial features of:
(a) Broad forehead
(b) Deep-set, widely spaced eyes
(c) An underdeveloped mandible
(d) All of the above

59. Cardiac causes of ascites:
(a) Inferior vena cava web
(b) Constrictive pericarditis
(c) Heart failure
(d) All of the above

60. Wilson disease (hepatolenticular degeneration) is characterized by:
(a) Autosomal recessive disorder
(b) Degenerative changes in the brain
(c) Kayser-Fleischer rings in the cornea
(d) All of the above

61. Which is site of the abnormal gene for Wilson disease?
(a) Long arm of chromosome 13
(b) Short arm of chromosome 13
(c) Long arm of chromosome 11
(d) Short arm of chromosome 11

62. Clinical manifestation of varies from Wilson disease:
(a) Asymptomatic hepatomegaly
(b) Subacute or chronic hepatitis
(c) Fulminant hepatic failure
(d) All of the above

63. Diet rich in copper food:
(a) Liver (b) Shell fish
(c) Chocolate (d) All of the above

64. Which condition is associated with hydrops of the gallbladder?
(a) Kawasaki disease (b) Ascariasis
(c) Threadworm (d) All of the above

65. Portal hypertension is when portal pressure is more than:
(a) 5-7 mmHg (b) 8-10 mmHg
(c) 10-12 mmHg (d) 12-14 mmHg

66. What is normal portal venous pressure?
(a) 5 mmHg (b) 7 mmHg
(c) 10 mmHg (d) 12 mmHg

67. Cause of extrahepatic portal hypertension:
(a) Splenic vein thrombosis
(b) Portal vein thrombosis
(c) Portal vein agenesis
(d) All of the above

68. Most common presentation of portal hypertension is:
(a) Malena
(b) Bleeding from esophageal varices
(c) Systemic hypotension
(d) None

69. Hepatic causes of ascites:
(a) Cirrhosis
(b) Budd-Chiari syndrome
(c) Portal vein obstruction
(d) All of the above

70. Renal causes of ascites:
(a) Nephrotic syndrome (b) Peritoneal dialysis
(c) Obstructive uropathy (d) All of the above

Answers

1. **(a)** 12
2. **(a)** 34
3. **(a)** 1 month
4. **(c)** At about 4 months of age
5. **(d)** All of the above
6. **(a)** 1st 48 hours
7. **(a)** Hirschsprung disease
8. **(d)** Cleidocranial dysplasia
9. **(b)** 0.05 mg/kg/day
10. **(b)** Neonatal hyperbilirubinemia
11. **(a)** Porphyria
12. **(c)** Tetracyclines
13. **(d)** All of the above
14. **(a)** Hyperthyroidism
15. **(d)** All of the above
16. **(a)** 3 months
17. **(d)** 1 year
18. **(d)** All of the above
19. **(a)** Buccal and lingual aspects of the mandibular ridges
20. **(b)** 8–10 cm
21. **(b)** 16–20 weeks
22. **(d)** 34 weeks
23. **(b)** Santmyer swallow
24. **(a)** Vater syndrome
25. **(a)** Cerebral palsy
26. **(d)** 4th week
27. **(b)** 270 cm
28. **(b)** 4 years
29. **(c)** Nonbilious vomiting
30. **(a)** Infantile hypertrophic pyloric stenosis
31. **(d)** All of the above
32. **(d)** All of the above
33. **(a)** Amoxicillin
34. **(d)** All of the above
35. **(a)** Type 1 diabetes
36. **(d)** All of the above
37. **(d)** All of the above
38. **(a)** Tryptophan
39. **(d)** All of the above
40. **(d)** All of the above
41. **(a)** 14 days
42. **(d)** 245
43. **(b)** 730
44. **(b)** 650
45. **(d)** All of the above
46. **(a)** 14 days
47. **(d)** All of the above
48. **(d)** All of the above
49. **(d)** All of the above
50. **(b)** 8th week
51. **(a)** 5th week
52. **(d)** All of the above
53. **(b)** Intestinal atresia
54. **(b)** 6th week
55. **(a)** 12th week
56. **(d)** 1.5–5.5 cm
57. **(d)** All of the above
58. **(d)** All of the above
59. **(d)** All of the above
60. **(d)** All of the above
61. **(a)** Long arm of chromosome 13
62. **(d)** All of the above
63. **(d)** All of the above
64. **(a)** Kawasaki disease
65. **(c)** 10–12 mm Hg
66. **(b)** 7 mm Hg
67. **(d)** All of the above
68. **(b)** Bleeding from esophageal varices
69. **(a)** Cirrhosis
70. **(d)** All of the above

Chapter 13

Central Nervous System

1. **A loss of skills (regression) over time strongly suggests an underlying:**
   (a) Degenerative disease of the CNS
   (b) Asperger syndrome
   (c) Autism
   (d) Heller's syndrome

2. **Milestones at the age of three months:**
   (a) Supports weight on forearms
   (b) Coos, laughs
   (c) Open hands spontaneously
   (d) All of the above

3. **Milestones at the age of six months:**
   (a) Sits momentarily (b) Transfers objects
   (c) Babbles (d) All of the above

4. **Milestones at the age of nine months:**
   (a) Pulls to stand
   (b) Plays pat-a-cake, peek-a-boo
   (c) Imitates sounds
   (d) All of the above

5. **Milestones at the age of twelve months:**
   (a) Walks with one hand held
   (b) Releases an object on command
   (c) 1-2 meaningful words
   (d) All of the above

6. **Milestones at the age of eighteen months:**
   (a) Feeds from a spoon
   (b) Mimics actions of others
   (c) Speaks at least 6 words
   (d) All of the above

7. **Milestones at the age of twenty four months:**
   (a) Runs
   (b) Speaks 2-3 word sentences
   (c) Plays with others
   (d) All of the above

8. **Musty smell of child is diagnostic of:**
   (a) Isovaleric academia
   (b) Tyrosenemia type II
   (c) Tetrahydrobiopterin deficiency
   (d) Phenylketonuria

9. **Sweaty feet smell is diagnostic of:**
   (a) Isovaleric academia
   (b) Phenylketonuria
   (c) Isovaleric academia
   (d) None

10. **A tower-head, or oxycephalic skull, suggestive of:**
    (a) Hydrocephalus
    (b) Thalassemia
    (c) Premature closure of sutures
    (d) Hematoma

11. **A broad forehead is sugestive of:**
    (a) Extra tentorial herniation
    (b) Hydrocephalus
    (c) Sutural dehiscence
    (d) None

12. **A square or a box-shaped skull is suggestive of:**
    (a) Anterior frontanelle prolapse
    (b) Thalassemia major
    (c) Osteoporosis
    (d) Chronic subdural hematomas

13. **Shape of anterior frontanelle is:**
    (a) Square window (b) Diamond
    (c) Star (d) Circular

14. **Fontanel that is situated in the midline at the junction of the coronal and sagittal sutures is known as:**
    (a) Anterior frontanelle (b) Posterior fontanel
    (c) Lateral fontanel (d) Metopic

15. **Fontanel between the intersection of the occipital and parietal bones is known as:**
(a) Anterior frontanelle (b) Posterior fontanel
(c) Lateral fontanel (d) None

16. **At what age posterior fontanel closes?**
(a) First 4 weeks (b) Mostly at birth
(c) At 18 weeks (d) At 18 months

17. **After what age posterior fontanel is usually closed and nonpalpable?**
(a) First 6-8 weeks (b) First 4 weeks
(c) At 18 months (d) After 5 years

18. **Persistence open posterior fontanel after first 6-8 weeks suggestive of:**
(a) Congenital hypothyroidism
(b) Rickets
(c) Achondroplasia
(d) Down's syndrome

19. **The average time of closure of anterior fontanel is:**
(a) First 4 weeks (b) At 18 weeks
(c) At 1 year (d) 18 months

20. **Approximate measurement of anterior fontanel is:**
(a) 0.5 cm (b) 4 by 4 cm
(c) 2 by 2 cm (d) 1 by 1 cm

21. **A very small or absent anterior fontanel at birth may indicate:**
(a) Microcephaly (b) Hypothyroidism
(c) Down's syndrome (d) Achondroplasia

22. **A bulging anterior fontanel is a reliable indicator of:**
(a) Extra tentorial herniation
(b) Increased intracranial pressure
(c) Chronic subdural hematomas
(d) None

23. **Ping-pong ball, softening of the parietal bone is called as:**
(a) Craniotabes (b) Chondromalacia
(c) Osteomalacia (d) None

24. **Craniotabes is commonly seen in:**
(a) Rickets (b) Hypothyroidism
(c) Subdural hematomas (d) Prematurity

25. **Skull bruit is heard in:**
(a) Increased intracranial pressure
(b) Anaemia
(c) Fever
(d) All of the above

26. **Increased intracranial pressure (ICP) results from:**
(a) Hydrocephalus (b) Tumor
(c) Subdural effusions (d) All of the above

27. **What is used for correct measurement of the head circumference?**
(a) Extensible plastic measuring tape
(b) Nondistensible plastic measuring tape
(c) Flexible synthetic tape
(d) Cotton tape

28. **The average rate of head growth in a premature infant is:**
(a) 0.5 mm in first two weeks
(b) 1 mm in first two weeks
(c) 1 cm in first two weeks
(d) 0.5 cm in the first 2 weeks

29. **The head circumference of a term infant at birth measures:**
(a) 50 cm (b) Less than 33 cm
(c) 44-45 cm (d) 34-35 cm

30. **Which is first cranial nerve?**
(a) Optic (b) Olfactory nerve
(c) Occulomotor (d) Trochlear

31. **Sense of smell can be tested reliably as early as:**
(a) 32nd weeks of gestation
(b) At birth
(c) After 4 weeks of life
(d) None

32. **Anosmia (loss of smell) is most commonly found in association with:**
(a) Upper respiratory tract infection
(b) Fracture of the base of the skull
(c) Frontal lobe tumor
(d) All of the above

33. **Diminished sense of smell in a child:**
(a) Purulent meningitis
(b) Nasal polyp
(c) Absence of olfactory nerve
(d) DNS

34. **How will you test sense of smell?**
(a) Peppermint (b) Strong acid
(c) Strong base (d) Urine

35. **Which is second cranial nerve?**
(a) Olfactory (b) Occulomotor
(c) Facial (d) Optic nerve

36. **For examination of the optic disc and retina dilation of the pupil is done by:**
(a) 1% çyclopentolate hydrochloride
(b) 2.5% phenylephrine hydrochloride
(c) 1% tropicamide
(d) Combination of all above

37. **Normal color of the optic nerve in child is:**
(a) Gray-white (b) Red
(c) Salmon-pink (d) None

38. **Normal color of the optic nerve in neonate is:**
(a) Gray-white (b) Salmon-pink
(c) Glistening purple (d) Almond cream

39. **Swelling of the optic disc due to raised intracranial pressure is called as:**
(a) Papilledema (b) Optic neuropathy
(c) Optic neuritis (d) Drusen

40. **Papilledema in an older child is recognized by:**
(a) The optic nerve becomes hyperemic
(b) Subhyaloid, flame-shaped hemorrhages appear in the retina surrounding the optic nerve
(c) The small capillaries that normally cross the optic nerve are no longer visualized as they become constricted
(d) All of the above

41. **Retinal hemorrhage occurs in how many percentages of full-term newborn infants?**
(a) 30-40% (b) <5%
(c) <1% (d) 50%

42. **Visual fixation and the ability to follow a brilliant target are present at what age of neonate?**
(a) 28 weeks (b) Term
(c) First 7 days (d) 28 days

43. **Optokinetic nystagmus is normal:**
(a) Newborn
(b) Optic neuritis
(c) Progressive infra nuclear palsy
(d) UV light induced

44. **Visual acuity in term infants approximates:**
(a) 6/60 (b) 20/150
(c) 20/20 (d) 6/150

45. **Visual acuity reaches the adult level of 20/20 by the age of:**
(a) At birth (b) 1 month
(c) 6 weeks (d) 6 months

46. **At what gestational age pupil reacts to light?**
(a) 24th week
(b) 29th-32nd week
(c) 34 to 36 weeks
(d) 36 to 42 weeks

47. **Pupillary equality, size and reaction to light is affected by:**
(a) A space-occupying brain lesion
(b) Metabolic disorders
(c) Abnormalities of the midbrain
(d) All of the above

48. **Horner syndrome is characterized by:**
(a) Miosis
(b) Ptosis
(c) Ipsilateral anhidrosis of the face
(d) All of the above

49. **Horner syndrome is caused by:**
(a) Congenital
(b) Lesion of sympathetic nervous system in the brainstem
(c) Lesion of sympathetic plexus in juxtaposition to the carotid artery
(d) All of the above

50. **Which is third cranial nerve?**
(a) Olfactory (b) Oculomotor
(c) Optic (d) Hypoglossal

51. **Which is fourth cranial nerve?**
(a) Trochlear (b) Occulomotor
(c) Trigeminal (d) Facial

52. **Which is fifth cranial nerve?**
(a) Trigeminal (b) Abducens nerves
(c) Trochlear (d) Auditory

53. **The oculomotor nerve innervates which muscles of the eye?**
(a) Medial rectus
(b) Inferior oblique
(c) Mevatorpalpebrae superioris muscles
(d) All of the above

54. **Complete paralysis of the oculomotor nerve causes:**
(a) Ptosis
(b) Pilation of the pupil
(c) Displacement of the eye outward and downward
(d) None

55. The trochlear nerve supplies which muscles of the eye?
(a) Superior oblique muscle
(b) Inferior oblique muscle
(c) Levator palpebrae superioris
(d) Lateral rectus

56. The abducens nerve supplieswhich muscles of the eye?
(a) Superior oblique muscle
(b) Inferior oblique muscle
(c) Levator palpebrae superioris
(d) Lateral rectus muscle

57. Horizontal nystagmus occurs due to:
(a) Abnormality of the peripheral labyrinth
(b) Lesion of the vestibular system in the brainstem
(c) Phenytoin
(d) All of the above

58. Vertical nystagmus occurs due to:
(a) Abnormality of the peripheral labyrinth
(b) Lesion of the vestibular system in the brainstem
(c) Phenytoin
(d) Brainstem dysfunction

59. Complete ocular movement may be demonstrated as early as_______________ using the doll's eye maneuver (week of gestation).
(a) 25 (b) 28
(c) 37 (d) 42

60. Name the fifth cranial nerve:
(a) Oculomotor (b) Trigeminal nerve
(c) Optic (d) Hypoglossal

61. What is sensory distribution of trigeminal nerve over the face?
(a) Ophthalmic area (b) Maxillary area
(c) Mandibular area (d) All of the above

62. Trigeminal nerve function test in premature neonates is done by:
(a) Puffing out cheeks (b) Facial grimacing
(c) Tongue protruding (d) Social smile

63. Which is seventh cranial nerve?
(a) Olfactory (b) Oculomotor
(c) Optic (d) Facial nerve

64. Innervation for taste for the anterior two thirds of the tongue:
(a) Facial nerve (b) Trochlear
(c) Hypoglossal (d) Glosopharyngeal

65. Which is eighth cranial nerve?
(a) Oculomotor (b) Trigeminal nerve
(c) Optic (d) Auditory nerve

66. At what age infant baby looks in the direction of the sound source?
(a) At birth (b) 1st week
(c) 3 months of age (d) 1year

67. What are risk factors that need evaluation of baby for hearing in first few months of life?
(a) Family history of deafness
(b) Severe asphyxia
(c) Hyperbilirubinemia
(d) All of the above

68. Which is ninth cranial nerve?
(a) Glossopharyngeal (b) Nerve facial nerve
(c) Trochlear (d) Hypoglossal

69. Which nerve supplies innervation to the stylopharyngeus muscle?
(a) Auditory
(b) Glossopharyngeal nerve
(c) Abducens nerves
(d) Trochlear

70. How will you test glossopharyngeal nerve?
(a) Facial grimace (b) Mouth puffing
(c) Deglution (d) Gag response

71. Taste sense for the posterior one third of the tongue is provided by:
(a) Glossopharyngeal nerve (b) Vagus
(c) Facial (d) Trochlear nucleus

72. Which is tenth cranial nerve?
(a) Vagus nerve
(b) Auditory
(c) Glossopharyngeal nerve
(d) Abducens nerves

73. A unilateral injury of the vagus nerve produces:
(a) Hoarse voice
(b) Total loss of speech
(c) Tongue protrusion
(d) Drooping of eyelid

74. Bilateral lesions of the vagus nerve produces:
(a) Vocal cord paralysis
(b) Nasal regurgitation of fluids
(c) Respiratory distress
(d) All of the above

75. Which is eleventh cranial nerve?
(a) Vagus nerve (b) Auditory
(c) Glossopharyngeal nerve (d) Accessory nerve

76. Paralysis and atrophy of the sternomastoid and trapezius muscles are due to lesion of:
(a) Vagus nerve
(b) Accessory nerve
(c) Glossopharyngeal nerve
(d) Auditory

77. Weakness and atrophy of sternomastoid muscle is due to:
(a) Motor neuron disease (b) Myotonic dystrophy
(c) Myasthenia gravis (d) All of the above

78. Which is twelth cranial nerve?
(a) Hypoglossal nerve (b) Accessory nerve
(c) Glossopharyngeal nerve (d) Auditory

79. The hypoglossal nerve innervates:
(a) Tongue (b) Pharynx
(c) Larynx (d) Vocal cords

80. What is the cause of hypoglossal nerve involvement?
(a) Pompe disease
(b) Werdnig-Hoffmann disease
(c) Hypothyroidism
(d) Danon disease

81. The components of the motor examination include testing of:
(a) Power
(b) Deep tendon reflexes
(c) Presence of primitive reflexes
(d) All of the above

82. What is grade of normal muscle power?
(a) Grade-6 (b) Grade-5
(c) Grade-4 (d) Grade-1

83. Spasticity is associated with:
(a) Brisk tendon reflexes
(b) Extensor plantar reflex, clonus
(c) Disuse atrophy
(d) All of the above

84. Spasticity results from a lesion that involves:
(a) Upper motor neuron tracts
(b) Lower motor neuron tracts
(c) Nerve nucleus
(d) Brainstem

85. Rigidity is manifested due to lesion of:
(a) Internal capsule (b) Medulla
(c) Spinal nerve nucleus (d) Basal ganglia

86. Decerebrate rigidity is due to injury to the:
(a) Brainstem (b) Medulla
(c) Basal ganglia (d) None

87. Ataxia may be demonstrated by:
(a) Finger-to-nose (b) Heel-to-shin tests
(c) Tandem walking (d) All of the above

88. What is feature of cerebellar abnormalities:
(a) Hypotonia (b) Dysarthria
(c) Decreased deep tendon (d) All of the above

89. Sensory ataxia is found with diseases of:
(a) Spinal cord (b) Cerebellum
(c) Medulla (d) None

90. Chorea is characterized by:
(a) Milkmaid sign (b) Explosive speech
(c) Hung upknee reflexes (d) All of the above

91. Chorea is due to lesion of:
(a) Medulla (b) Basal ganglia
(c) Pons (d) Spinal cord

92. Athetosis is due to lesion of:
(a) Basal ganglia (b) Thalamus
(c) Putaman (d) Caudate nucleus

93. Which is common motor tic?
(a) Eye blinking
(b) Grimacing
(c) Rapid movements of shoulders
(d) All of the above

94. Deep tendon reflex is absent or decreased in:
(a) Myopathy
(b) Neuropathy
(c) Abnormalities of cerebellum
(d) All of the above

95. Deep tendon reflex increased in:
(a) Lower motor neuron lesion
(b) Brainstem lesion
(c) Cerebellar lesion
(d) Upper motor neuron lesions

96. Abnormal Babinski reflex indicates:
(a) Upper motor neuron lesion
(b) Lower motor neuron lesion
(c) Brainstem lesion
(d) Cerebellar lesions

97. Which primitive reflex reappears during old age?
(a) Sucking (b) Moro's
(c) Atonic neck reflex (d) Rooting reflex

98. An asymmetric Moro reflex response may signify:
(a) A fractured clavicle (b) Brachial plexus injury
(c) Hemiparesis (d) All of the above

99. Contraindications for performing a lumbar puncture:
(a) Suspected mass lesion of the brain or spinal cord
(b) Skin infection at the site of the LP
(c) Thrombocytopenia
(d) All of the above

100. What is color of normal CSF is the color?
(a) Like water (b) Turbid
(c) Yellow green (d) Similar to blood

101. Normally CSF contains up to ________ WBCs.
(a) $5/mm^3$ (b) $15/mm^3$
(c) $20/mm^3$ (d) $25/mm^3$

102. An elevated PMN count in CSF suggestive of:
(a) TBM (b) Meningitis
(c) Hydrocephalous (d) SLE

103. CSF lymphocytosis indicates:
(a) Meningitis
(b) Demyelinating diseases
(c) Collagen vascular diseases
(d) All of the above

104. Normal CSF contains how much RBC?
(a) Nil (b) 5 to 10
(c) 15 to 20 (d) 25 to 30

105. CSF Xanthochromia may result from:
(a) Hyperbilirubinemia
(b) Carotenemia
(c) Markedly elevated CSF protein
(d) All of the above

106. The normal CSF protein in child is:
(a) 10 to 40 mg/dL (b) 20 to 80 mg/dL
(c) <10 mg/dL (d) 80 to 120 mg/dL

107. The normal CSF protein in neonate is:
(a) Upto 120 mg/dL (b) 10 to 40 mg/dL
(c) 20 to 80 mg/dL (d) <10 mg/dL

108. The CSF protein falls to the normal childhood range by the age of:
(a) 1 month (b) 2 months
(c) 10 weeks (d) 3 months

109. Elevation of CSF immunoglobulin G (IgG) is observed in:
(a) Subacute sclerosing panencephalitis
(b) Post infectious encephalomyelitis
(c) Multiple sclerosis
(d) All of the above

110. Increase in convolutional markings on skull X-ray is suggestive of:
(a) SLE
(b) Tuberous sclerosis
(c) Meningitis
(d) Long-standing intracranial hypertension

111. Magnetic resonance imaging is ideally advised for:
(a) Cerebral edema
(b) Acute stroke
(c) Congenital anomalies of the posterior fossa
(d) All of the above

112. Waves of EEG:
(a) Delta (1-3/sec) (b) Theta (4-7/sec)
(c) Alpha (8-12/sec) (d) All of the above

113. Neural tube to close spontaneously between _____ of in utero development.
(a) 3rd and 4th week
(b) 6th and 8th week
(c) 10th and 12th week
(d) Never closes in intrauterine life

114. Neural tube defects include:
(a) Dermal sinus (b) Tethered cord
(c) Syringomyelia (d) All of the above

115. Which is biochemical markers for a neural tube defect?
(a) CRP (b) α-fetoprotein
(c) ESR (d) CA-125

116. At which week of gestation prenatal screening of maternal serum for AFP for identifying pregnancies at risk for fetuses with neural tube defects in utero is done?
(a) 16th-18th week (b) 3rd - 4th week
(c) 6th and 8th week (d) 10th and 12th week

117. At what intrauterine age rostral end of the neural tube closes?
(a) 1st week (b) 2nd week
(c) 23rd day (d) 86th day

118. Which is nonepileptic paroxysmal disorder in neonate?
(a) Jitteriness
(b) Bruxism
(c) Temper tandrum
(d) Clonic neck movements

119. Cause of prolonged fever (>10 days) is:
(a) Drug reaction
(b) Secondary bacterial infection
(c) To intercurrent viral infection
(d) All of the above

120. Which is nonepileptic paroxysmal disorder in infant?
(a) Cyanotic breath-holding spells
(b) Rumination
(c) Masturbation
(d) All of the above

121. Benign paroxysmal vertigo commonly occurs at what age ?
(a) Toddler
(b) Infancy
(c) School going children
(d) Adolescents

122. What is drug of choice for benign paroxysmal vertigo?
(a) Meclizine (b) Diphenhydramine
(c) Dimenhydrinate (d) Dramamine

123. Night terror is associated with:
(a) Dilated pupils (b) Tachycardia
(c) Hyperventilation (d) All of the above

124. A cyanotic breath-holding spell is usually provoked by:
(a) Cry (b) Clonic jerks
(c) Scolding a child (d) Tension

125. A cyanotic breath-holding spell has component of:
(a) Shrill cry (b) Forced expiration
(c) Apnea (d) All of the above

126. A cyanotic breath-holding spell is usually associated with:
(a) Clonic jerks (b) Opisthotonos
(c) Bradycardia (d) All of the above

127. Breath-holding spells abates at what age?
(a) 1 year (b) 5 years
(c) 12 years (d) 18 years

128. Pallid spells are typically initiated by:
(a) Painful experience (b) Emotional drive
(c) Tension (d) None

129. Drug of choice for pallid breath-holding spells is:
(a) Glycopyrrolate (b) Atropine sulfate
(c) Theophylline (d) All of the above

130. MELAS syndrome constitutes:
(a) Mitochondrial myopathy
(b) Encephalopathy
(c) Lactic acidosis
(d) All of the above

131. Neurofibromatosis (von Recklinghausen disease) is inherited as:
(a) Autosomal dominant
(b) Autosomal recessive
(c) X-linked recessive
(d) Non-genetic disorder

132. What is hallmark of neurofibromatosis?
(a) Acoustic neuromas (b) Schwannomas
(c) Café au-lait spots (d) Angiofibromas

133. Neurofibromatosis type 2 gene is located on:
(a) Long arm of chromosome 11
(b) Long arm of chromosome 9
(c) Long arm of chromosome 22
(d) Short arm of chromosome 22

134. Enlargement of the 4th ventricle at the junction between the midbrain and medulla (molar tooth sign) on MRI is seen in:
(a) Tuberous sclerosis
(b) Diamond Blackfan syndrome
(c) Joubert syndrome
(d) Syndrome X

135. Drug that can induce chorea:
(a) L-dopa (b) Lithium
(c) Theophylline (d) All of the above

136. Infectious cause of ataxia include:
(a) Cerebellar abscess (b) Acute labyrinthitis
(c) Acute cerebellar ataxia (d) All of the above

137. Viral origin of acute cerebellar ataxia occurs in:
(a) Varicella (b) Coxsackievirus
(c) Echovirus (d) All of the above

138. Toxic causes of ataxia is:
(a) Alcohol (b) Thallium
(c) Phenytoin (d) All of the above

139. Metabolic disorder which gives rise to ataxia is:
(a) Abetalipoproteinemia
(b) Arginosuccinicaciduria
(c) Hartnup disease
(d) All of the above

140. Degenerative diseases of the central nervous which are associated with ataxia:
(a) Roussy-Levy disease
(b) Ramsay Hunt syndrome
(c) Olivopontocerebellar atrophies
(d) All of the above

141. Which vitamin deficiency gives rise to progressive cerebellar ataxia?
(a) Vit A (b) Vit E
(c) Vit C (d) Vit K

142. Historical static encephalopathy means:
(a) Cerebral palsy
(b) Down's syndrome
(c) Marfan's syndrome
(d) Cerebellar ataxia

143. What is the first indication of spastic diplegia?
(a) Muscular atrophy
(b) Bicycling of legs
(c) Distal muscle weakness
(d) Commando crawl

144. The inherited neurodegenerative disorder is:
(a) Neuronal ceroidlipofuscinoses
(b) Adrenoleukodystrophy
(c) Sialidosis
(d) All of the above

145. Prenatal diagnosis of GM_1 gangliosidoses is done by the measurement of___________ in cultured amniotic cells.
(a) Acid β-galactosidase (b) Glucocerebrosidase
(c) Sphingomyelinase (d) None

146. Hurler syndrome has facial feature of:
(a) Prominent forehead
(b) Depressed nasal bridge
(c) Macroglossia
(d) All of the above

147. Tay-Sachs disease is gene located on chromosome:
(a) 15 (b) 5
(c) 25 (d) X chromosome

148. Sandhoff disease gene located on chromosome:
(a) -5q1 (b) 5q13
(c) -13q5 (d) 5p13

149. Krabbe disease gene is located on chromosome:
(a) 4q24.3-q32.1 (b) 24q24.3-q32.1
(c) 13q24.3-q32.1 (d) 14q24.3-q32.1

150. Metachromatic leukodystrophy (MLD) gene is located on chromosome:
(a) 22q13 (b) 22p13
(c) 9q13 (d) 22q1

151. Most common cause of neonatal meningitis is:
(a) Group B streptococcus
(b) E. coli
(c) H. influenzae
(d) Staphylococcus aureus

152. What is an acute complication of bacterial meningitis?
(a) Communicating hydrocephalus
(b) Hearing loss
(c) Cerebral palsy
(d) Encephalitis

Answers

1. (a) Degenerative disease of the CNS
2. (d) All of the above
3. (d) All of the above
4. (d) All of the above
5. (d) All of the above
6. (d) All of the above
7. (d) All of the above
8. (d) Phenylketonuria
9. (a) Isovaleric academia
10. (c) Premature closure of sutures
11. (b) Hydrocephalus
12. (d) Chronic subdural hematomas

    (Nelson 18th edition)

    Because the long-standing presence of fluid in the subdural space causes enlargement of the middle fossa.
13. (b) Diamond
14. (a) Anterior frontanelle
15. (b) Posterior fontanel
16. (b) Mostly at birth
17. (a) First 6–8 weeks
18. (a) Congenital hypothyroidism
19. (d) 18 monhts
20. (c) 2 by 2 cm
21. (a) Microcephaly
22. (b) Increased intracranial pressure
23. (a) Craniotabes
24. (d) Prematurity
25. (d) All of the above
26. (d) All of the above
27. (b) Nondistensible plastic measuring tape

    The tape is placed over the midforehead and is extended circumferentially to include the most prominent portion of the occiput so that the greatest volume of the cranium is measured.
28. (d) 0.5 cm in the first 2 weeks

    Average rate of head growth in a healthy premature infant

0.5 cm in the 1st 2 weeks
0.75 cm during the 3rd week
1.0 cm in the 4th week

29. (d) 34–35 cm

    Head circumference of a term baby

Birth	34–35 cm
6 months	44 cm by
1 year of age	47 cm

30. (b) Olfactory nerve
31. (a) 32nd weeks of gestation
32. (d) All of the above
33. (a) Purulent meningitis
34. (a) Peppermint
35. (d) Optic nerve
36. (d) Combination of all above
37. (c) Salmon-pink
38. (a) Gray-white
39. (a) Papilledema
40. (d) All of the above
41. (a) 30–40%

    Retinal hemorrhages occur in 30–40% of all full-term newborn infants. The hemorrhages are more common after vaginal delivery than after cesarean section and are not associated with birth injury or with neurologic complications. They disappear spontaneously by 1–2 weeks of age.
42. (b) Term

    Normal 28 weeks old premature infants blink when a bright light is directed to the eyes and, by 32 weeks, infants maintain eye closure until the light source is removed. At 37 weeks, normal premature infants turn the head and the eyes to a soft light and, by term, visual fixation and the ability to follow a brilliant target are present.
43. (a) Newborn
44. (b) 20/150
45. (d) 6 months
46. (b) 29th–32nd week

47. **(d)** All of the above
48. **(d)** All of the above
49. **(d)** All of the above
50. **(b)** Oculomotor
51. **(a)** Trochlear
52. **(b)** Abducens nerves
53. **(d)** All of the above
54. **(a)** Ptosis
55. **(a)** Superior oblique muscle
56. **(d)** Lateral rectus muscle
57. **(d)** All of the above
58. **(d)** Brainstem dysfunction
59. **(a)** 25
60. **(b)** Trigeminal nerve
61. **(d)** All of the above
62. **(b)** Facial grimacing
63. **(d)** Facial nerve
64. **(a)** Facial nerve
65. **(d)** Auditory nerve
66. **(c)** 3 months of age
67. **(d)** All of the above
68. **(a)** Glossopharyngeal nerve
69. **(b)** Glossopharyngeal nerve
70. **(d)** Gag response
71. **(a)** Glossopharyngeal nerve
72. **(a)** Vagus nerve
73. **(a)** Hoarse voice
74. **(d)** All of the above
75. **(d)** Accessory nerve
76. **(b)** Accessory nerve
77. **(d)** All of the above
78. **(a)** Hypoglossal nerve
79. **(a)** Tongue
80. **(b)** Werdnig-Hoffmann disease
81. **(d)** All of the above
82. **(b)** Grade 5

    Muscle power in a cooperative child is graded on a scale of 0–5 as follows: 0 = no contraction; 1 = flicker or trace of contraction; 2 = active movement, with gravity eliminated; 3 = active movement against gravity; 4 = active movement against gravity and resistance; 5 = normal power.
83. **(d)** All of the above
84. **(a)** Upper motor neuron tracts
85. **(d)** Basal ganglia
86. **(a)** Brainstem
87. **(d)** All of the above
88. **(d)** All of the above
89. **(a)** Spinal cord
90. **(d)** All of the above
91. **(b)** Basal ganglia
92. **(a)** Basal ganglia
93. **(d)** All of the above
94. **(d)** All of the above
95. **(d)** Upper motor neuron lesions
96. **(a)** Upper motor neuron lesion
97. **(d)** Rooting reflex
98. **(d)** All above
99. **(d)** All of the above
100. **(a)** Like water
101. **(a)** 5/mm^3
102. **(b)** Meningitis
103. **(d)** All of the above
104. **(a)** Nil
105. **(d)** All of the above
106. **(a)** 10 to 40 mg/dL
107. **(a)** Upto 120 mg/dL
108. **(d)** 3 months
109. **(d)** All of the above
110. **(d)** Long-standing intracranial hypertension
111. **(d)** All of the above
112. **(d)** All of the above
113. **(a)** 3rd and 4th week
114. **(d)** All of the above
115. **(b)** ∝-fetoprotein
116. **(a)** 16th–18th week
117. **(c)** 23rd day
118. **(a)** Jitteriness
119. **(d)** All of the above
120. **(d)** All of the above

121. **(a)** Toddler
122. **(b)** Diphenhydramine
123. **(d)** All of the above
124. **(c)** Scolding a child
125. **(d)** All of the above
126. **(d)** All of the above
127. **(b)** 5 years
128. **(a)** Painful experience
129. **(b)** Atropine sulfate
130. **(d)** All of the above
131. **(a)** Autosomal dominant
132. **(c)** Café au-lait spots
133. **(c)** Long arm of chromosome 22
134. **(c)** Joubert syndrome
135. **(d)** All of the above
136. **(d)** All of the above
137. **(d)** All of the above
138. **(d)** All of the above
139. **(d)** All of the above
140. **(d)** All of the above
141. **(b)** Vitamin E
142. **(a)** Cerebral palsy
143. **(d)** Commando crawl
144. **(d)** All of the above
145. **(a)** Acid β-galactosidase
146. **(d)** All of the above
147. **(a)** 15
148. **(b)** 5q13
149. **(d)** 14q24.3–q32.1
150. **(a)** 22q13–13
151. **(a)** Group B streptococcus
152. **(a)** Communicating hydrocephalus

Chapter 14

Neuromuscular Disorders

1. **Which peripheral neuropathy gives acute flaccid paralysis?**
   (a) Guillain-Barré syndrome
   (b) Acute intermittent porphyria
   (c) Post-rabies vaccine neuropathy
   (d) All of the above

2. **Which muscle disorder gives acute flaccid paralysis?**
   (a) Acute rhabdomyolysis (b) Hypophosphatemia
   (c) Hypokalemia (d) All of the above

3. **Creatine kinase is found in:**
   (a) Skeletal muscle (b) Cardiac muscle
   (c) Brain (d) All of the above

4. **Inheritance pattern of Duchenne and Becker muscular dystrophy:**
   (a) X-linked recessive (b) X-linked dominant
   (c) Autosomal recessive (d) Autosomal dominant

5. **Duchenne muscular dystrophy is characterised by:**
   (a) Progressive weakness
   (b) Intellectual impairment
   (c) Hypertrophy of the calves
   (d) All of the above

6. **The abnormal gene of Duchenne muscular dystrophy is located at:**
   (a) Xp21 (b) Xp23
   (c) Xp25 (d) Xp27

7. **The abnormal cytoskeletal protein of Duchenne muscular dystrophy is known as:**
   (a) Laminin (b) Dystrophin
   (c) Myosin (d) Fibrilin

8. **Which is the first sign of weakness in Duchenne muscular dystrophy?**
   (a) Eyelid drooping (b) Leg weakness
   (c) Poor head control (d) Respiratory distress

9. **What is earliest age at which Gowers sign is often evident in Duchenne muscular dystrophy?**
   (a) 1 year (b) 2 years
   (c) 5 years (d) 3 years

10. **What is earliest age at which Gowers sign is fully expressed in Duchenne muscular dystrophy?**
    (a) 5 or 6 years (b) 7 or 8 years
    (c) 9 or 10 years (d) 11-12 years

11. **Pseudohypertrophy in Duchenne muscular dystrophy in seen following muscle?**
    (a) Calves (b) Tongue
    (c) Muscles of the forearm (d) All of the above

12. **Which drug causes toxic myopathies?**
    (a) L-Dopa
    (b) Chloroquine
    (c) Cholesterol-lowering drugs
    (d) All of the above

13. **The main pathology of myasthenia gravis is related with:**
    (a) Acetylcholine (b) Methylcholine
    (c) Adrenaline (d) Nor-adrenalin

14. **What is a characteristic feature of myasthenia gravis?**
    (a) Pain in abdomen
    (b) Headache
    (c) Rapid fatigue of muscles
    (d) All of the above

15. Which is drug of choice in myasthenia gravis?
(a) Neostigmine methylsulfate
(b) Neostigmine bromide
(c) Pyridostigmine
(d) All of the above

16. Peroneal muscular atrophy is characterised by:
(a) Autosomal dominant
(b) Footdrop
(c) Palpably enlarged nerves
(d) All of the above

17. Which type of paralysis occurs in Guillain-Barré syndrome?
(a) Ascending paralysis (b) Descending paralysis
(c) Quadriplegia (d) Paraplegia

18. Miller-Fisher syndrome consists of:
(a) Acute external ophthalmoplegia
(b) Ataxia
(c) Areflexia
(d) All of the above

19. Congenital Guillain-Barré syndrome presents as:
(a) Generalized hypotonia (b) Weakness
(c) Areflexia (d) All of the above

20. What is cause of acute peripheral facial palsy?
(a) Herpes simplex virus type 1
(b) Varicella-Zoster virus
(c) Epstein-Barr virus
(d) All of the above

Answers

1. **(d)** All of the above
2. **(d)** All of the above
3. **(d)** All of the above
4. **(a)** X-linked recessive
5. **(d)** All of the above
6. **(a)** Xp21
7. **(b)** Dystrophin
8. **(c)** Poor head control
9. **(d)** 3 years
10. **(a)** 5 or 6 years
11. **(d)** All of the above
12. **(d)** All of the above
13. **(a)** Acetylcholine
14. **(c)** Rapid fatigue of muscles
15. **(d)** All of the above
16. **(d)** All of the above
17. **(a)** Ascending paralysis
18. **(d)** All of the above
19. **(d)** All of the above
20. **(d)** All of the above

Chapter 15

Blood

1. **What are anatomic stages for Developmental hematopoiesis?**
   (a) Mesoblastic (b) Hepatic
   (c) Myeloid (d) All of the above

2. **Mesoblastic hematopoiesis occurs in extraembryonic structures principally in:**
   (a) Chorion (b) Yolk sac
   (c) Liver (d) Lungs

3. **Mesoblastic hematopoiesis begins between ______ days of gestation.**
   (a) 4th and 6th (b) 6th and 8th
   (c) 8th and 10th (d) 10th and 14th

4. **Hepatic hematopoiesis is predominant at the gestation of:**
   (a) 8-10 weeks (b) 10-14 weeks
   (c) 16-18 weeks (d) 20-24 weeks

5. **At what gestational age neutrophils are first observed in the human fetus?**
   (a) 3 weeks (b) 5 weeks
   (c) 7 weeks (d) 9 weeks

6. **At what gestational age fetal bone marrow space begins to develop?**
   (a) 2nd week (b) 4th week
   (c) 6th week (d) 8th week

7. **At what intrauterine age granulocytic neutrophil cells found in the fetal bone marrow space?**
   (a) 10 weeks (b) 14 weeks
   (c) 16 weeks (d) 18 weeks

8. **At what intrauterine age granulocyte and macrophage colony-stimulating factors are expressed in developing fetal bone?**
   (a) 6 weeks (b) 8 weeks
   (c) 10 weeks (d) 12 weeks

9. **Who is the physiologic regulator of platelet production?**
   (a) Thromboplastin (b) Thrombopoietin
   (c) Thrombomodulin (d) Erythropoietin

10. **The gene that encodes the thrombopoietin is located on the:**
    (a) Long arm of chromosome 6
    (b) Long arm of chromosome 3
    (c) Short arm of chromosome 6
    (d) Short arm of chromosome 3

11. **Thrombopoietin -mRNA is expressed primarily in:**
    (a) Liver (b) Kidney
    (c) Bone marrow (d) All of the above

12. **Which factor controls the erythropoiesis in utero?**
    (a) Fibroblast growth factor
    (b) Insulin growth factor
    (c) Erythroid growth factor
    (d) Platelet derived growth factor

13. **Can erythropoietin (EPO) cross the placenta in humans?**
    (a) No (b) Yes
    (c) Both (d) None

14. **Normal adult hemoglobin (Hb A) is made up of:**
    (a) $\alpha_2 \partial_2$ (b) $\propto_2 \beta_2$
    (c) $\partial_2 \beta_2$ (d) $\alpha_2\gamma_2$

15. **Genes for the α chains are located on human chromosome:**
    (a) 11 (b) 16
    (c) 13 (d) 15

16. **Genes for the β, γ, δ genes are located on chromosome:**
    (a) 11 (b) 16
    (c) 13 (d) 15

17. **Name the embryonic hemoglobin:**
(a) Gower-1 (b) Gower-2
(c) Portland (d) All of the above

18. **In embryos, Gower hemoglobins predominate at:**
(a) 2-4 weeks gestation
(b) 4-8 weeks gestation
(c) 10-12 weeks gestation
(d) After 12 weeks gestation

19. **After which gestational age Hb F is the predominant hemoglobin?**
(a) 4th week (b) 6th week
(c) 8th week (d) 10th week

20. **At what gestational age, earliest a prenatal diagnosis of major β-chain hemoglobinopathies, such as thalassemia major is possible?**
(a) 16-20 weeks (b) 18-22 weeks
(c) 24-26 weeks (d) 26-28 weeks

21. **What is the normal ratio of Hb A to A_2 throughout life?**
(a) 15:1 (b) 30:1
(c) 45:1 (d) 60:1

22. **Name the condition where small amounts of the Gower hemoglobins are detectable in a newborn?**
(a) Trisomy 11 (b) Trisomy 21
(c) Trisomy 13 (d) Trisomy 5

23. **Raised levels of Hb Portland have been found in cord blood of stillborn infants with:**
(a) Homozygous α-thalassemia
(b) Heterozygous α-thalassemia
(c) Homozygous β-thalassemia
(d) Heterozygous β-thalassemia

24. **Raised levels of Hb F occurs in:**
(a) Hemolytic anemias (b) Leukemia
(c) Aplastic anemia (d) All of the above

25. **Raised levels of Hb A_2 are found in:**
(a) Iron deficiency anaemia
(b) Megaloblastic anemias secondary to vitamin B_{12} and folic acid deficiency
(c) Hemolytic anaemia
(d) None

26. **Decreased Hb A_2 levels are found in:**
(a) Iron-deficiency anemia
(b) Megaloblastic anemias secondary to vitamin B_{12} and folic acid deficiency
(c) Hemolytic anaemia
(d) None

27. **Average life span for a neonatal RBC is:**
(a) 60-90 days (b) 90-120 days
(c) 120-140 days (d) More than 140 days

28. **At what level hemoglobin level pallor becomes evident in the mucous membranes?**
(a) Under 7-8 g/d (b) 8-9 g/d
(c) 10-11 g/d (d) 11-12 g/d

29. **Normal mean level of hemoglobin in cord blood:**
(a) 11.2 Gm/Dl (b) 12.6 Gm/Dl
(c) 14.8 Gm/Dl (d) 16.8 Gm/Dl

30. **Normal mean level of hemoglobin in 2 weeks age:**
(a) 11.2 Gm/Dl (b) 16.5 Gm/Dl
(c) 12.6 Gm/Dl (d) 14.8 Gm/Dl

31. **Normal mean level of hemoglobin in 3 months:**
(a) 12 Gm/Dl (b) 14 Gm/Dl
(c) 16Gm/Dl (d) 18Gm/Dl

32. **Normal mean level of hemoglobin in 6 months-6 years:**
(a) 18 Gm/Dl (b) 16 Gm/Dl
(c) 14Gm/Dl (d) 12Gm/Dl

33. **Normal mean level of hemoglobin in 7-12 years:**
(a) 13 Gm/Dl (b) 11 Gm/Dl
(c) 15Gm/Dl (d) 18Gm/Dl

34. **Features of β-thalassemia:**
(a) Pathologic bone fractures
(b) Marked hepatosplenomegaly
(c) Hypersplenism
(d) All of the above

35. **Normal mean level of hemoglobin in adult female:**
(a) 10 Gm/Dl (b) 11 Gm/Dl
(c) 14Gm/Dl (d) 16Gm/Dl

36. **Child with anemia and reticulocytopenia is suggestive of:**
(a) Iron deficiency (b) Thalassemia trait
(c) Hemoglobin E disorders (d) All of the above

37. **Congenital Hypoplastic Anemia (Diamond-Blackfan Anemia) is characterized by:**
(a) Macrocytic anemia
(b) Reticulocytopenia
(c) High levels of erythropoietin (EPO) are present in serum and urine
(d) All of the above

38. **Diamond-Blackfan anemia is characterized by:**
(a) Short stature
(b) Craniofacial dysmorphism

(c) Triphalangeal thumbs
(d) All of the above

39. **Pearson Marrow-Pancreas syndrome is characterised by:**
(a) Macrocytic anemia
(b) Elevated hemoglobin F level
(c) Vacuolated erythroblasts in the marrow
(d) All of the above

40. **Transient erythroblastopenia of childhood is associated with:**
(a) Acquired red cell aplasia
(b) Occurs between 6 months and 3 years of age
(c) Transient immunologic suppression of erythropoiesis
(d) All of the above

41. **Physiologic anemia of infancy appears at:**
(a) 4-6 weeks (b) 6-8 weeks
(c) 8-10 weeks (d) 10-12 weeks

42. **Physiologic anemia in premature infants develops at:**
(a) 3-6 weeks of age (b) 6-8 weeks of age
(c) 8-10 weeks of age (d) 10-12 weeks of age

43. **The megaloblastic anemias is characterised by:**
(a) Increased mean corpuscular volume
(b) Hypersegmented neutrophils
(c) Result from a deficiency of folic acid or vitamin B_{12}
(d) All of the above

44. **Adolescents are more susceptible to iron deficiency because:**
(a) Growth spurt (b) Dietary deficiencies
(c) Menstrual blood loss (d) All of the above

45. **What is response to iron therapy within 24 hours in iron-deficiency anemia?**
(a) Subjective improvement
(b) Decreased irritability
(c) Increased appetite
(d) All of the above

46. **What is response to iron therapy in 36-48 hours in iron-deficiency anemia?**
(a) Erythroid hyperplasia (b) Reticulocytosis
(c) Increased HB levels (d) Repletion of stores

47. **What is response to iron th erapy in 48-72 hours in iron-deficiency anemia?**
(a) Erythroid hyperplasia (b) Reticulocytosis
(c) Increased HB levels (d) Repletion of stores

48. **What is response to iron therapy in 4-30 days in iron-deficiency anemia?**
(a) Erythroid hyperplasia (b) Reticulocytosis
(c) Increased HB levels (d) Repletion of stores

49. **What is response to iron therapy in1-3 months in iron-deficiency anemia?**
(a) Erythroid hyperplasia (b) Reticulocytosis
(c) Increased HB levels (d) Repletion of stores

50. **Sideroblastic anemias result from:**
(a) Disorders of heme synthesis
(b) Hypochromic microcytic red blood cells
(c) Dimorphic population of erythrocytes
(d) All of the above

51. **What is normal RBC survival time?**
(a) 80-90 days (b) 90-100 days
(c) 100-110 days (d) 110-120 days

52. **What is characteristic of hereditary pyropoikilocytosis?**
(a) Inherited as a dominant disorder
(b) Microspherocytosis
(c) Poikilocytosis
(d) All of the above

53. **What is the shape of the red blood cells in hereditary stomatocytosis?**
(a) Cup-shaped (b) Tear-shaped
(c) Oval (d) Round

54. **Paroxysmal nocturnal hemolysis is associated with:**
(a) Chronic hemolysis (b) Thrombocytopenia
(c) Leukopenia (d) All of the above

55. **Which is the diagnostic test of choice for paroxysmal nocturnal hemolysis?**
(a) Flow cytometry (b) Sugar test
(c) Reticulocyte (d) Ham's test

56. **Acanthocytosis is seen with:**
(a) Congenital abetalipoproteinemia associated with malabsorption
(b) Retinitis pigmentosa
(c) X-linked McLeod syndrome
(d) All of the above

57. **What is a prophylactic drug for children with sickle cell anemia?**
(a) Oral penicillin V (b) Penicillin G
(c) Procaine penicillin (d) All of the above

58. Feature of acute splenic sequestration is:
(a) Engorgement of the spleen
(b) Hypovolemia
(c) Decline in hemoglobin
(d) All of the above

59. Drugs causing acquired methemoglobinemia:
(a) Chloroquine (b) Metoclopramide
(c) Primaquine (d) All of the above

60. In β-thalassemias which chain is responsible for anemia and increased erythroid production?
(a) Excess of α-globin chain
(b) Excess of β -globin chain
(c) Excess of γ -globin chain
(d) Excess of δ -globin chain

61. In β-thalassemias, which chain is responsible for an elevated Hb F ($\alpha_2\gamma_2$)?
(a) α-globin (b) β -globin
(c) γ-globin (d) δ-globin

62. In β-thalassemias which chain is responsible for elevated Hb $A_2(\alpha_2\delta_2)$?
(a) α-globin (b) δ-globin
(c) β-globin (d) δ-globin

63. What is feature of α-thalassemia?
(a) Fewer α-globin chains
(b) Excess of β- and γ-globin chains
(c) Bart's hemoglobin (γ_4) in fetal life
(d) All of the above

64. Normal mean level of hemoglobin in adult female:
(a) 11 Gm/Dl (b) 14 Gm/Dl
(c) 16 Gm/Dl (d) 18 Gm/Dl

65. What is typical facies in β-thalassemia?
(a) Maxillary hyperplasia
(b) Flat nasal bridge
(c) Frontal bossing
(d) All of the above

66. Which is features of ineffective erythropoiesis in β-thalassemia?
(a) Expanded medullary spaces
(b) Extramedullary hematopoiesis
(c) Huge caloric need
(d) All of the above

67. Which is the contributing factor to produce a greenish brown complexion in beta thalassemia?
(a) Pallor (b) Hemosiderosis
(c) Jaundice (d) All of the above

68. Complications of β-thalassemia treatment:
(a) Hypothyroidism (b) Diabetes mellitus
(c) Cardiac arrhythmias (d) All of the above

69. Laboratory findings of β-thalassemia is:
(a) Severe anemia
(b) Numerous nucleated red cells
(c) Low reticulocyte count
(d) All of the above

70. Transfusional hemosiderosis can be prevented by the use of:
(a) Deferoxamine (b) Deferiprone
(c) ICL670 (d) All of the above

71. Which is the precaution to be taken for splenectomy in beta-thalassemia?
(a) Immunized against encapsulated bacteria before splenectomy
(b) Receive long-term penicillin prophylaxis
(c) Fever management
(d) All of the above

72. α-thalassemia is identified in the newborn period by:
(a) Raised Bart's hemoglobin (γ_4)
(b) Raised β hemoglobin
(c) Raised α hemoglobin
(d) Raised δ hemoglobin

73. Drugs precipitating hemolysis in glucose-6-phosphate dehydrogenase deficiency:
(a) Chloramphenicol (b) Chloroquine
(c) Vitamin K analogs (d) All of the above

74. What is the cause of drug-induced immune hemolytic anemia?
(a) Penicillin (b) Quinine
(c) Methyldopa (d) All of the above

75. Polycythemia is diagnosed with:
(a) Increased red blood cell count
(b) Raised hemoglobin level
(c) Increased total RBC volume
(d) All of the above

76. Which is major criteria for diagnosis of polycythemia vera?
(a) Increased red cell mass
(b) Arterial O_2 saturation of ≥92%
(c) Palpable splenomegaly
(d) All of the above

77. Viruses which give rise to aplastic anemia:
(a) Cytomegalovirus
(b) Epstein-Barr
(c) Human immunodeficiency
(d) All of the above

78. Drugs which give rise to aplastic anemia:
(a) Gold (b) Antiepileptics
(c) Chloramphenicol (d) All of the above

79. Hemophilia A (classic hemophilia) is due to deficiency of clotting factor:
(a) VIII (b) VII
(c) IX (d) X

80. Hemophilia B is due to deficiency of clotting factor:
(a) Christmas factor (b) Stuart factor
(c) Tissue factor (d) TPA

81. Hemophilia C is due to deficiency of clotting factor:
(a) V (b) XI
(c) X (d) XII

82. Parahemophilia is due to deficiency of clotting factor:
(a) V (b) XI
(c) X (d) XII

83. In full term neonate prothrombine time is:
(a) 13.0 sec (b) 15.0 sec
(c) 17.0 sec (d) 19.0 sec

84. Hallmark of hemophilia is:
(a) Hemaetemesis (b) Malena
(c) Hemarthrosis (d) Gum bleeding

85. von Willebrand disease has features of:
(a) Hereditary bleeding disorder
(b) Long bleeding time
(c) Long partial thromboplastin time
(d) All of the above

86. Vitamin K-dependent clotting factor is:
(a) II (b) VII
(c) IX (d) All of the above

87. Thrombotic thrombocytopenic purpura is characterised by:
(a) Fever
(b) Microangiopathic hemolytic anemia
(c) Thrombocytopenia
(d) All of the above

88. TAR syndrome consists of:
(a) Thrombocytopenia
(b) Hypoplasia of megakaryocytes
(c) Limb shortening
(d) All of the above

89. Wiskott-Aldrich syndrome (WAS) is characterized by:
(a) Tiny platelets (b) Eczema
(c) Recurrent infection (d) All of the above

90. Glanzmann thrombasthenia is characterised by:
(a) Severe platelet dysfunction
(b) Prolonged bleeding time
(c) Normal platelet count
(d) All of the above

91. Gray platelet syndrome has features of:
(a) Absence of platelet α granules
(b) Platelets that appear gray on Wright stain
(c) Aggregation and release are absent with most agonists other than thrombin and ristocetin
(d) All of the above

92. At what gestational age splenic precursor is recognizable?
(a) 2 weeks (b) 4 weeks
(c) 8 weeks (d) 5 weeks

93. What is approximate weight of spleen at birth?
(a) 5 gm (b) 9 gm
(c) 11 gm (d) 22 gm

94. What is weight of spleen at puberty?
(a) 90 g (b) 110 g
(c) 155 g (d) 135 g

95. Functional or anatomic hyposplenia is characterized by:
(a) Howell-Jolly bodies
(b) Heinz bodies
(c) Debris in RBCs
(d) All of the above

96. How much percentage of normally spleen is palpable?
(a) 15% of neonates
(b) 10% of normal children
(c) 5% of adolescents
(d) All true

Answers

1. **(d)** All of the above
2. **(b)** Yolk sac
3. **(d)** 10th and 14th
4. **(d)** 20–24 weeks
5. **(b)** 5 weeks
6. **(d)** 8th week
7. **(b)** 14 weeks
8. **(a)** 6 weeks
9. **(b)** Thrombopoietin
10. **(b)** Long arm of chromosome 3
11. **(d)** All of the above
12. **(c)** Erythroid growth factor
13. **(a)** No
14. **(d)** $\alpha_2\gamma_2$
15. **(b)** 16
16. **(a)** 11
17. **(d)** All of the above
18. **(b)** 4–8 weeks gestation
19. **(c)** 8th week
20. **(a)** 16–20 weeks
21. **(b)** 30:1
22. **(c)** Trisomy 13
23. **(a)** Homozygous α-thalassemia
24. **(d)** All of the above
25. **(b)** Megaloblastic anemias secondary to vitamin B_{12} and folic acid deficiency
26. **(a)** Iron-deficiency anemia
27. **(a)** 60–90 days
28. **(a)** Under 7–8 g/d
29. **(d)**16.8 Gm/Dl
30. **(b)** 16.5 Gm/Dl
31. **(a)** 12 Gm/Dl
32. **(d)** 12 Gm/Dl
33. **(a)** 13 Gm/Dl
34. **(d)** All of the above
35. **(d)** 16 Gm/Dl
36. **(d)** All of the above
37. **(d)** All of the above
38. **(d)** All of the above
39. **(d)** All of the above
40. **(d)** All of the above
41. **(b)** 6–8 weeks
42. **(a)** 3–6 weeks of age
43. **(d)** All of the above
44. **(d)** All of the above
45. **(d)** All of the above
46. **(a)** Erythroid hyperplasia
47. **(b)** Reticulocytosis
48. **(c)** Increased HB levels
49. **(d)** Repletion of stores
50. **(d)** All of the above
51. **(d)** 110–120 days
52. **(d)** All of the above
53. **(a)** Cup-shaped
54. **(d)** All of the above
55. **(a)** Flow cytometry
56. **(d)** All of the above
57. **(a)** Oral penicillin
58. **(d)** All of the above
59. **(d)** All of the above
60. **(a)** Excess of α-globin chain
61. **(c)** γ-globin

62. **(b)** δ-globin
63. **(d)** All of the above
64. **(b)** 14 Gm/Dl
65. **(d)** All of the above
66. **(d)** All of the above
67. **(d)** All of the above
68. **(d)** All of the above
69. **(d)** All of the above
70. **(d)** All of the above
71. **(d)** All of the above
72. **(a)** Raised Bart's hemoglobin (γ_4)
73. **(d)** All of the above
74. **(d)** All of the above
75. **(a)** All of the above
76. **(d)** All of the above

Diagnosis of Polycythemia Vera

Major Criteria
1. Increased red cell mass (see text) 2. Arterial O2 saturation of ≥ 92%[*] 3. Palpable splenomegaly
Minor Criteria
1. Platelet count of >400 × 109/L 2. Leukocytosis of >12 × 109/L 3. Increased leukocyte alkaline phosphatase 4. Increased vitamin B12 (>900 pg/mL) or unbound B12 binding capacity (>2,200 pg/mL)
Diagnosis
All 3 major criteria
1, 2 and 2 minor criteria

77. **(d)** All of the above
78. **(d)** All of the above
79. **(a)** VIII
80. **(a)** Christmas factor
81. **(b)** XI
82. **(a)** V

Coagulation Factors

Clotting factor	Synonym	Disorder
I	Fibrinogen	Congenital deficiency (afibrinogenemia) or dysfunction (dysfibrinogenemia)
II	Prothrombin or dysfunction	Congenital deficiency
V	Labile factor, proaccelerin	Congenital deficiency (parahemophilia)
VII	Stable factor or proconvertin	Congenital deficiency
VIII	Antihemophilic factor	Congenital deficiency is hemophilia A (classic hemophilia)
IX	Christmas factor	Congenital deficiency is hemophilia B
X	Stuart-Prower factor	Congenital deficiency
XI	Plasma thromboplastin antecedent	Congenital deficiency, sometimes referred to as hemophilia C
XII	Hageman factor	Congenital deficiency is not associated with clinical symptoms
XIII	Fibrin-stabilizing factor	Congenital deficiencyte

83. **(a)** 13.0 sec
84. **(c)** Hemarthrosis
85. **(d)** All of the above
86. **(d)** All of the above
87. **(d)** All of the above
88. **(d)** All of the above
89. **(d)** All of the above
90. **(d)** All of the above
91. **(d)** All of the above
92. **(d)** 5 weeks
93. **(c)** 11 gm
94. **(d)** 135 g
95. **(d)** All of the above
96. **(d)** All true

Chapter 16

Endocrine System (1)

1. **Adenohypophysis develops from:**
(a) Endoderm (b) Mesoderm
(c) Neural crest cell (d) Oral ectoderm

2. **Craniopharyngiomas arise from remnant of:**
(a) Connection between oropharynx and Rathke's pouch
(b) From hypothalamus
(c) From median eminence
(d) From neurohypophysis

3. **Ant. pituitary produces how many peptide hormones?**
(a) 5 (b) 7
(c) 6 (d) 8

4. **In the Hall-Pallister syndrome all of the following seen *except:***
(a) Normal pituitary gland
(b) Hypothalamic hamartoblastoma
(c) Bifid epiglottis
(d) Imperforate anus

5. **In congenital hypopituitarism all is seen *except:***
(a) Severe hypoglycemia
(b) Microphalus in boys
(c) Prolonged neonatal jaundice
(d) Normal glucose level

6. **Wolfram syndrome includes all *except:***
(a) Diabetes mellitus (b) Optic atrophy
(c) Deafness (d) Ataxia

7. **Marfan's syndrome include all *except:***
(a) Tall stature
(b) Decreased upper to lower segment ratio
(c) Increased arm span
(d) Increased upper to lower segment ratio

8. **Mc Cune Albright syndrome includes all *except:***
(a) Precocious puberty
(b) Fibrous dysplasia
(c) Café au lait spots
(d) Petechial haemorrhage

9. **Sotos syndrome include all of the following *except:***
(a) Precocious puberty
(b) Rapid growth
(c) Macrocrania at birth
(d) Clumsiness and awkward gait

10. **The most common cause of infants who are large for gestational age (LGA):**
(a) Maternal diabetes mellitus
(b) Cerebral gigantism (Sotos syndrome)
(c) Weaver syndrome
(d) Beckwith-Wiedemann syndrome

11. **Beckwith Wiedeman syndrome includes all *except:***
(a) Hepatosplenomegaly
(b) Macroglossia
(c) Nephromegaly
(d) Hyperglycemia

12. **Children with Beckwith-Wiedemann syndrome (BWS) are predisposed to which neoplasm?**
(a) Wilm's tumour (b) ALL
(c) GIST (d) Malignant melanoma

13. **The first sign of puberty in female is:**
(a) Thelarche (b) Pubic hair
(c) Axillary hair (d) Menarche

14. **The first sign of puberty in male is:**
(a) Axillary hair (b) Pubic hair
(c) Growth of penis (d) Growth of the testes

15. Most common cause of thyroid disease in children is:
(a) Hashimotos thyroiditis
(b) Suppurative thyroiditis
(c) Riedels thyroiditis
(d) Congenital hypothyroidism

16. Most common organism responsible for acute suppurative thyroiditis is:
(a) Streptococcus viridans
(b) Staphylococcus aureus
(c) Pneumococcus
(d) Diphtheria

17. For thyroid function test which of the following radioisotopes used?
(a) I-131 (b) I-132
(c) Tc-99m (d) Cr-51

18. Feature of Pendred syndrome is:
(a) Hyperthyroidism and conductive deafness
(b) Hypothyroidism and sensorineural hearing loss
(c) Hypothyroidism and conductive deafness
(d) Hyperthyroidism and sensorineural hearing loss

19. All are the features of hyperthyroidism *except:*
(a) Palpitations
(b) Weight loss with increased appetite
(c) Heat intolerance and increased sweating
(d) Menorrhagia

20. Most common thyroid neoplasm is:
(a) Medullary carcinoma (b) Follicular carcinoma
(c) Papillary carcinoma (d) Anaplastic carcinoma

21. The tumour associated with thyroglossal duct remnant is:
(a) Papillary carcinoma (b) Follicular carcinoma
(c) Anaplastic carcinoma (d) Medullary carcinoma

22. The most helpful diagnostic test in the case of a solitary nodule is:
(a) USG (b) FNAC
(c) TFT (d) Thyroid scan

23. Multiple Endocrine Neoplasia (MEN) IIA include all of the following *except:*
(a) Phaechromocytoma
(b) Papillary carcinoma thyroid
(c) Medullary carcinoma thyroid
(d) Parathyroid hyperplasia

24. Mucosal Neuroma Syndrome, is the occurrence of all *except:*
(a) Medullary carcinoma thyroid
(b) Phaechromocytoma
(c) Parathyroid hyperplasia
(d) Neuromas on the tongue

25. DiGeorge syndrome include all of the following *except:*
(a) Neonatal hypocalcemia
(b) Conotruncal defects of the heart
(c) Velopharyngeal insufficiency
(d) Neonatal hyperglycemia

26. HDR syndrome includes all of the following *except:*
(a) Sensorineural deafness
(b) Renal anomaly
(c) Hypoparathyroidism
(d) Reiter's thyroiditis

27. In 21 α hydroxylase deficiency all of the following is seen *except:*
(a) Female pseudohermaphrotidism
(b) Menstrual irregularity
(c) Excessive reabsorption of salt and water
(d) Postnatal virilization in males and female

28. In 17 α hydroxylase all of the following seen *except:*
(a) Male pseudohermaphrotidism
(b) Sexual infantilism
(c) Hypertension
(d) Hypotension

29. Most common cause of congenital adrenal hyperplasia is:
(a) 21 α hydroxylase
(b) 17 α hydroxylase
(c) 11 β hydroxlase
(d) 3β-Hydroxysteroid dehydrogenase deficiency

30. Antley-Bixler syndrome all of the following seen *except:*
(a) Craniosynostosis
(b) Humeroradial synostosis
(c) Narrow iliac wings
(d) Absence of radius and ulna

31. Infants with aldosterone synthase deficiency have all electrolyte abnormalities *except:*
(a) Hyponatremia (b) Hyperkalemia
(c) Metabolic acidosis (d) Metabolic alkalosis

Answers

1. **(d)** Oral ectoderm

(Nelson Textbook of Pediatrics, 18th ed.)

The anterior pituitary gland originates from the Rathke's pouch as an invagination of the oral ectoderm. It then detaches from the oral epithelium and becomes an individual structure of rapidly proliferating cells. By 6 weeks gestation, the connection between the Rathke's pouch and the oropharynx is completely obliterated and the pouch establishes a direct connection with the downward extension of the hypothalamus, which gives rise to the pituitary stalk.

2. **(a)** Connection between oropharynx and Rathke's pouch

(Nelson Textbook of Pediatrics, 18th ed.)

Persistent remnants of the original connection between the Rathke's pouch and the oral cavity can develop into craniopharyngiomas, the most common type of tumor in this area.

3. **(c)** 6

(Nelson Textbook of Pediatrics, 18th ed.)

Five cell types in the anterior pituitary produce 6 peptide hormones. Somatotropes produce growth hormone (GH); lactotropes produce prolactin (PRL); thyrotropes make thyroid-stimulating hormone (TSH); corticotropes express pro-opiomelanocortin (POMC), the precursor of adrenocorticotropic hormone (ACTH); and gonadotropes express both luteinizing hormone (LH) and follicle-stimulating hormone (FSH).

4. **(a)** Normal pituitary gland

(Nelson Textbook of Pediatrics, 18th ed.)

In the Hall-Pallister syndrome, absence of the pituitary gland is associated with hypothalamic hamartoblastoma, postaxial polydactyly, nail dysplasia, bifid epiglottis, imperforate anus, and anomalies of the heart, lungs and kidneys.

5. **(d)** Normal glucose level

(Nelson Textbook of Pediatrics, 18th ed.)

Infants with congenital defects of the pituitary or hypothalamus usually present with neonatal emergencies such as apnea, cyanosis, or severe hypoglycemia with or without seizures. Microphallus in boys provides an additional diagnostic clue. Deficiency of GH may be accompanied by hypoadrenalism and hypothyroidism. Prolonged neonatal jaundice is common. It involves elevation of conjugated and unconjugated bilirubin and may be mistaken for neonatal hepatitis.

6. **(d)** Ataxia

(Nelson Textbook of Pediatrics, 18th ed.)

Wolfram syndrome, which includes DI, diabetes mellitus, optic atrophy, and deafness, also results in vasopressin deficiency.

7. **(d)** Increased upper to lower segment ratio

(Nelson Textbook of Pediatrics, 18th ed.)

Marfan syndrome is an autosomal dominant connective tissue disorder consisting of tall stature, increased arm span, and decreased upper to lower body segment ratio.

8. **(d)** Petechial haemorrhage

(Nelson Textbook of Pediatrics, 18th ed.)

Mc Cune Albright syndrome commonly consisting of a triad of precocious puberty, café-au-lait spots, and fibrous dysplasia.

9. **(a)** Precocious puberty

(Nelson Textbook of Pediatrics, 18th ed.)

Cerebral gigantism (Sotos syndrome): Children with cerebral gigantism (Sotos syndrome) are above the 90th percentile for both length and weight at birth; macrocrania may also be noted at that time. Sotos syndrome is caused by haploinsufficiency of the NSD1 gene (nuclear receptor SET domain–containing gene–1). Although it is characterized by rapid growth, there is no evidence that Sotos syndrome is an endocrine disorder. A hypothalamic defect has been suggested as a cause, but none has been demonstrated functionally or at necropsy. Growth is rapid, and by 1 yr of age, affected infants are greater than the 97th percentile in height. Accelerated growth continues for the first 4–5 years and then returns to a normal rate. Puberty usually occurs at the normal time but may occur slightly early. Adult height is usually in the upper normal range. The hands and feet are large, with thickened subcutaneous tissue. The head is large and dolichocephalic, the jaw is prominent, there is hypertelorism, and the eyes have an antimongoloid slant. Clumsiness and awkward gait are characteristic, and affected children have great difficulty in sports, in learning to ride a bicycle, and in other tasks requiring coordination. Some degree of mental retardation affects most patients; in some children, perceptual deficiencies may predominate. Osseous maturation is compatible with the patient's height.

10. **(a)** Maternal diabetes mellitus

(Nelson Textbook of Pediatrics, 18th ed.)

Maternal diabetes constitutes the most common cause of infants who are large for gestational age (LGA). Even in the absence of clinical symptoms or a family history, the birth of an excessively large infant should lead to evaluation for maternal (or gestational) diabetes.

11. **(d)** Hyperglycemia

(Nelson Textbook of Pediatrics, 18th ed.)

A group of disorders associated with excessive somatic growth and growth of specific organs has been described and is collectively referred to as overgrowth syndromes. These disorders appear to be caused by excess availability of insulin-like growth factor-II (IGF-II) encoded by the gene *Igf2*. The best described of these syndromes is the Beckwith-Wiedemann syndrome (BWS), which is an overgrowth malformation syndrome that occurs with an incidence of 1 : 13,700 births. It manifests as a fetal overgrowth syndrome in which hypertrophy dominates the clinical picture. Typically, macroglossia, hepatosplenomegaly, nephromegaly, and hypoglycemia secondary to hyperinsulinemia due to pancreatic β-cell hyperplasia in an LGA baby make up the clinical picture at birth. These children are predisposed to a specific subset of childhood neoplasms, including Wilm's tumor and adrenocortical carcinoma.

12. **(a)** Wilm's tumour

(Nelson Textbook of Pediatrics, 18th ed.)

The children of Beckwith-Wiedemann syndrome are predisposed to a specific subset of childhood neoplasms, including Wilm's tumor and adrenocortical carcinoma.

13. **(a)** Thelarche

(Nelson Textbook of Pediatrics, 18th ed.)

The age of onset of puberty varies and is more closely correlated with osseous maturation than with chronological age.In females, the breast bud is usually the first sign of puberty (10–11 years), followed by the appearance of pubic hair 6–12 months later. The interval to menarche is usually 2–2½ years but may be as long as 6 years.

14. **(d)** Growth of the testes

(Nelson Textbook of Pediatrics, 18th ed.)
In males, growth of the testes (>3 mL in volume or 2.5 cm in longest diameter) and thinning of the scrotum are the first signs of puberty. These are followed by pigmentation of the scrotum and growth of the penis. Pubic hair then appears. Appearance of axillary hair usually occurs in mid-puberty. In males, unlike in females, acceleration of growth begins after puberty is well under way and is maximal at genital stage IV–V (typically between 13 and 14 years of age). In males, the growth spurt occurs approximately 2 years later than in females, and growth may continue beyond 18 years of age.

15. **(a)** Hashimotos thyroiditis

(Nelson Textbook of Pediatrics, 18th ed.)

Lymphocytic thyroiditis is the most common cause of thyroid disease in children and adolescents and accounts for many of the enlarged thyroids formerly designated "adolescent" or "simple" goiter. It is also the most common cause of acquired hypothyroidism, with or without goiter.

Characteristics of Thyroiditis Syndromes

Characteristic	Hashimoto's thyroiditis	Painless postpartum thyroiditis	Painless sporadic thyroiditis	Painful subacute thyroiditis	Suppurative thyroiditis	Riedel's thyroiditis
Sex ratio (F : M)	8–9 : 1	—	2 : 1	5 : 1	1 : 1	3–4 : 1
Cause	Autoimmune	Autoimmune	Autoimmune	Unknown	Infectious	Unknown
Pathologic findings	Lymphocytic infiltration, germinal centers, fibrosis	Lymphocytic infiltration	Lymphocytic infiltration	Giant cells, granulomas	Abscess formation	Dense fibrosis
Thyroid function	Hypothyroidism	Thyrotoxicosis, hypothyroidism, or both	Thyrotoxicosis, hypothyroidism, or both	Thyrotoxicosis, hypothyroidism, or both	Usually euthyroidism	Usually euthyroidism
TPO antibodies	High titer, persistent	High titer, persistent	High titer, persistent	Low titer, or absent, or transient	Absent	Usually present
ESR	Normal	Normal	Normal	High	High	Normal
24-hour ^{123}I uptake	Variable	<5%	<5%	<5%	Normal	Low or normal

16. **(a)** Streptococcus viridans

(Nelson Textbook of Pediatrics, 18th ed.)

Acute suppurative thyroiditis is uncommon; it is usually preceded by a respiratory infection. The left lower lobe is affected predominantly. Abscess formation may occur. Anaerobic organisms, with or without aerobes, are the typical infectious agent. The most common organism is *Streptococcus viridans,* followed by *Staphylococcus aureus* and pneumococcus.

17. **(c)** Tc-99m

(Nelson Textbook of Pediatrics, 18th ed.)

In vivo Radionuclide Studies

The iodine trapping or concentrating mechanism of the thyroid can be evaluated by measuring the uptake of radioactive isotope ^{123}I (half-life of 13 hours). The technology allows doses of radioiodine (0.1–0.5 mCi) that are only a fraction of those formerly used with ^{131}I. Technetium (^{99m}Tc) is a particularly useful radioisotope for children, because in contrast to iodine, it is trapped but not organified by the thyroid and has a half-life of only 6 hours.

18. **(b)** Hypothyroidism and sensorineural hearing loss

(Nelson Textbook of Pediatrics, 18th ed.)

Patients with, a disorder comprising sensorineural deafness and goiter, have a positive perchlorate discharge. Pendred syndrome is due to a defect in a sulfate transport protein common to the thyroid gland and the cochlea.

19. **(d)** Menorrhagia

(Nelson Textbook of Pediatrics, 18th ed.)

Manifestations of Hyperthyroidism

Symptoms

- Hyperactivity, irritability, altered mood, insomnia, anxiety
- Heat intolerance, increased sweating
- Palpitations
- Fatigue, weakness
- Dyspnea
- Weight loss with increased appetite (weight gain in 10% of patients)
- Pruritus
- Increased stool frequency
- Thirst and polyuria
- Oligomenorrhea or amenorrhea, loss of libido

Signs

- Sinus tachycardia, atrial fibrillation (rare in children), supraventricular tachycardia
- Fine tremor, hyperkinesis, hyperreflexia
- Warm, moist skin
- Palmar erythema, onycholysis
- Hair loss
- Osteoporosis
- Hypercalcemia

Contd.

Contd.

- Muscle weakness and wasting
- High-output heart failure
- Chorea
- Periodic (hypokalemic) paralysis (primarily in Asian men)
- Psychosis (rare)

20. **(c)** Papillary carcinoma

(Nelson Textbook of Pediatrics, 18th ed.)

Histologically, the carcinomas are papillary (80%), follicular (17%), medullary (2%), or mixed differentiated tumors. These are usually slow-growing tumors and may remain dormant for years. The type of tumor and the natural course of disease in irradiated and nonirradiated patients are the same except that multicentricity is more frequent in irradiation-induced cancer. Undifferentiated (anaplastic) thyroid neoplasms are rare in children and usually have a rapidly fatal course. Thyroid cancer, most commonly papillary cancer, has been reported in thyroglossal duct remnants in children. Lymphomas and teratomas of the thyroid are also reported in children.

21. **(a)** Papillary carcinoma

(Nelson Textbook of Pediatrics, 18th ed.)

Thyroid cancer, most commonly papillary cancer, has been reported in thyroglossal duct remnants in children. Lymphomas and teratomas of the thyroid are also reported in children.

22. **(b)** FNAC

(Nelson Textbook of Pediatrics, 18th ed.)

The most helpful diagnostic test in the case of a solitary nodule is fine-needle aspiration (FNA). An ultrasonographic examination of the thyroid can provide information on the consistency of the nodule (solid vs cystic) and whether other nonpalpable nodules are present. A thyroid scan, preferably using ^{123}I or ^{99m}Tc-pertechnetate, can provide information on trapping function and whether the nodule is "cold", "warm", or "hot". The majority of cold nodules are benign. Neither ultrasound nor a thyroid scan can differentiate between a benign or malignant lesion. FNA specimens may be interpreted as benign tumor, malignant tumor, indeterminate, or inadequate specimen. Tests of thyroid function are normal, but Hashimoto's thyroiditis has been associated with thyroid cancer.

23. **(b)** Papillary carcinoma thyroid

(Nelson Textbook of Pediatrics, 18th ed.)

When hyperplasia or carcinoma of C cells is associated with adrenal medullary hyperplasia or pheochromocytoma and parathyroid hyperplasia, it is known as multiple endocrine neoplasia (MEN) IIA.

The inheritance pattern for MEN IIA is autosomal dominant, with a high degree of penetrance and variable expressivity. C-cell hyperplasia or tumors usually appear earlier than pheochromocytoma. Pheochromocytomas are frequently bilateral and may be multiple. Adrenal medullary hyperplasia is known to precede pheochromocytoma, but the detectable latent period is short. Hypercalcemia is a late manifestation and indicates hyperparathyroidism. The parathyroid glands may reveal chief-cell hyperplasia or only hypercellularity.

24. **(c)** Parathyroid hyperplasia

(Nelson Textbook of Pediatrics, 18th ed.)

Multiple Endocrine Neoplasia, Type IIB

The distinguishing feature of MEN IIB, also called the mucosal neuroma syndrome, is the occurrence of multiple neuromas and a characteristic phenotype associated with medullary carcinoma and pheochromocytoma. This condition is also autosomal dominant, and 93% of families have a missense mutation of the *RET* proto-oncogene. However, the mutation is in exon 16, the tyrosine catalytic domain of *RET;* all patients have had the same point mutation.The neuromas most often occur on the tongue, buccal mucosa, lips, and conjunctivae. Peripheral neurofibromas and café-au-lait patches may be present, and intestinal ganglioneuromatosis is common. Diffuse proliferation of nerves and ganglion cells is found in mucosal, submucosal, myenteric, and subserosal plexus involving the small and large bowel as well as the esophagus. The patients may be tall, with arachnodactyly and a Marfan-like appearance. Scoliosis, pectus excavatum, pes cavus, and muscular hypotonia are common. The eyelids may be thickened and everted, the lips patulous and blubbery, the jaw prognathic. Feeding difficulties, poor sucking, diarrhea, constipation, and failure to thrive may begin in infancy or early childhood, many years before the appearance of neuromas or endocrine symptoms.

25. **(d)** Neonatal hyperglycemia

(Nelson Textbook of Pediatrics, 18th ed.)

Aplasia or Hypoplasia of the parathyroid gland is often associated with the DiGeorge/velocardiofacial syndrome. In 90% of patients, the condition is caused by a deletion of chromosome 22q11.2. Approximately 25% of these patients inherit the chromosomal abnormality from a parent. Neonatal hypocalcemia occurs in 60% of affected patients, but it is transitory in the majority; hypocalcemia may recur or may have its onset later in life. Associated abnormalities of the 3rd and 4th pharyngeal pouches are common; these include conotruncal defects of the heart in 25%, velopharyngeal insufficiency in 32%, cleft palate in 9%, renal anomalies in 35%, and aplasia of the thymus with severe immunodeficiency in 1%.

26. **(d)** Reiter's thyroiditis

(Nelson Textbook of Pediatrics, 18th ed.)

HDR Syndrome: Hypoparathyroidism, sensorineural deafness, and renal anomaly occur owing to mutations of the *GATA3* gene. The protein encoded by this gene is essential in the development of the parathyroids, auditory system and kidneys.

27. **(c)** Excessive reabsorption of salt and water (see the following Table)

Diagnosis and Treatment of Congenital Adrenal Hyperplasia (Nelson 18th Edition)

Disorder	Affected gene and chromosome	Signs and symptoms	Laboratory findings	Therapeutic measures
21-Hydroxylase deficiency, classical form	*CYP21*	Glucocorticoid deficiency	↓ Cortisol, ↑ ACTH	Glucocorticoid (hydrocortisone) replacement
	6p21.3		↑↑ Baseline and ACTH-stimulated 17-hydroxy-progesterone	
		Mineralocorticoid deficiency (salt-wasting crisis)	Hyponatremia, hyperkalemia	Mineralocorticoid (fludrocortisone) replacement; sodium chloride supplementation
			↑ Plasma renin	
		Female pseudohermaphroditism	↑ Serum androgens	Vaginoplasty and clitoral recession
		Postnatal virilization in males and females	↑ Serum androgens	Suppression with glucocorticoids
21-Hydroxylase deficiency, nonclassical form	*CYP21*	Precocious adrenarche, menstrual irregularity, hirsutism, acne, infertility	↑ Baseline and ACTH-stimulated 17-hydroxyprogesterone	Suppression with glucocorticoids

Contd.

Contd.

Disorder	Affected gene and chromosome	Signs and symptoms	Laboratory findings	Therapeutic measures
	6p21.3		↑ Serum androgens	
11b-Hydroxylase deficiency	*CYP11B1*	Glucocorticoid deficiency	↓ Cortisol, ↑ ACTH	Glucocorticoid (hydrocortisone) administration
	8q24.3		↑↑ Baseline and ACTH-stimulated 11-deoxycortisol and deoxycorticosterone	
		Female pseudohermaphroditism	↑ Serum androgens	Vaginoplasty and clitoral recession
		Postnatal virilization in males and females	↑ Serum androgens	Suppression with glucocorticoids
		Hypertension	↓ Plasma renin, hypokalemia	Suppression with glucocorticoids
17α-Hydroxylase/17, 20-lyase deficiency	*CYP17*	Cortisol deficiency (corticosterone is an adequate glucocorticoid)	↓ Cortisol, ↑ ACTH	Glucocorticoid (hydrocortisone) administration
	10q24.3		↑ DOC, corticosterone response to ACTH Low 17α-hydroxylated steroids; poor	
		Male pseudohermaphroditism	↓ Serum androgens; poor response to hCG	Orchidopexy or removal of intra-abdominal testes; sex hormone replacement consonant with sex of rearing
		Sexual infantilism	↓ Serum androgens or estrogens	Sex hormone replacement consonant with sex of rearing
		Hypertension	↓ Plasma renin; hypokalemia	Suppression with glucocorticoids

28. **(d)** Hypotension

(Nelson, 18th Edition)

Same as above.

29. **(a)** 21 α hydroxylase

More than 90% of CAH cases are caused by 21-hydroxylase deficiency. This P450 enzyme (CYP21, P450c21) hydroxylates progesterone and 17-hydroxyprogesterone (17-OHP) to yield 11-deoxycorticosterone (DOC) and 11-deoxycortisol, respectively. These conversions are required for synthesis of aldosterone and cortisol, respectively. Both hormones are deficient in the most severe, "salt wasting" form of the disease.

30. **(d)** Absence of radius and ulna

(Nelson, 18th Edition)

Antley-Bixler syndrome: Occurs due to deficiency of P450 oxidoreductase. The syndrome include craniosynostosis; brachycephaly; frontal bossing; severe midface hypoplasia with proptosis and choanal stenosis or atresia; humeroradial synostosis; medial bowing of ulnas; long, slender fingers with camptodactyly; narrow iliac wings; anterior bowing of femurs; and malformations of the heart and kidneys.

31. **(d)** Metabolic alkalosis

(Nelson, 18th Edition)

This is a rare autosomal recessive disorder in which conversion of corticosterone to aldosterone is impaired. The majority of cases result from mutations in the *CYP11B2* gene coding for aldosterone synthase. Infants with aldosterone synthase deficiency may have severe electrolyte abnormalities with hyponatremia, hyperkalemia, and metabolic acidosis. However, because cortisol synthesis is unaffected, infants rarely become as ill as untreated infants with salt-losing forms of congenital adrenal hyperplasia such as 21-hydroxylase deficiency. Thus, some infants escape diagnosis. Later in infancy or in early childhood they may exhibit failure to thrive and poor growth. Adults often are asymptomatic, although they may develop electrolyte abnormalities when depleted of sodium through procedures such as bowel preparation for a barium enema.

Chapter 17

Endocrine System (2)

1. **Which gland in the human body is designated as the "master gland"?**
(a) Pineal gland (b) Adrenal gland
(c) Pituitary gland (d) Hypothalamus

2. **The pituitary gland is located in:**
(a) Sella turcica (b) Anterior fossa
(c) Tympanic fossa (d) Posterior fossa

3. **The anterior lobe (adenohypophysis) of pituitary gland constitutes about __________ of the gland.**
(a) 80% (b) 70%
(c) 60% (d) 50%

4. **The anterior pituitary gland originates from:**
(a) Sella turcica (b) Rathke's pouch
(c) Thalamus (d) Hypothalamus

5. **Persistent remnants of the original connection between the Rathke's pouch and the oral cavity can develop into:**
(a) Tuberculoma (b) Thymoma
(c) Craniopharyngiomas (d) Leukoplakia

6. **Which is an anterior pituitary hormone?**
(a) Growth hormone
(b) Prolactin
(c) Thyroid-stimulating hormone
(d) All of the above

7. **Growth hormone is secreted by:**
(a) Hypothalamus (b) Thalamus
(c) Anterior pituitary (d) Posteror pituitary

8. **Growth hormone secretion is stimulated by which hormone?**
(a) Growth hormone releasing hormone
(b) Somatostatin
(c) Somatomedin
(d) GnRH

9. **Growth hormone secretion is inhibited by which hormone?**
(a) Somatomedin (b) Somatostatin
(c) GHRH (d) GnRH

10. **Which is physiologic factor that stimulates growth hormone production?**
(a) Sleep (b) Exercise
(c) Puberty (d) All of the above

11. **Which is physiologic factor that inhibits growth hormone production?**
(a) Hyperglycemia (b) Hypothyroidism
(c) Glucocorticoids (d) All of the above

12. **Which is biologic effect of growth hormone?**
(a) Increases in linear growth
(b) Protein synthesis
(c) Insulin resistance
(d) All of the above

13. **Prolactin hormone is secreted by:**
(a) Thalamus (b) Hypothalamus
(c) Anterior pituitary (d) Posterior pituitary

14. **In which condition there is increased production of prolactin occurs?**
(a) Dopamine antagonists
(b) Pituitary tumors
(c) Physiologic stress
(d) All of the above

15. **Which decreases the production of prolactin?**
(a) Dopamine agonists
(b) Dopamine antagonist
(c) Serotonin agonist
(d) Serotonin antagonist

16. **What is the primary physiologic role of prolactin?**
(a) Initiation and maintenance of lactation
(b) Production of milk
(c) Ejaculation of milk
(d) All of the above

17. **Which hormone prepares the breasts for lactation and stimulates milk production in postpartum period?**
(a) Oxytocin (b) Prolactin
(c) GH (d) ADH

18. **During pregnancy which hormone stimulates the development of the milk secretory apparatus?**
(a) Prolactin (b) Oxytocin
(c) GH (d) ADH

19. **Thyroid-stimulating hormone is secreted by:**
(a) Anterior pituitary (b) Posterior pituitary
(c) Thalamus (d) Hypothalamus

20. **Thyrotrophic-releasing hormone is produced by:**
(a) Anterior pituitary (b) Posterior pituitary
(c) Thalamus (d) Hypothalamus

21. **Release of thyroxin (T_4) and triiodothyronine (T_3) from the thyroid gland occurs because of:**
(a) Thyroid-stimulating hormone
(b) Thyrotropin releasing hormone
(c) Follicle stimulating hormone
(d) GnRH

22. **Thyroid-stimulating hormone production is inhibited by:**
(a) Dopamine (b) Somatostatin
(c) Glucocorticoids (d) All of the above

23. **ACTH is secreted by:**
(a) Anterior pituitary (b) Posterior pituitary
(c) Thalamus (d) Hypothalamus

24. **Secretion of ACTH is regulated by:**
(a) Corticotrophin releasing hormone
(b) Thyroid-stimulating hormone
(c) Thyrotropin releasing hormone
(d) Follicle stimulating hormone

25. **Which hormone acts on the adrenal cortex to stimulate cortisol synthesis and secretion?**
(a) ADH (b) ACTH
(c) TRH (d) FSH

26. **At what time of day ACTH and cortisol levels are highest?**
(a) Afternoon (b) Evening
(c) Early night (d) Morning

27. **Which physiologic conditions stimulate the release of CRH and ACTH?**
(a) Stress (b) Fasting
(c) Hypoglycemia (d) All of the above

28. **Luteinizing hormone and follicle-stimulating Hormone is secreted by:**
(a) Posterior pituitary (b) Hypothalamus
(c) Thalamus (d) Anterior pituitary

29. **Receptors for follicle-stimulating hormone on the ovary is:**
(a) Corona cells (b) Sertoli cells
(c) Leydig's cells (d) Granulosa cells

30. **Receptors for follicle-stimulating hormone on testis is:**
(a) Corona cells (b) Sertoli cells
(c) Leydig's cells (d) Granulosa cells

31. **Luteinization of the ovary and Leydig cell function of the testis is promoted by:**
(a) Follicle stimulating hormone
(b) GnRH
(c) Luteinizing hormone
(d) ADH

32. **Hormone released from the posterior pituitary:**
(a) Arginine vasopressin (b) Antidiuretic hormone
(c) Oxytocin (d) All of the above

33. **Which hormone regulates water conservation at the level of the kidney?**
(a) ACTH
(b) Antidiuretic hormone
(c) TRH
(d) Oxytocin

34. **Which hormone stimulates uterine contractions at the time of labor and delivery?**
(a) ACTH
(b) Antidiuretic hormone
(c) TRH
(d) Oxytocin

35. Underproduction of growth hormone alone or in combination with deficiencies of other pituitary hormones gives rise to a clinical condition of:
(a) Hypothyroidism (b) Hypopituitarism
(c) Hyperpituitarism (d) Hyperthyroidism

36. Hall-Pallister syndrome is associated with:
(a) Hypothalamic hamartoblastoma
(b) Postaxial polydactyly
(c) Bifid epiglottis
(d) All of the above

37. Hall-Pallister syndrome is due to:
(a) Absence of the pituitary gland
(b) McKusick Kaufman syndrome
(c) Bardel Biedl syndrome
(d) Orofacial digital syndrome

38. Microphallus in boys provides an additional diagnostic clue to the diagnosis of:
(a) Congenital hypopituitarism
(b) Klineffelter's syndrome
(c) Smith-Lemli Opitz syndrome
(d) Hypothyroidism

39. Adverse effect of growth hormone therapy:
(a) Pseudotumor cerebri
(b) Slipped capital femoral epiphysis
(c) Gynecomastia
(d) All of the above

40. Development of antibodies to administered growth hormone give rise to:
(a) Encephalitis
(b) Alzheimer's disease
(c) Hashimoto encephalopathy
(d) Creutzfeldt-Jakob disease

41. Diabetes insipidus may result from:
(a) Vasopressin deficiency
(b) Adrenalin deficiency
(c) Oxytocin deficiency
(d) Somatostatin deficiency

42. Extracellular volume of body is regulated by:
(a) Potassium (b) Chlorides
(c) Magnesium (d) Sodium

43. Plasma tonicity of human body is regulated by:
(a) Vasopressin (b) Adrenalin
(c) Oxytocin (d) Somatostatin

44. Vasopressin is synthesized in:
(a) Thalamus (b) Pons
(c) Medulla (d) Hypothalamus

45. Sensation of thirst is regulated by:
(a) Adrenalin (b) Vasopressin
(c) Oxytocin (d) Somatostatin

46. Wolfram syndrome consists of:
(a) Diabetes insipidus (b) Diabetes mellitus
(c) Optic atrophy (d) All of the above

47. In children hyponatremia is labelled when serum sodium is below:
(a) 110 mEq/L (b) 120 mEq/L
(c) 125 mEq/L (d) 130 mEq/L

48. Syndrome of inappropriate antidiuretic hormone secretion (SIADH) occurs with:
(a) Encephalitis (b) Brain tumors
(c) Head trauma (d) All of the above

49. Drugs that give rise to hyponatremia:
(a) Oxcarbazepine (b) Chlorpropamide
(c) Vinblastine (d) All of the above

50. Cerebral type of salt wasting is seen in:
(a) Brain tumors (b) Head trauma
(c) Hydrocephalus (d) All of the above

51. Fetal overgrowth occurs in:
(a) Maternal diabetes mellitus
(b) Sotos syndrome
(c) Beckwith-Wiedemann syndrome
(d) All of the above

52. Cause of postnatal overgrowth leading to childhood tall stature is:
(a) Marfan syndrome (b) Fragile X syndrome
(c) Homocystinuria (d) All of the above

53. Cause of postnatal overgrowth leading to adult tall stature is:
(a) Pituitary gigantism
(b) Testicular feminization
(c) Marfan's syndrome
(d) All of the above

54. XXY syndrome means:
(a) Down's syndrome
(b) Klinefelter syndrome
(c) Turner's syndrome
(d) Noonan's syndrome

55. Klinefelter syndrome is associated with:
(a) Tall stature
(b) Gynecomastia
(c) Decreased upper to lower body segment ratio
(d) All of the above

56. XYY syndrome is associated with:
(a) Tall stature (b) Behavioral
(c) Mental problems (d) All of the above

57. Marfan syndrome is associated with:
(a) Tall stature
(b) Increased arm span
(c) Decreased upper to lower body segment ratio
(d) All of the above

58. Prolactinoma having clinical manifestations of:
(a) Headache (b) Amenorrhea
(c) Galactorrhea (d) All of the above

59. Overproduction of growth hormone with open epiphyses results in:
(a) Acromegaly (b) Cretinism
(c) Gigantism (d) Dwarfism

60. Overproduction of growth hormone with closed epiphyses results in:
(a) Acromegaly (b) Cretinism
(c) Gigantism (d) Dwarfism

61. Acromegalic features consists of:
(a) Increased skull circumference
(b) Broad nose
(c) Enlarged tongue
(d) All of the above

62. McCune-Albright syndrome consists of:
(a) Precocious puberty (b) Café-au-lait spots
(c) Fibrous dysplasia (d) All of the above

63. Sotos syndrome (cerebral gigantism) having features of:
(a) Dolichocephalic head
(b) Hypertelorism
(c) Antimongoloid slant
(d) All of the above

64. Most common cause of overgrowth in the fetus is:
(a) TORCH
(b) Maternal diabetes
(c) Maternal toxoplasmosis
(d) Gestational hypertension

65. Beckwith-Wiedemann syndrome consists of:
(a) Macroglossia
(b) Hepatosplenomegaly
(c) Nephromegaly
(d) All of the above

66. What is first sign of puberty in females?
(a) Breast bud (b) Axillary hairs
(c) Pubic hairs (d) Menarch

67. What is first sign of puberty in males?
(a) Axillary hairs (b) Pubic hairs
(c) Musculine voice (d) Growth of the testes

68. Precocious puberty in girls is defined as the onset of secondary sexual characteristics before_______ of age.
(a) 8 years (b) 9 years
(c) 12 years (d) 14 years

69. Precocious puberty in boys is defined as the onset of secondary sexual characteristics before ______ of age.
(a) 4 years (b) 9 years
(c) 12 years (d) 14 years

70. Which condition give rise to precocious puberty?
(a) Hypothalamic hamartoma
(b) Hydrocephalus
(c) Prolonged and untreated hypothyroidism
(d) All of the above

71. McCune-Albright syndrome consists of:
(a) Precocious puberty
(b) Polyostotic fibrous dysplasia
(c) Abnormal pigmentation
(d) All of the above

72. At what intrauterine life bilobed thyroid shape is recognized?
(a) 6-8 weeks (b) 12 weeks
(c) 8-10 weeks (d) 7 weeks

73. At what intrauterine life thyroid follicle cell and colloid formation is seen?
(a) 10 weeks (b) 6-8 weeks
(c) 12 weeks (d) 7 weeks

74. At what intrauterine life thyroglobulin synthesis occurs?
(a) 6-8 weeks (b) 12 weeks
(c) 8-10 weeks (d) 4 weeks

75. At what intrauterine life iodine trapping occurs?
(a) 6-8 weeks (b) 8-10 weeks
(c) 12 weeks (d) 4 weeks

76. At what intrauterine life and thyroxine (T_4) and triiodothyronine (T_3) synthesis and secretion occur?
(a) 6-8 weeks (b) 8-10 weeks
(c) 12 weeks (d) 4 weeks

77. At what intrauterine life hypothalamic neurons synthesizes thyrotropin-releasing hormone?
(a) 6-8 weeks (b) 12 weeks
(c) 8-10 weeks (d) 4 weeks

78. At what intrauterine life thyroid-stimulating hormone secretion occurs?
(a) 6-8 weeks (b) 12 weeks
(c) 8-10 weeks (d) 4 weeks

79. What is recommended dietary allowance of iodine in infants?
(a) 150 μg/24 hr (b) 130 μg/kg/24 hr
(c) 90-12 μg/24 hr (d) 30 μg/kg/24 hr

80. What is recommended dietary allowance of iodine in children?
(a) 150 μg/24 hr (b) 130 μg/kg/24 hr
(c) 90-120 μg/24 hr (d) 30 μg/kg/24 hr

81. What is recommended dietary allowance of iodine in adolescents?
(a) 150 μg/24 hr
(b) 130 μg/kg/24 hr
(c) 90-120 μg/24 hr
(d) 30 μg/kg/24 hr

82. What is role of thyroid hormones?
(a) Increases oxygen consumption
(b) Stimulate protein synthesis
(c) Influence growth and differentiation
(d) All of the above

83. The function of thyroid gland is regulated by:
(a) TRH (b) T3
(c) TSH (d) T4

84. Which is neonatal manifestation of hypothyroidism?
(a) Prolongation of physiologic jaundice
(b) Feeding difficulties
(c) Lack of interest
(d) All of the above

85. Which is cardiac manifestation of hypothyroidism?
(a) Pulse is slow (b) Heart murmurs,
(c) Cardiomegaly (d) All of the above

86. Clinical features of hypothyroidism:
(a) Stunted growth
(b) Anterior and posterior fontanels widely open
(c) Thick, broad tongue protrudes
(d) All of the above

87. Clinical features of hypothyroidism:
(a) Delayed dentition
(b) Myxedema
(c) Coarse, brittle and scanty hair
(d) All of the above

88. Radiological features of hypothyroidism:
(a) Wormian bones in skull
(b) Absent distal femoral epiphysis
(c) Beaking of the 12th thoracic or 1st or 2nd lumbar vertebra
(d) All of the above

89. Oral drug of choice for hypothyroid management is:
(a) TSH (b) Levothyroxine
(c) Propylthiouracil (d) Lugol's iodine

90. Dose of levothyroxine in neonates is:
(a) 10-15 μg/kg /24 hr (b) 5-10 μg/kg/24 hr
(c) 1-4 μg/kg/24 hr (d) 15-20 μg/kg/24 hr

91. Dose of levothyroxine in children is:
(a) 4 μg/kg/24 hr (b) 0.5 μg/kg/24 hr
(c) 1 μg/kg/24 hr (d) 2 μg/kg/24 hr

92. Dose of levothyroxine in adolescent is:
(a) 0.2 μg/kg/24 hr (b) 0.5 μg/kg/24 hr
(c) 1 μg/kg/24 hr (d) 2 μg/kg/24 hr

93. Overtreatment of levothyroxine leads to:
(a) Craniosynostosis
(b) Temperament disorders
(c) Pseudotumor cerebri
(d) All of the above

94. The most common cause of acquired hypothyroidism is:
(a) Chronic lymphocytic thyroiditis
(b) Lodine deficiency goitre
(c) Hashimoto's thyroiditis
(d) Multinodular goitre

95. **Autoimmune thyroid disease occurs in:**
(a) Down's syndrome (b) Turner's syndrome
(c) Klinefelter syndrome (d) All of the above

96. **Hypothyroidism is a part of:**
(a) Sjögren syndrome (b) Multiple sclerosis
(c) Pernicious anemia (d) All of the above

97. **Protracted ingestion of which medications give rise to hypothyroidism?**
(a) Amiodarone (b) Lithium carbonate
(c) Thalidomide (d) All of the above

98. **Grave's disease is associated with:**
(a) Enlargement of the thymus
(b) Splenomegaly
(c) Lymphadenopathy
(d) All of the above

99. **Which is a manifestation of Grave's disease?**
(a) Heat intolerance (b) Palpitations
(c) Fatigue (d) All of the above

100. **Which is a sign of Grave's disease?**
(a) Fine tremor (b) Osteoporosis
(c) Muscle wasting (d) All of the above

101. **Which is a manifestation of Grave's disease?**
(a) Exophthalmos (b) Diffuse goiter
(c) Lymphoid hyperplasia (d) All of the above

102. **Thyroid storm is manifested as:**
(a) Hyperthermia (b) Severe tachycardia
(c) Restlessness (d) All of the above

103. **Masked hyperthyroidism is characterized by-**
(a) Extreme listlessness (b) Apathy
(c) Cachexia (d) All of the above

104. **Treatment of neonate having congenital hypothyroidism:**
(a) Propranolol (b) Propylthiouracil
(c) Lugol solution (d) All of the above

105. **Cause of parathyroid hormone deficiency leading to hypocalcemia:**
(a) Wilson's disease
(b) DiGeorge syndrome
(c) Conotruncal-face syndrome
(d) All of the above

106. **HDR syndrome consists of:**
(a) Hypoparathyroidism
(b) Sensorineural deafness
(c) Renal anomaly
(d) All of the above

107. **Kenny-Caffey syndrome is associated with:**
(a) Symptomatic hypocalcemia
(b) Short stature
(c) Delayed closure of the fontanel
(d) All of the above

108. **Multiple endocrine neoplasia (MEN) syndromes is characterized by:**
(a) Neoplasia of pancreatic
(b) Neoplasia of anterior pituitary
(c) Neoplasia of parathyroid glands
(d) All of the above

109. **Hormone secreted by the adrenal medulla:**
(a) Dopamine (b) Norepinephrine
(c) Epinephrine (d) All of the above

110. **Smith-Lemli-Opitz syndrome is characterized by:**
(a) Facial anomalies
(b) Limb anomalies
(c) Developmental delay
(d) All of the above

111. **Wolman disease is characterized by:**
(a) Hepatosplenomegaly (b) Steatorrhea
(c) Abdominal distention (d) All of the above

112. **Drug causing adrenal insufficiency:**
(a) Ketoconazole (b) Rifampicin
(c) Phenytoin (d) All of the above

113. **Antley-Bixler syndrome has features of:**
(a) Craniosynostosis (b) Brachycephaly
(c) Humeroradial synostosis (d) All of the above

114. **Cushing's syndrome has feature of:**
(a) Moon facies
(b) Generalized obesity
(c) Hirsutism
(d) All of the above

115. **Cushing's syndrome has feature of:**
(a) Short stature
(b) Delayed pubertal development
(c) Osteoporosis
(d) All of the above

116. **Cortisol level in the blood is normally elevated at:**
(a) 4 A.M. (b) 8 A.M.
(c) 6 A.M. (d) 10 A.M.

117. Most common site of origin of pheochromocytomas is:
(a) Adrenal cortex (b) Carotid bodies
(c) Thoracic duct (d) Adrenal medulla

118. Antimüllerian hormone is secreted in males during both fetal and postnatal life by:
(a) Granulosa cells (b) Leydig's cells
(c) Corona radiata (d) Sertoli cells

119. Antimüllerian hormone is secreted in females during both fetal and postnatal life by:
(a) Granulosa cells (b) Leydig's cells
(c) Corona radiata (d) Sertoli cells

120. At what age serum concentration of antimüllerian hormone in males is highest?
(a) Puberty (b) Prepubertal period
(c) Birth (d) Adolescent

121. At what age serum concentration of antimüllerian hormone in females is highest ?
(a) Birth (b) Puberty
(c) Prepubertal period (d) Adolescent

122. Which is the median age of sperm production (spermarche)?
(a) 14 years (b) 12 years
(c) 16 years (d) 18 years

123. The average age at menarche in girls is:
(a) 8-10 years (b) 10-12 years
(c) 14-16 years (d) 12.5-13 years

124. Primary hypogonadism is manifested as:
(a) Testes and penis are abnormally small at birth
(b) Failure of secondary sex characteristics to develop
(c) Delayed closure of epiphyses
(d) All of the above

125. Clinical features of Noonan syndrome:
(a) Short stature (b) Webbing of the neck
(c) Cubitus valgus (d) All of the above

126. Characteristic facies of Noonan syndrome:
(a) Hypertelorism
(b) Downward slanted palpebral fissures
(c) Micrognathia
(d) All of the above

127. Chromosomal pattern of Klinefelter syndrome is:
(a) 46 XY (b) 47 XXY
(c) 21 trisomy (d) 45X

128. Clinical features of Klinefelter syndrome is:
(a) Tall, slim and underweight child
(b) Smaller phallus
(c) Small for age testes
(d) All of the above

129. Clinical features of XX males:
(a) Small testes and phallus (b) Hypogonadism
(c) Gynecomastia (d) All of the above

130. What is cause of hereditary mental retardation and macro-orchidism?
(a) Fanconi's anaemia
(b) Xeroderma pigmentosa
(c) Bloom's syndrome
(d) Fragile X syndrome

131. Which is the pathological cause of gynacomastia?
(a) 11β-hydroxylase deficiency
(b) Leydig cell tumors of the testis
(c) Peutz-Jeghers syndrome
(d) All of the above

132. Which is the pharmacological cause of gynacomastia?
(a) Spironolactone (b) Methyldopa
(c) Digitalis (d) All of the above

133. What is chromosomal complement pattern in Turner's syndrome?
(a) 46 XY (b) 47 XXY
(c) 21 trisomy (d) 45 X

134. Which is constituent of Turner's syndrome in adult females?
(a) Sexual infantilism (b) Webbed neck
(c) Cubitus valgus (d) All of the above

135. What is feature of Turner's syndrome at birth?
(a) Edema of the dorsa of the hands and feet
(b) Loose skinfolds at the nape of the neck
(c) Low birthweight
(d) All of the above

136. Denys-Drash syndrome is characterised by:
(a) Nephropathy (b) Ambiguous genitals
(c) Bilateral Wilm's tumor (d) All of the above

137. WAGR syndrome is characterised by:
(a) Wilm's tumor
(b) Aniridia
(c) Genitourinary malformations
(d) All of the above

138. WAGR syndrome is characterised by:
(a) Obesity (b) Wilm's tumor
(c) Retardation (d) All of the above

139. Reifenstein syndrome is characterised by:
(a) Hypogonadism (b) Severe hypospadias
(c) Gynecomastia (d) All of the above

140. Smith-Lemli-Opitz syndrome is characterised by:
(a) Growth retardation
(b) Syndactyly of the 2nd-3rd toes
(c) Severe mental retardation
(d) All of the above

141. Endocrinopathies giving rise to diabetes mellitus:
(a) Cushing's disease (b) Pheochromocytoma
(c) Hyperthyroidism (d) All of the above

142. Drugs causing diabetes mellitus:
(a) Pentamidine (b) Nicotinic acid
(c) Thiazides (d) All of the above

143. Genetic syndromes sometimes associated with diabetes:
(a) Down's syndrome
(b) Klinefelter syndrome
(c) Prader-Willi syndrome
(d) All of the above

144. A reliable index of long-term glycemic control is provided by measurement of:
(a) Blood glucose level
(b) Urine glucose level
(c) Liver glycogen store
(d) Glycosylated hemoglobin

145. Dawn phenomenon consists of:
(a) Overnight growth hormone secretion
(b) Increased insulin clearance
(c) Normal physiologic process seen in most nondiabetic adolescents
(d) All of the above

146. Somogyi phenomenon consists of:
(a) High morning glucose
(b) Rebound from late night or early morning hypoglycemia
(c) Due to an exaggerated counter-regulatory response
(d) All of the above

147. Criteria for diagnosis of Type 2 diabetes in children:
(a) Overweight (BMI > 85th percentile for age and sex)
(b) Family history of type 2 diabetes in 1st- or 2nd-degree relative
(c) Signs of insulin resistance or conditions associated with insulin resistance
(d) All of the above

148. Impaired glucose tolerance is a replacement term for:
(a) Asymptomatic diabetes (b) Chemical diabetes
(c) Subclinical diabetes (d) All of the above

149. Wolfram syndrome is characterized by:
(a) Diabetes insipidus (b) Optic atrophy
(c) Deafness (d) All of the above

150. Which is abnormalities in transient neonatal DM?
(a) Chromosome 11 (b) Chromosome 9
(c) Chromosome 6 (d) Chromosome 13

151. Rabson-Mendenhall syndrome is characterized by:
(a) Extreme insulin resistance
(b) Acanthosis nigricans
(c) Pineal hyperplasia
(d) All of the above

Answers

1. **(c)** Pituitary gland
2. **(a)** Sella turcica
3. **(a)** 80%
4. **(b)** Rathke's pouch
5. **(c)** Craniopharyngiomas
6. **(d)** All of the above
7. **(c)** Anterior pituitary
8. **(a)** Growth hormone releasing hormone
9. **(b)** Somatostatin
10. **(d)** All of the above
11. **(d)** All of the above
12. **(d)** All of the above
13. **(c)** Anterior pituitary
14. **(d)** All of the above
15. **(a)** Dopamine agonists
16. **(a)** Initiation and maintenance of lactation
17. **(b)** Prolactin
18. **(a)** Prolactin
19. **(a)** Anterior pituitary
20. **(d)** Hypothalamus
21. **(a)** Thyroid-stimulating hormone
22. **(d)** All of the above
23. **(a)** Anterior pituitary
24. **(a)** Corticotrophin releasing hormone
25. **(b)** ACTH
26. **(d)** Morning
27. **(d)** All of the above
28. **(d)** Anterior pituitary
29. **(d)** Granulosa cells
30. **(b)** Sertoli cells
31. **(c)** Luteinizing hormone
32. **(d)** All of the above
33. **(b)** Antidiuretic hormone
34. **(d)** Oxytocin
35. **(b)** Hypopituitarism
36. **(d)** All of the above
37. **(a)** Absence of the pituitary gland
38. **(a)** Congenital hypopituitarism
39. **(d)** All of the above
40. **(d)** Creutzfeldt-Jakob disease
41. **(a)** Vasopressin deficiency
42. **(d)** Sodium
43. **(a)** Vasopressin
44. **(d)** Hypothalamus
45. **(b)** Vasopressin
46. **(d)** All of the above
47. **(d)** 130 mEq/L
48. **(d)** All of the above
49. **(d)** All of the above
50. **(d)** All of the above
51. **(d)** All of the above
52. **(d)** All of the above
53. **(d)** All of the above
54. **(b)** Klinefelter syndrome
55. **(d)** All of the above
56 **(d)** All of the above
57. **(d)** All of the above
58. **(d)** All of the above
59. **(c)** Gigantism
60. **(a)** Acromegaly
61. **(d)** All of the above
62. **(d)** All of the above
63. **(d)** All of the above
64. **(b)** Maternal diabetes
65. **(d)** All of the above
66. **(a)** Breast bud
67. **(d)** Growth of the testes
68. **(a)** 8 years
69. **(b)** 9 years
70. **(d)** All of the above
71. **(d)** All of the above
72. **(d)** 7 weeks

73. **(a)** 10 weeks
74. **(d)** 4 weeks
75. **(b)** 8–10 weeks
76. **(c)** 12 weeks
77. **(a)** 6–8 weeks
78. **(b)** 12 weeks
79. **(d)** 30 μg/kg/24 hr
80. **(c)** 90–120 μg/24 hr
81. **(a)** 150 μg/24 hr
82. **(d)** All of the above
83. **(c)** TSH
84. **(d)** All of the above
85. **(d)** All of the above
86. **(d)** All of the above
87. **(d)** All of the above
88. **(d)** All of the above
89. **(b)** Levothyroxine
90. **(a)** 10–15 μg/kg /24 hr
91. **(a)** 4 μg/kg/24 hr
92. **(d)** 2 μg/kg/24 hr
93. **(d)** All of the above
94. **(a)** Chronic lymphocytic thyroiditis
95. **(d)** All of the above
96. **(d)** All of the above
97. **(d)** All of the above
98. **(d)** All of the above
99. **(d)** All of the above
100. **(d)** All of the above
101. **(d)** All of the above
102. **(d)** All of the above
103. **(d)** All of the above
104. **(d)** All of the above
105. **(d)** All of the above
106. **(d)** All of the above
107. **(d)** All of the above
108. **(d)** All of the above
109. **(d)** All of the above
110. **(d)** All of the above
111. **(d)** All of the above
112. **(d)** All of the above
113. **(d)** All of the above
114. **(d)** All of the above
115. **(d)** All of the above
116. **(b)** 8 A.M.
117. **(d)** Adrenal medulla
118. **(d)** Sertoli cells
119. **(a)** Granulosa cells
120. **(c)** Birth
121. **(b)** Puberty
122. **(a)** 14 years
123. **(d)** 12.5–13 years
124. **(d)** All of the above
125. **(d)** All of the above
126. **(d)** All of the above
127. **(b)** 47 XXY
128. **(d)** All of the above
129. **(d)** All of the above
130. **(d)** Fragile X syndrome
131. **(d)** All of the above
132. **(d)** All of the above
133. **(d)** 45 X
134. **(d)** All of the above
135. **(d)** All of the above
136. **(d)** All of the above
137. **(d)** All of the above
138. **(d)** All of the above
139. **(d)** All of the above
140. **(d)** All of the above
141. **(d)** All of the above
142. **(d)** All of the above
143. **(d)** All of the above
144. **(d)** Glycosylated hemoglobin
145. **(d)** All of the above
146. **(d)** All of the above
147. **(d)** All of the above
148. **(d)** All of the above
149. **(d)** All of the above
150. **(c)** Chromosome 6
151. **(d)** All of the above

Chapter 18

Genitourinary System (1)

1. **Which is the most important part of immune system involved in immune mediated glomerular injury?**
(a) Cell mediated
(b) Humoral
(c) Complement
(d) Humoral + cell mediated

2. **False-positive results may be seen, in dipstick test of urine for hematuria, in all of the following conditions *except:***
(a) After exercise
(b) Presence of formalin
(c) Contamination with oxidizing agents
(d) Presence of menstrual blood

3. **False-negative results may be seen, in dipstick test of urine for hematuria, in this following condition:**
(a) High urinary concentrations of ascorbic acid
(b) Alkaline urine with a pH >9
(c) Fever
(d) Presence of menstrual blood

4. **Red urine without RBCs is seen in:**
(a) Hemoglobinuria
(b) Postinfectious GN
(c) Alport syndrome
(d) Henoch-Schönlein purpura nephritis

5. **Myoglobinuria is seen in all of the following conditions *except:***
(a) Viral myositis
(b) Crush injury
(c) DIC
(d) Henoch-Schönlein purpura nephritis

6. **Drug causing red coloured urine:**
(a) Amphetamine (b) Chloroquine
(c) Paracetamol (d) Amoxicillin

7. **Following is feature of lower urinary tract haematuria:**
(a) Proteinuria >100 mg/dL
(b) Terminal hematuria
(c) Paracetamol
(d) Urinary microscopic findings of RBC casts

8. **Tea or cola-colored urine, facial/body edema, hypertension and oliguria suggest:**
(a) Acute nephritic syndrome
(b) Coagulopathy
(c) Urinary tract infection
(d) Trauma

9. **IgA nephropathy is seen with:**
(a) Tuberculosis
(b) Hepatic cirrhosis
(c) Sarcoidosis
(d) Enteric fever

10. **Glomerular filtration begins around the ___ weeks of fetal life.**
(a) 6 (b) 12
(c) 9 (d) 16

11. **The GFR may be best estimated by measurement of this endogenous substance:**
(a) Inulin (b) Cystatin C
(c) Urea (d) Creatinine

12. **____ is the most common cause of glomerular injury.**
(a) Genetic (b) Idiopathic
(c) Coagulation (d) Immunologic

13. **Deposition of immune complexes in glomeruli shows _____ appearance on immunofluorescence microscopy.**
(a) Tram tract (b) Normal
(c) Lumpy-bumpy (d) Any of the above

14. All of the following conditions are associated with hematuria with history of recent respiratory infection:

(a) Acute glomerulonephritis
(b) HUS
(c) SLE
(d) HSP nephritis

15. Most common chronic glomerular disease worldwide:

(a) Acute glomerulonephritis
(b) HUS
(c) SLE
(d) IgA nephropathy

16. IgA nephropathy is seen more often in:

(a) Male (b) Female
(c) Both (d) No such correlation

17. Suresh, a 2 years boy, came with complaints of gross hematuria. His mother gives history of cough and cold since 2-3 days, no fever. What is the most probable diagnosis?

(a) Acute glomerulonephritis
(b) HUS
(c) SLE
(d) IgA nephropathy

18. All of the following are poor prognostic factors in IgA nephropathy *except:*

(a) Persistent hypertension
(b) Heavy or prolonged proteinuria
(c) Diminished renal function
(d) Age of child

19. In membranous nephropathy _______ cells are affected.

(a) Epithelial cell (b) Mesangial cells
(c) Endothelial cells (d) Macula densa cell

20. A worse prognosis in IgA nephropathy is suggested by all of the following *except:*

(a) Diffuse mesangial proliferation
(b) Extensive glomerular crescents
(c) Glomerulosclerosis
(d) Tubular necrosis

21. The primary treatment of IgA nephropathy is_____.

(a) Alternate day corticosteroid
(b) Chemotherapy
(c) ACE inhibitors
(d) Conservative treatment

22. In post streptococcal glomerulonephritis ____ complement level is mostly decreased.

(a) C1 (b) C2
(c) C3 (d) C4

23. Post streptococcal glomerulonephritis in warm weather is caused following Group A β hemolytic streptococcal_________ infection.

(a) Throat (b) Skin
(c) Kidney (d) Lungs

24. Most common organism causing post-infectious glomerulonephritis_______.

(a) Group A β hemolytic streptococci
(b) Staph. aureus
(c) Pseudomonas
(d) E. coli

25. Deposition of immune complexes in glomeruli are:

(a) On endothelial side (b) On epithelial side
(c) Mesangial cells (d) All three type of cells

26. Which complement pathway is activated in post streptococcal glomerulonephritis?

(a) Classical pathway
(b) Alternative pathway
(c) Both
(d) None

27. Post streptococcal glomerulonephritis is uncommon before the age of_____.

(a) 1 year (b) 2 years
(c) 3 years (d) 4 years

28. Post streptococcal glomerulonephritis is most common in children aged:

(a) 1-3 years (b) 5-12 years
(c) 3-5 years (d) 12-14 years

29. A 10-year-old boy came with history of haematuria since 3 days. Doctors are suspecting post infectious glomerulonephritis. What relevant past history do you expect from mother?

(a) History of sore throat 1-2 weeks back
(b) History of skin infection 3-6 weeks back
(c) Either (a) or (b)
(d) None

30. In a case of post streptococcal glomerulonephritis persistent microscopic hematuria may persist for ____.

(a) 6 months (b) 1-2 years
(c) 3-4 years (d) 4-5 years

31. Serum c3 level becomes normal in ____ in post streptococcal glomerulonephritis.

(a) 2-4 weeks (b) 4-6 weeks
(c) 6-8 weeks (d) 8-10 weeks

32. Conformation of diagnosis of post streptococcal glomerulonephritis is done by:

(a) Antistreptolysin O titer
(b) Anti-deoxyribonuclease (DNase) B level
(c) Streptozyme test
(d) Streptokinase level

33. A 6 years boy known case of post-streptococcal glomerulonephritis is having hematuria and proteinuria and low C3 level since last two months after onset of disease. What will be your next line of management?

(a) Start with corticosteroid treatment
(b) Do renal biopsy
(c) Do IVP
(d) Switch to III generation cephalosporines

34. Renal biopsy should be considered in cases of all of the following *except:*

(a) Post streptococcal glomerulonephritis
(b) Nephrotic syndrome
(c) Presence of acute renal failure
(d) Post streptococcal glomerulonephritis with normal complement levels

35. Post streptococcal glomerulonephritis is associated with one of the following HLA type:

(a) HLA-Bw 35
(b) HLA-DR4
(c) HLA-B12
(d) HLA-DR2

36. Chances of developing nephrotic syndrome are least in:

(a) Poststreptococcal glomerulonephritis
(b) IgA nephropathy
(c) RPGN
(d) None

37. Raise ASO titer is used for diagnosis of:

(a) Post streptococcal infection (sore throat)
(b) Post streptococcal infection (skin infection)
(c) IgA nephropathy
(d) Goodpasture syndrome

38. In post streptococcal glomerulonephritis ______ complement level is always normal.

(a) C1 (b) C2
(c) C3 (d) C4

39. Crescents are more commonly seen in:

(a) PIGN (b) RPGN
(c) MPGN (d) IgA nephropathy

40. Immune deposits are seen in all of the following *except:*

(a) Post streptococcal glomerulonephritis
(b) IgA nephropathy
(c) RPGN
(d) Goodpasture syndrome

41. Membranous glomerulopathy in children may be associated with all of the following *except:*

(a) Penicillamine therapy
(b) Immune thrombocytopenic purpura
(c) Systemic lupus erythematosus
(d) Enteric fever

42. Neonatal-onset membranous glomerulopathy is suspected in a baby. What will you suspect in mother?

(a) Anti nuclear antibody in maternal serum
(b) Anti neutral endopeptidase (NEP)
(c) ANCA
(d) Anti double stranded DNA antibodies

43. In children with membranous glomerulopathy c3 level are normal *except:*

(a) With cases of immune thrombocytopenic purpura
(b) With cases of systemic lupus erythematosus
(c) With cases of sarcoidosis
(d) With cases of gonadoblastoma

44. ________ is the most common cause of chronic glomerulonephritis in older children.

(a) Membranoproliferative glomerulonephritis (MPGN)
(b) RPGN
(c) PSGN
(d) HUS

45. Most common form of MPGN is:

(a) Type I (b) Type II
(c) Type III (d) Type IV

46. What is the diagnosis?

(a) RPGN

(b) PSGN

(c) Membranous glomerulopathy

(d) IgA nephropathy

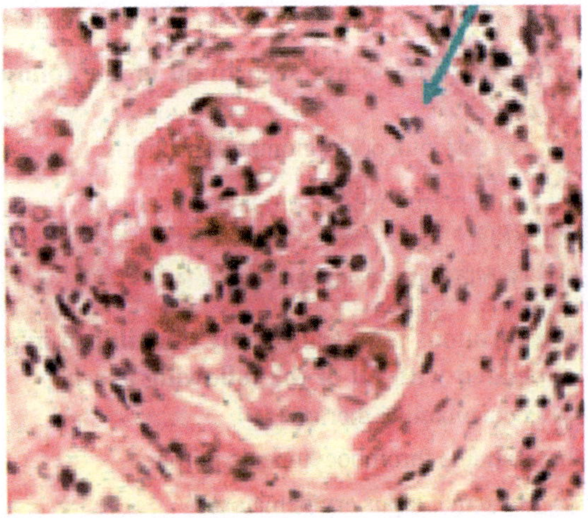

47. Tram tract appearance is seen in:

(a) RPGN

(b) PSGN

(c) Membranous glomerulopathy

(d) MPGN

48. _____ is the most common and most severe form of lupus nephritis.

(a) Class I lupus nephritis

(b) Class II lupus nephritis

(c) Class III lupus nephritis

(d) Class IV lupus nephritis

49. "Wire-loop" lesion is seen in:

(a) PSGN (b) SLE

(c) IgA nephropathy (d) MPGN

50. The majority of children with SLE are:

(a) Male less than 6 years

(b) Female less than 6 years

(c) Adolescent male

(d) Adolescent female

51. Least common lupus nephropathy is:

(a) Type II (b) Type III

(c) Type V (d) Type IV

52. A 13 years female came with complaints of hematuria. Her urine analysis was done. It showed proteinuria of range 700 mg in 24 hours sample. Her renal functions are normal. Pediatrician are suspecting SLE. What will be your investigation of choice?

(a) IVP (b) Renal biopsy

(c) MCU (d) Renal angiography

Answers

1. **(c)** Complement

(Nelson Textbook of Pediatrics, 18th ed.)

The inflammatory reaction that follows immunologic injury results from activation of one or more mediator pathways. The most important of these is the complement system, which has two initiating sequences: (1) the classic pathway, which is activated by antigen-antibody immune complexes, and (2) the alternative or properdin pathway, which is activated by polysaccharides and endotoxin. These pathways converge at C3; from that point on, the same sequence leads to lysis of cell membranes. The major noxious products of complement activation are produced after activation of C3 and include anaphylatoxin (which stimulates contractile proteins within vascular walls and increases vascular permeability) and chemotactic factors (C5a) that direct neutrophils and perhaps macrophages to the site of complement activation, where the cells release substances that damage vascular cells and basement membranes.

2. **(b)** Presence of formalin

(Nelson Textbook of Pediatrics, 18th ed.)

In the clinical setting, qualitative estimates are provided by a urinary "dipstick" that uses a very sensitive peroxidase-like chemical reaction between hemoglobin (or myoglobin) and a chemical indicator compound impregnated on the dipstick. Chemstrip (Boehringer Mannheim), a common commercially available dipstick, is capable of detecting 3–10 RBCs/μL of unspun urine with significant hematuria suggested by the presence of >50 RBCs/μL. False-negative results may occur in the presence of formalin (used as a urine preservative) or high urinary concentrations of ascorbic acid. False-positive results may be seen in a child with fever or after exercise or in the presence of menstrual blood or alkaline urine with a pH >9 or contamination with oxidizing agents such as hydrogen peroxide used to clean the perineum before obtaining a specimen.

3. **(a)** High urinary concentrations of ascorbic acid

(Nelson Textbook of Pediatrics, 18th ed.)

See explanation of Question No. 2.

4. **(c)** Hemoglobinuria

(Nelson Textbook of Pediatrics, 18th ed.)

Red urine without RBCs is seen in a number of conditions. Heme-positive urine without RBCs is caused by the presence of either hemoglobin or myoglobin. Hemoglobinuria without hematuria may occur in the presence of hemolysis. Myoglobinuria without hematuria occurs in the presence of rhabdomyolysis syndrome resulting from skeletal muscle injury and is generally associated with a five-fold increase in the plasma concentration of creatine kinase. Rhabdomyolysis may occur secondary to viral myositis, crush injury, severe electrolyte abnormalities (hypernatremia, hypophosphatemia), hypotension, disseminated intravascular coagulation, toxins (drugs, venom), and prolonged seizures. Heme-negative urine may appear red, cola colored, or burgundy, owing to ingestion of various drugs, foods (blackberries, beets), or food dyes, whereas dark brown (or black) urine may result from various urinary metabolites.

5. **(d)** Henoch-Schönlein purpura nephritis

(Nelson Textbook of Pediatrics, 18th ed.)

For explanation see Question No. 4

6. **(b)** Chloroquine

(Nelson Textbook of Pediatrics, 18th ed.)

Drugs causing red coloured urine–Chloroquine, Deferoxamine, Ibuprofen, Iron, Sorbitol, Metronidazole, Nitrofurantoin, Phenazopyridine, Phenolphthalein, Phenothiazines, Rifampin, Salicylates, Sulfasalazine.

7. **(b)** Terminal hematuria

(Nelson Textbook of Pediatrics, 18th ed.)

Upper urinary tract sources of hematuria originate within the nephron (glomerulus, convoluted/collecting tubules and interstitium). Lower urinary tract sources of hematuria originate from the pelvocalyceal system, ureter, bladder, or urethra. Hematuria from within the glomerulus is frequently associated with brown, cola-colored, or burgundy urine, proteinuria >100 mg/dL via dipstick, urinary microscopic findings of RBC casts, and deformed urinary RBCs (particularly acanthocytes). Hematuria originating within the convoluted or collecting tubules may be associated with the presence of leukocyte or renal tubular epithelial cell casts. Lower urinary tract sources of hematuria may be associated with gross hematuria, terminal hematuria (onset of gross hematuria occurring at the end of the urine stream), blood clots, normal urinary RBC morphology, by microscopy, and minimal proteinuria on dipstick (<100 mg/dL).

8. **(a)** Acute nephritic syndrome

(Nelson Textbook of Pediatrics, 18th ed.)

Tea or cola-colored urine, facial/body edema, hypertension, and oliguria suggest the acute nephritic syndrome. Diseases commonly presenting as acute nephritic syndrome include post-infectious glomerulonephritis, IgA nephropathy, membrano-proliferative glomerulonephritis, Henoch-Schönlein purpura (HSP) nephritis, systemic lupus erythematosus (SLE) nephritis, Wegener granulomatosis, microscopic polyarteritis nodosa, Goodpasture syndrome, and hemolytic-uremic syndrome.

9. **(c)** Hepatic cirrhosis

(Nelson Textbook of Pediatrics, 18th ed.)

IgA nephropathy is the most common chronic glomerular disease worldwide. It is characterized by a predominance of IgA within mesangial deposits of the glomerulus in the absence of systemic diseases such as systemic lupus erythematosus or Henoch-Schönlein purpura. Other diseases with prominent IgA mesangial deposition include rheumatoid arthritis, ankylosing spondylitis, reactive arthritis, inflammatory bowel disease, celiac disease, dermatitis herpetiformis, HIV, and hepatic cirrhosis.

10. **(c)** 9

(Nelson Textbook of Pediatrics, 18th ed.)

Although glomerular filtration begins around the 9th week of fetal life, kidney function is not necessary for normal intrauterine homeostasis because the placenta serves as the major fetal excretory organ.

11. **(b)** Cystatin C

(Nelson Textbook of Pediatrics, 18th ed.)

Cystatin C, a 13.6-kd protease inhibitor produced by nucleated cells, is an endogenous marker that may be more reliable than serum creatinine measurements in estimating the GFR since serum levels are unaffected by gender, height, muscle mass, bilirubin, or red blood cell hemolysis.

12. **(d)** Immunologic

(Nelson Textbook of Pediatrics, 18th ed.)

Glomerular injury may be a result of genetic, immunologic, or coagulation disorders. Immunologic injury is the most common cause and results in glomerulonephritis, which is a generic term for several diseases and a histopathologic term signifying inflammation of the glomerular capillaries.

13. **(c)** Lumpy-bumpy

(Nelson Textbook of Pediatrics, 18th ed.)

With deposition of immune complexes in glomeruli, rabbits develop an acute proliferative glomerulonephritis. Immunofluorescence microscopy demonstrates granular ("lumpy-bumpy") deposits containing immunoglobulin and complement in the glomerular capillary wall. Electron microscopic studies show these deposits to be on the epithelial side of the GBM and in the mesangium. For the next few days, as additional antibody enters the circulation, the antigen is ultimately removed from the circulation and the glomerulonephritis subsides.

14. **(c)** SLE

(Nelson Textbook of Pediatrics, 18th ed.)

A history of recent upper respiratory, skin, or gastrointestinal infection suggests acute glomerulonephritis, hemolytic-uremic syndrome, or HSP nephritis.

15. **(d)** IgA nephropathy

(Nelson Textbook of Pediatrics, 18th ed.)

IgA nephropathy is the most common chronic glomerular disease worldwide. It is characterized by a predominance of IgA within mesangial deposits of the glomerulus in the absence of systemic diseases such as systemic lupus erythematosus or Henoch-Schönlein purpura. Other diseases with prominent IgA mesangial deposition include rheumatoid arthritis, ankylosing spondylitis, reactive arthritis, inflammatory bowel disease, celiac disease, dermatitis herpetiformis, HIV, and hepatic cirrhosis.

16. **(a)** Male

(Nelson Textbook of Pediatrics, 18th ed.)

IgA nephropathy is seen more often in males than in females.

17. **(d)** IgA nephropathy

(Nelson Textbook of Pediatrics, 18th ed.)

A majority of children with IgA nephropathy in the United States and Europe present with gross hematuria, whereas microscopic hematuria and/or proteinuria is a more common presentation in Japan. Other types of presentation include acute nephritic syndrome, nephrotic syndrome, or a combined nephritic-nephrotic syndrome. IgA nephropathy is seen more often in males than in females. Gross hematuria often occurs in association with an upper respiratory or gastrointestinal infection and may be associated with loin pain. Proteinuria is frequently less than 1000 mg/24 hr in patients with asymptomatic microscopic hematuria. Mild to moderate hypertension is most often seen in patients with nephritic or nephrotic syndrome but is rarely severe enough to result in hypertensive emergencies. Normal serum levels of C3 in IgA nephropathy help to distinguish this disorder from poststreptococcal glomerulonephritis. Serum IgA levels have no diagnostic value because they are elevated in only 15% of patients.

18. **(d)** Age of child

(Nelson Textbook of Pediatrics, 18th ed.)

Poor prognostic indicators include persistent hypertension, diminished renal function, and heavy or prolonged proteinuria.

19. **(a)** Epithelial cell

(Nelson Textbook of Pediatrics, 18th ed.)

Glomerular cells	Type of disease
Mesangial cells	IgA Nephropathy IgM Nephropathy Mesangioproliferative glomerulonephritis Class II lupus nephritis Diabetic nephropathy
Epithelial cells	Membranous nephropathy Minimal change nephropathy Focal and segmental glomerulosclerosis Class V lupus nephritis Diabetic nephropathy
Endothelial cells	Infection associate glomerulonephritis Mesangiocapillary glomerulonephritis Class III and IV lupus nephritis Antiglomerular basement membrane disease Vasculitis and cryoglobulinemia HUS

20. **(d)** Tubular necrosis

(Nelson Textbook of Pediatrics, 18th ed.)

A worse prognosis is suggested by histologic evidence of diffuse mesangial proliferation, extensive glomerular crescents, glomerulosclerosis, and tubulointerstitial changes, including inflammation and fibrosis.

21. **(c)** ACE inhibitors

(Nelson Textbook of Pediatrics, 18th ed.)

The primary treatment of IgA nephropathy is proper blood pressure control. Fish oil, which contains anti-inflammatory omega-3 polyunsaturated fatty acids, decreases the rate of renal progression in adults. Immunosuppressive therapy with alternate day corticosteroids or more intensive multidrug regimens may be beneficial in some patients. Angiotensin-converting enzyme inhibitors and angiotensin II receptor antagonists are effective in reducing proteinuria and retarding the rate of renal progression when used as single agents or in combination. Tonsillectomy may reduce the frequency of gross hematuria and the rate of renal disease progression. Patients with IgA nephropathy may undergo successful renal transplantation. Although recurrent disease is frequent, allograft loss caused by IgA nephropathy occurs in only 15-30% of patients.

22. **(c)** C3

(Nelson Textbook of Pediatrics, 18th ed.)

Although morphologic studies and a depression in the serum complement (C3) level strongly suggest that poststreptococcal glomerulonephritis is mediated by immune complexes, the precise mechanisms by which nephritogenic streptococci induce complex formation remain to be determined. Despite clinical and histologic similarities to acute serum sickness in rabbits, the finding of circulating immune complexes in poststreptococcal glomerulonephritis is not uniform and complement activation is primarily through the alternative rather than the classic (immune complex–activated) pathway.

23. **(b)** Skin

(Nelson Textbook of Pediatrics, 18th ed.)

Acute poststreptococcal glomerulonephritis follows infection of the throat or skin by certain "nephritogenic" strains of group A β-hemolytic streptococci. The factors that allow only certain strains of streptococci to be nephritogenic remain unclear. Poststreptococcal glomerulonephritis commonly follows streptococcal pharyngitis during cold weather months and streptococcal skin infections or pyoderma during warm weather months. Although epidemics of nephritis have been described in association with both throat (serotype 12) and skin (serotype 49) infections, this disease is most commonly sporadic.

24. **(a)** Group A hemolytic streptococci

(Nelson Textbook of Pediatrics, 18th ed.)

For explanation refer Question No. 23.

25. **(b)** On epithelial side

(Nelson Textbook of Pediatrics, 18th ed.)

Immunofluorescence microscopy reveals lumpy-bumpy deposits of immunoglobulin and complement on the glomerular basement membrane (GBM) and in the mesangium. On electron microscopy, electron-dense deposits, or 'humps', are observed on the epithelial side of the GBM.

26. **(b)** Alternative pathway

(Nelson Textbook of Pediatrics, 18th ed.)

Although morphologic studies and a depression in the serum complement (C3) level strongly suggest that poststreptococcal glomerulonephritis is mediated by immune complexes, the precise mechanisms by which nephritogenic streptococci induce complex formation remain to be determined. Despite clinical and histologic similarities to acute serum sickness in rabbits, the finding of circulating immune complexes in poststreptococcal glomerulonephritis is not uniform and complement activation is primarily through the alternative rather than the classic (immune complex–activated) pathway.

27. **(c)** 3 years

(Nelson Textbook of Pediatrics, 18th ed.)

Poststreptococcal glomerulonephritis is most common in children aged 5-12 years and uncommon before the age of 3 years.

28. **(b)** 5-12 years

(Nelson Textbook of Pediatrics, 18th ed.)

29. **(c)** Either (a) or (b)

(Nelson Textbook of Pediatrics, 18th ed.)

Poststreptococcal glomerulonephritis is most common in children aged 5–12 years and uncommon before the age of 3 years. The typical patient develops an acute nephritic syndrome 1-2 weeks after an antecedent streptococcal pharyngitis or 3-6 weeks after a streptococcal pyoderma.

30. **(b)** 1-2 years

(Nelson Textbook of Pediatrics, 18th ed.)

The acute phase generally resolves within 6-8 weeks. Although urinary protein excretion and hypertension usually normalize by 4-6 weeks after onset, persistent microscopic hematuria may persist for 1-2 years after the initial presentation.

31. **(c)** 6-8 weeks

(Nelson Textbook of Pediatrics, 18th ed.)

Urinalysis demonstrates red blood cells (RBCs), frequently in association with RBC casts, proteinuria, and polymorphonuclear leukocytes. A mild normochromic anemia may be present from hemodilution and low-grade hemolysis. The serum C3 level is usually reduced in the acute phase and returns to normal 6–8 weeks after onset.

32. **(c)** Streptozyme test

(Nelson Textbook of Pediatrics, 18th ed.)

Confirmation of the diagnosis requires clear evidence of invasive streptococcal infection. A positive throat culture report may support the diagnosis or may simply represent the carrier state. On the other hand, a rising antibody titer to streptococcal antigen(s) confirms a recent streptococcal infection. Importantly, the antistreptolysin O titer is commonly elevated after a pharyngeal infection but rarely increases after streptococcal skin infections. The best single antibody titer to document cutaneous streptococcal infection is the anti-deoxyribonuclease (DNase) B level. The Streptozyme test (Wampole Laboratories, Stamford, CT) is a useful and simple diagnostic test that detects antibodies to streptolysin O, DNase B, hyaluronidase, streptokinase, and nicotinamide-adenine dinucleotidase using a slide agglutination test.

33. **(b)** Do renal biopsy

(Nelson Textbook of Pediatrics, 18th ed.)

The clinical diagnosis of poststreptococcal glomerulonephritis is quite likely in a child presenting with acute nephritic syndrome, evidence of recent streptococcal infection, and a low C3 level. However, it is important to consider other diagnoses such as systemic lupus erythematosus and an acute exacerbation of chronic glomerulonephritis. Renal biopsy should be considered only in the presence of acute renal failure, nephrotic syndrome, absence of evidence of streptococcal infection, or normal complement levels. In addition, renal biopsy is considered when hematuria and proteinuria, diminished renal function, and/or a low C3 level persist more than 2 months after onset.

34. **(a)** Poststreptococcal glomerulonephritis

(Nelson Textbook of Pediatrics, 18th ed.)

The clinical diagnosis of poststreptococcal glomerulonephritis is quite likely in a child presenting with acute nephritic syndrome, evidence of recent streptococcal infection, and a low C3 level. However, it is important to consider other diagnoses such as systemic lupus erythematosus and an acute exacerbation of chronic glomerulonephritis. Renal biopsy should be considered only in the presence of acute renal failure, nephrotic syndrome, absence of evidence of streptococcal infection, or normal complement levels. In addition, renal biopsy is considered when hematuria and proteinuria, diminished renal function, and/or a low C3 level persist more than 2 months after onset.

35. **(c)** HLA-B_{12}

(Nelson Textbook of Pediatrics, 18th ed.)

Diseases	Poststreptococcal glomerulonephritis	IgA nephropathy	Goodpasture syndrome	Idiopathic rapidly progressive glomerulonephritis (RPGN)
Clinical manifestations				
Age and sex	All ages, mean 7 years,	10–35 years,	15–30 years,	Adults,
	2 : 1 male	2 : 1 male	6 : 1 male	2 : 1 male
Acute nephritic syndrome	90%	50%	90%	90%
Asymptomatic hematuria	Occasionally	50%	Rare	Rare
Nephrotic syndrome	10–20%	Rare	Rare	10–20%
Hypertension	70%	30–50%	Rare	25%
Acute renal failure	50% (transient)	Very rare	50%	60%
Other	Latent period of 1-3 weeks	Follows viral syndromes	Pulmonary hemorrhage; iron deficiency anemia	None
Laboratory findings	↑ ASO titers (70%)	↑ Serum IgA (50%)	Positive anti-GBM antibody	Positive ANCA in some
	Positive streptozyme (95%)		IgA in dermal capillaries	
	↓ C3–C9; normal C1, C4			
Immunogenetics	HLA-B12, D "EN" (9)[*]	HLA-Bw 35, DR4 (4)[*]	HLA-DR2 (16)[*]	None established
Renal pathology				
Light microscopy	Diffuse proliferation	Focal proliferation	Focal → diffuse proliferation with crescents	Crescentic GN
Immunofluorescence	Granular IgG, C3	Diffuse mesangial IgA	Linear IgG, C3	No immune deposits
Electron microscopy	Subepithelial humps	Mesangial deposits	No deposits	No deposits
Prognosis	95% resolve spontaneously	Slow progression in 25–50%	75% stabilize or improve if treated early	75% stabilize or improve if treated early
	5% RPGN or slowly progressive			
Treatment	Supportive	Uncertain (options include steroids, fish oil, and ACE inhibitors)	Plasma exchange, steroids, cyclophosphamide	Steroid pulse therapy

36. **(c)** RPGN

(Nelson Textbook of Pediatrics, 18th ed.)

37. **(a)** Poststreptococcal infection (sore throat)

(Nelson Textbook of Pediatrics, 18th ed.)

38. **(a)** C1

(Nelson Textbook of Pediatrics, 18th ed.)

39. **(b)** RPGN

(Nelson Textbook of Pediatrics, 18th ed.)

40. **(c)** RPGN

(Nelson Textbook of Pediatrics, 18th ed.)

41. **(d)** Enteric fever

(Nelson Textbook of Pediatrics, 18th ed.)

Although membranous glomerulopathy is the most common cause of nephrotic syndrome in adults, it is an uncommon cause of hematuria in children. Membranous glomerulopathy typically presents as an isolated renal disease. However, it may be associated with systemic illnesses, including autoimmune diseases such as systemic lupus erythematosus or chronic immune thrombocytopenic purpura, sarcoidosis, neuroblastoma, gonadoblastoma, gold or penicillamine therapy, syphilis, and hepatitis B and C virus infections.

These secondary causes of membranous glomerulopathy are more common in children compared to adults. Furthermore, identification of these secondary causes of membranous glomerulopathy is important because treatment of these diseases may lead to resolution of the glomerular lesions.

42. **(b)** Anti neutral endopeptidase (NEP)

(Nelson Textbook of Pediatrics, 18th ed.)

Genetic factors may influence disease susceptibility and/or disease progression. Neonatal-onset membranous glomerulopathy is characterized by maternal anti–neutral endopeptidase (NEP) antibodies, which cross the placenta from mothers genetically deficient in the NEP antigen. NEP is a membrane metalloendopeptidase that is absent in antibody-producing mothers. Alloimmunization by fetal NEP produces maternal antibodies that cross the placenta, initiating membranous glomerulopathy.

43. **(b)** With cases of systemic lupus erythematosus

(Nelson Textbook of Pediatrics, 18th ed.)

In children, membranous glomerulopathy is most common in the 2nd decade of life. The disease usually presents as nephrotic syndrome and accounts for 2–6% of childhood nephrotic syndrome cases. Most patients have microscopic hematuria and occasionally demonstrate gross hematuria. Approximately 20% of children present with hypertension. C3 levels are normal except in cases of systemic lupus erythematosus, in which levels may be depressed.

44. **(b)** Membranoprolifcrative glomerulonephritis (MPGN)

(Nelson Textbook of Pediatrics, 18th ed.)

The term chronic glomerulonephritis implies continuing glomerular injury that frequently leads to glomerular destruction and end-stage renal failure. Membranoproliferative glomerulonephritis (MPGN) is the most common cause of chronic glomerulonephritis in older children and young adults.

45. **(a)** Type I

(Nelson Textbook of Pediatrics, 18th ed.)

Type I MPGN is the most common form. The glomeruli reveal an accentuation of the lobular pattern owing to a generalized increase in mesangial cells and matrix.

46. **(a)** RPGN

(Glomerular pictures flashcards | Quizlet [quizlet.com])

47. **(d)** MPGN

(http://en.wikipedia.org)

The term "tram-tracks" is also used to describe the basement membrane duplication found on light microscopy that is characteristic of membranoproliferative glomerulonephritis (MPGN) type I.

48. **(d)** Class IV lupus nephritis

(Nelson Textbook of Pediatrics, 18th ed.)

The clinical manifestations of SLE are mediated by immune complexes. Aberrations in both B- and T-cell function are noted. The classification of lupus nephritis of the World Health Organization (WHO) is based on a combination of light microscopy, immunofluorescence, and electron microscopy features. In patients with WHO class I nephritis, no histologic abnormalities are detected. In WHO class II nephritis (mesangial lupus nephritis), glomeruli demonstrate mesangial deposits containing immunoglobulin and complement; light microscopy may show mild (class II-A) or moderate mesangial hypercellularity and increased matrix (class II-B).

In WHO class III nephritis (focal segmental lupus glomerulonephritis), mesangial deposits occur in almost all glomeruli and subendothelial deposits are noted between the endothelial cells and glomerular basement membrane. In addition to focal and segmental mesangial proliferation, occasional glomeruli show capillary wall necrosis, crescent formation and sclerosis.

WHO class IV nephritis (diffuse proliferative lupus nephritis) is the most common and most severe form of lupus nephritis. All glomeruli contain significant mesangial and subendothelial deposits of immunoglobulin and complement. All glomeruli show mesangial proliferation. The capillary walls are frequently thickened secondary to subendothelial deposits (creating the "wire-loop" lesion) and often demonstrate necrosis, crescent formation and scarring.

WHO class V nephritis (membranous lupus nephritis) is the least common. It histologically resembles idiopathic membranous glomerulopathy, except for the presence of mild to moderate mesangial proliferation.

Transformation of the histologic lesion from one class to another is common. This is more likely to occur among inadequately treated patients and usually results in progression to a more severe histologic lesion.

49. **(b)** SLE

(Nelson Textbook of Pediatrics, 18th ed.)

50. **(d)** Adolescent female

(Nelson Textbook of Pediatrics, 18th ed.)

The majority of children with SLE are adolescent females.

51. **(c)** Type V

(Nelson Textbook of Pediatrics, 18th ed.)

WHO class V nephritis (membranous lupus nephritis) is the least common. It histologically resembles idiopathic membranous glomerulopathy, except for the presence of mild to moderate mesangial proliferation.

52. **(b)** Renal biopsy

(Nelson Textbook of Pediatrics, 18th ed.)

The majority of children with SLE are adolescent females. Clinical evidence of renal disease occurs in 30–70% of children. The clinical findings in patients having the milder forms (all class II, some class III) of lupus nephritis include hematuria, normal renal function, and proteinuria of <1 g/24 hours. Some patients with class III and all patients with class IV nephritis have hematuria and proteinuria, reduced renal function, nephrotic syndrome, or acute renal failure. In rare patients with proliferative glomerulonephritis, the urinalysis may be completely normal. Patients with class V nephritis commonly present with nephrotic syndrome.

Chapter 19

Genitourinary System (2)

1. **What is the approximate length of kidney at birth?**
   (a) 4 cm (b) 6 cm
   (c) 8 cm (d) 10 cm

2. **What is the approximate length of kidney in adults?**
   (a) 10 cm (b) 12 cm
   (c) 14 cm (d) 18 cm

3. **What is the approximate weight of kidney at birth?**
   (a) 20 gm (b) 24 gm
   (c) 28 gm (d) 34 gm

4. **What is the approximate weight of kidney in adults?**
   (a) 120 gm (b) 150 gm
   (c) 175 gm (d) 220 gm

5. **What are the components of an outer layer (cortex) of the kidney?**
   (a) Glomeruli
   (b) Proximal and distal convoluted tubules
   (c) Collecting ducts
   (d) All of the above

6. **What are the components of an inner layer (medulla) of the kidney?**
   (a) Straight portions of the tubules
   (b) Loops of Henle
   (c) Vasa recta
   (d) All of the above

7. **At what intrauterine age glomerular filtration begins?**
   (a) 7th week (b) 9th week
   (c) 12th week (d) 18th week

8. **Hematuria is defined as the presence of at least ___________ red blood cells (RBCs) per microliter of urine.**
   (a) 5 (b) 7
   (c) 11 (d) 15

9. **Cola-colored urine, facial/body edema, hypertension and oliguria are suggestive of:**
   (a) Phenylketonuria
   (b) Acute nephritic syndrome
   (c) Nephrotic syndrome
   (d) All of the above

10. **Which drug gives false positive tests for hematuria?**
    (a) Chloroquine
    (b) Deferoxamine
    (c) Metronidazole
    (d) All of the above

11. **Which metabolite gives false positive tests for hematuria?**
    (a) Porphyrin (b) Methemoglobin
    (c) Porphyrin (d) All of the above

12. **Which glomerular cause gives hematuria?**
    (a) Postinfectious GN
    (b) Goodpasture syndrome
    (c) Sickle cell glomerulopathy
    (d) All of the above

13. **Which extra glomerular cause gives hematuria?**
    (a) Heavy exercise (b) Cystitis
    (c) Meatal stenosis (d) All of the above

14. **Common causes of gross hematuria:**
    (a) IgA nephropathy
    (b) Urinary tract infection
    (c) Trauma
    (d) All of the above

15. **Acute nephritic syndrome characterized by:**
    (a) Sudden onset of gross hematuria
    (b) Edema
    (c) Hypertension
    (d) All of the above

16. Urinalysis in acute nephritic syndrome shows:
(a) Red blood cells
(b) Proteinurea
(c) Polymorphonuclear leukocytes
(d) All of the above

17. Complication of acute nephritic syndrome:
(a) Hypertensive encephalopathy
(b) Hyperkalemia
(c) Uremia
(d) All of the above

18. A characteristic feature of hemolytic uremic syndrome is:
(a) Microangiopathic hemolytic anemia
(b) Thrombocytopenia
(c) Uremia
(d) All of the above

19. Urinary protein concentration of 4+ by dipstick is reported as:
(a) 10-20 mg/Dl (b) 30 mg/dL
(c) 100 mg/Dl (d) 1000-2000 mg/dL

20. False-positive test for protein urea is seen in:
(a) Gross hematuria
(b) Urinary pH >7.0
(c) Phenazopyridine therapy
(d) All of the above

21. What is cause of transient proteinuria?
(a) Temperature >38.3°C (b) Exercise
(c) Seizures (d) All of the above

22. What is cause of isolated proteinuria in glomerular diseases?
(a) Membranous nephropathy
(b) Diabetic nephropathy
(c) Amyloidosis
(d) All of the above

23. What is the cause of idiopathic nephrotic syndrome?
(a) Minimal change disease
(b) Mesangial proliferation
(c) Focal segmental glomerulosclerosis
(d) All of the above

24. What is drug induced cause of nephrotic syndrome?
(a) Penicillamine
(b) Nonsteroidal anti-inflammatory drugs
(c) Interferon
(d) All of the above

25. Fanconi syndrome is characterized by:
(a) Proteinuria (b) Glycosuria
(c) Phosphaturia (d) All of the above

26. Lowe syndrome is characterized by:
(a) Congenital cataracts (b) Mental retardation
(c) X-linked disorder (d) All of the above

27. Bartter syndrome is characterized by:
(a) Hypokalemic metabolic alkalosis
(b) Hypercalciuria
(c) Autosomal recessive pattern of inheritance
(d) All of the above

28. Dent disease is characterized by:
(a) Recurrent stone formation
(b) X-linked recessive inheritance
(c) Seen almost exclusively in males
(d) All of the above

29. Common cause of prerenal acute renal failure:
(a) Dehydration (b) Cardiac failure
(c) Hemorrhage (d) All of the above

30. Common cause of renal acute renal failure:
(a) Glomerulonephritis
(b) Henoch-Schönlein purpura
(c) Hemolytic uremic syndrome
(d) All of the above

31. Common cause of post renal acute renal failure:
(a) Posterior urethral valves
(b) Neurogenic bladder
(c) Ureterocele
(d) All of the above

32. The volume of urine production at term is:
(a) 25 mL/hr (b) 30 mL/hr
(c) 40 mL/hr (d) 51 mL/hr

33. Mayer-Rokitansky-Kuster-Hauser syndrome refers to:
(a) Unilateral renal agenesis
(b) Ipsilateral müllerian defects
(c) Vaginal agenesis.
(d) All of the above

34. Ask-Upmark kidney constitutes:
(a) Small kidneys (b) Large kidney
(c) Both (d) None

35. What is risk factor for urinary tract infection?
(a) Female gender
(b) Vesicoureteral reflux
(c) Pinworm infestation
(d) All of the above

36. Prune-Belly syndrome (Eagle-Barrett syndrome) is characterized by:
(a) Deficient abdominal muscles
(b) Undescended testes
(c) Urinary tract abnormalities
(d) All of the above

37. Nocturnal enuresis means the occurrence of involuntary voiding at night after what age?
(a) 5 years (b) 7 years
(c) 9 years (d) 13 years

38. Cause of urinary incontinence in childhood?
(a) Behavioral
(b) Detrusor-sphincter dyssynergia
(c) Uninhibited bladder
(d) All of the above

39. What is cause of micropenis?
(a) Hypogonadotropic hypogonadism
(b) Hypergonadotropic hypogonadism
(c) Idiopathic micropenis
(d) All of the above

40. Conditions associated with micropenis:
(a) Kallmann syndrome
(b) Prader-Willi syndrome
(c) Lawrence-Moon-Biedl syndrome
(d) All of the above

41. The complication of cryptorchidism include:
(a) Infertility
(b) Testicular malignancy
(c) Torsion of the cryptorchid testis
(d) All of the above

42. Which is the indications for pelvic examination in adolescent girl?
(a) Age 21, not sexually active
(b) Menstrual irregularities, acute phase
(c) Unexplained abdominal pain
(d) All of the above

43. Complete absence of breast is associated with:
(a) Noonan's syndrome
(b) Poland syndrome
(c) Turner's syndrome
(d) Whipple syndrome

44. Poland syndrome has component of:
(a) Aplasia of the pectoralis muscles
(b) Rib deformities
(c) Webbed fingers
(d) All of the above

45. Drugs which give rise to galactorrhea:
(a) Amitriptyline (b) Reserpine
(c) Metoclopramide (d) All of the above

46. Normal ovarian volume at birth:
(a) 0.5 cm^3 (b) 0.7 cm^3
(c) 0.9 cm^3 (d) 1.1 cm^3

47. Normal ovarian volume at postpuberty:
(a) 0.2-0.5 cm^3 (b) 0.7-1.5 cm^3
(c) 1.8-5.7 cm^3 (d) 7.6-8.2 cm^3

48. Normal uterine length at birth:
(a) 0.6-0.8 cm (b) 1.2-1.8 cm
(c) 2.3-4.6 cm (d) 5.2-6.8 cm

49. Normal uterine length at postpuberty:
(a) 6 cm (b) 8 cm
(c) 10 cm (d) 12 cm

Answers

1. (b) 6 cm
2. (b) 12 cm
3. (b) 24 gm
4. (b) 150 gm
5. (d) All of the above
6. (d) All of the above
7. (b) 9th week
8. (a) 5
9. (b) Acute nephritic syndrome
10. (d) All of the above
11. (d) All of the above
12. (d) All of the above
13. (d) All of the above
14. (d) All of the above
15. (d) All of the above
16. (d) All of the above
17. (d) All of the above
18. (d) All of the above
19. (d) 1000–2000 mg/dL
20. (d) All of the above
21. (d) All of the above
22. (d) All of the above
23. (d) All of the above
24. (d) All of the above
25. (d) All of the above
26. (d) All of the above
27. (d) All of the above
28. (d) All of the above
29. (d) All of the above
30. (d) All of the above
31. (d) All of the above
32. (d) 51 mL/hour
33. (d) All of the above
34. (a) Small kidneys
35. (d) All of the above
36. (d) All of the above
37. (a) 5 years
38. (d) All of the above
39. (d) All of the above
40. (d) All of the above
41. (d) All of the above
42. (d) All of the above
43. (b) Poland syndrome
44. (d) All of the above
45. (d) All of the above

Medications that Cause Galactorrhea

- Amitriptyline
- Amphetamines
- Androgens
- Anesthetics
- Chlorpromazine
- Cimetidine
- Domperidone
- Estrogens
- Fluphenazine
- Haloperidol
- Meprobamate
- Methyldopa
- Metoclopramide
- Monoamine oxidase inhibitors
- Narcotics
- Prostaglandins
- Reserpine
- Sulpiride
- Trifluoperazine

46. (b) 0.7 cm^3
47. (c) 1.8–5.7 cm^3
48. (c) 2.3–4.6 cm
49. (a) 6 cm

Chapter 20

Rheumatic Diseases in Childhood

1. **Age of onset of JRA is before:**
(a) 16 years (b) 13 years
(c) 12 years (d) 8 years

2. **Autoimmune arthritis is seen in:**
(a) Rheumatoid arthritis (b) Osteoarthritis
(c) Psoriatic arthritis (d) Suppurative

3. **The etiology of rheumatoid arthritis is:**
(a) Presence of cell destructive elements
(b) Increase in cellular growth
(c) Decrease immunoglobulins
(d) Altered cell mediated immunity

4. **Eye changes in juvenile rheumatoid arthritis are all *except:***
(a) Cataract (b) Uveitis
(c) Scleritis (d) Keratopathy

5. **All of the following are features of systemc juvenile rheumatoid arthritis *except:***
(a) Uveitis
(b) Rash
(c) Fever
(d) Hepatosplenomegaly

6. **About juvenile RA all are true *except:***
(a) Pericarditis
(b) Rheumatoid factor positive
(c) Subcutaneous nodule
(d) Pyrexia

7. **Heart lesion in rheumatoid arthritis:**
(a) Pancarditis (b) Pericarditis
(c) Myocarditis (d) Endocarditis

8. **Butterfly rash is seen in:**
(a) SLE (b) OA
(c) Gout (d) Lupus vulgaris

9. **Which of the following condition is associated with Coomb's positive hemolytic anemia?**
(a) TTP (b) Systemic sclerosis
(c) SLE (d) PAN

10. **Not a complication of SLE:**
(a) Meningitis (b) MI
(c) Nephritis (d) None

11. **Most sensitive test for SLE:**
(a) Anti Ds DNA (b) ANA
(c) Anti Histone (d) Anti Sm

12. **Drug induced lupus caused by:**
(a) Procainamide (b) OCP
(c) Rifampicin (d) Ranitidine

13. **Anti Smith antibodies include:**
(a) Systemic sclerosis (b) SLE
(c) Polymyositis (d) RA

14. **Indications of steroid in SLE in all *except:***
(a) Chronic skin lesions (b) Glomerulonephritis
(c) CNS involvement (d) Thrombocytopenia

15. **Antibodies most specific for drug induced lupus:**
(a) Anti ds DNA (b) Anti Sm
(c) ANA (d) Anti histone

16. **Following is called the pulseless disease:**
(a) PAN
(b) Kawasaki's disease
(c) Takayasu's arteritis
(d) Wegener's granulomatosis

17. **True about Takayasu's arteritis is:**
(a) Most common in male
(b) Reno-vascular hypertension
(c) Aortic intima necrosis
(d) Ascending aorta is most commonly involved

18. Mucocutaneous lymph node disease is known as:
(a) Kawasaki disease (b) Takayasu's arteritis
(c) PAN (d) SLE

19. Strawberry tongue is seen in:
(a) Takayasu's arteritis
(b) SLE
(c) Henoch-Schönlein purpura
(d) Kawasaki's disease

20. Kawasaki's disease is associated with all *expect:*
(a) Thrombocytopenia
(b) Conjunctivitis
(c) Truncal rash
(d) Posterior cervical lymphadenopathy

21. Which amyloidosis affects children commonly?
(a) AL amyloidosis
(b) AA amyloidosis
(c) Both
(d) None

22. Which of the following statements regarding Kawasaki disease is true?
(a) Associated with coronary artery aneurysm in upto 25% of untreated cases
(b) It is the most common cause of vasculitis in children
(c) IV immunoglobulins are recommended only if coronary artery is involved
(d) Lymph node biopsy is used for diagnosis

23. A child with an obvious rash presents with recurrent infections. Investigation revealed decreased platelet count and reduced IgM. Which of the following is the most likely diagnosis?
(a) Idiopathic thrombocytopenic purpura
(b) Thrombotic thrombocytopenic purpura
(c) Wiskott-Aldrich syndrome
(d) Di George anomaly

24. A 4-year-old child is admitted with fever, non-purulent conjunctivitis, rashes, cervical lymph-adenopathy, hepatomegaly and desquamation of fingers and toes. Echocardiography shows coronary artery aneurysm. What is the most likely diagnosis?
(a) Measles
(b) German measles
(c) Progeria
(d) Kawasaki disease

25. Biochemical screening of newborn infants by heelprick blood samples is performed by using the:
(a) Tay-Sachs card (b) Duchenne card
(c) Guthrie card (d) Maple card

26. The most common leukoctoclastic vasculitis affectcting children is:
(a) Takayasu disease
(b) Mucocutaneous lymph node syndrome
(c) Henoch-Schönlein purpura
(d) Polyarthritis nodosa

27. Palpable purpura is seen in all *except:*
(a) H.S. purpura
(b) Mixed cryoglobulinemia
(c) Giant cell arthritis
(d) Drug induced vasculitis

28. Treatment of Kawasaki disease in children is:
(a) Oral steroid
(b) IV steroid
(c) IV Ig
(d) Mycophenolate mefentil

29. Kawasaki disease is associated with all the clinical features *except:*
(a) Thrombocytopenia
(b) Truncal rash
(c) Conjunctivitis
(d) Posterior cervical lymphadenopathy

30. All are true about PAN *except:*
(a) Hypertension
(b) Microaneurysm
(c) Neurological disorders
(d) Associated with hepatitis

31. PAN most commonly involves:
(a) Large vessels
(b) Medium and small size vessels
(c) Arterioles
(d) Venules

32. Hypersensitivity angitis is seen in:
(a) SLE
(b) PAN
(c) H.S. purpura
(d) Buerger's disease

33. Which of the following disease is associated with antibody against nuclear ribonucleoprotein Ag?

(a) SLE

(b) Osteogenesis imperfecta

(c) Mixed connective tissue disease

(d) Systemic sclerosis

34. True about Perthes' disease:

(a) Common in boys

(b) Common in girls

(c) Common in elders

(d) Common in all age groups

35. Earliest detection of Perthes' disease is by:

(a) Radionuclide scan

(b) Clinical examination

(c) MRI

(d) Arthroscopy

36. The late radiographic changes seen in active Perthes' disease are all *except:*

(a) Narrow joint space

(b) Widened femoral neck

(c) Flattened head

(d) Irregular epiphysial line

Answers

1. **(a)** 16 years

   (Nelson, 18th edition)

   Arthritis of one or more joints with onset below the age of 16 years and persisting for atleast 6weeks with explicit exclusion of other specific diseases.

2. **(a)** Rheumatoid arthritis

   (Nelson, 18th edition)

3. **(d)** Altered cell mediated immunity

   (Nelson, 18th edition)

   Although the etiology of juvenile arthritis is unknown, studies suggest an exaggerated immune reactivity in immunogenetically predisposed children. Studies of T cell receptor expression confirm recruitment of T cells specific for synovial non-self antigens.

4. **(c)** Scleritis

   (Nelson, 18th edition)

5. **(a)** Uveitis

   (Nelson, 18th edition)

   Systemic onset diseases is characterised by arthritis and prominent visceral involvement that includes hepatosplenomegaly, lymphadenopathy, serositis such as pericardial effusion, quotidian fever with temperature more than 39 degree Celsius; each febrile episode frequently accompanied by faint erythematous macular rash, these salmon coloured lesions may be linear or circular 2-5 mm in size and often distributed in groups, mostly over trunk and proximal extremities.

6. **(b)** Rheumatoid factor positive

   (Nelson, 18th edition)

7. **(b)** Pericarditis

   (Nelson, 18th edition)

8. **(a)** SLE

   (Nelson, 18th edition)

   "Butterfly rash" is seen in patients of SLE that involves nasal bridge, cheeks and varies from erythematous blush to thickened epidermis to scaly patches.

9. **(c)** SLE

   (Nelson, 18th edition)

   Hematological abnormalities in SLE may include a Coomb's positive hemolytic anemia, leucopenia, lymphopenia and thrombocytopenia.

10. **(a)** Meningitis

    (Nelson, 18th edition)

    The major cause of death in lupus patients are: Nephritis, MI, Pulmonary haemorrage.

11. **(b)** ANA

    (Nelson, 18th edition)

12. **(a)** Procainamide

    (Nelson, 18th edition)

    Drugs associated with lupus chlorpromazine, hydralazine, isoniazide, methyldopa, quinidine, procainamide.

13. **(b)** SLE

    (Nelson, 18th edition)

    SLE includes elevated ESR, CRP; decreased C3, C4; ANA; anti Ds DNA antibody.

14. **(a)** Chronic skin lesions

    (Nelson, 18th edition)

    Systemic steroids are usually not given for minor arthritis, skin rashes, leucopenia, anaemia associated with chronic diseases. Glomerulonephritis, hemolytic anaemia, pericarditis, myocarditis, alveolar haemorrhage, CNS involvement, TTP all require steroid treatement.

15. **(d)** Anti histone

    (Nelson, 18th edition)

16. **(c)** Takayasu's arteritis

    (Nelson, 18th edition)

17. **(b)** Reno-vascular hypertension

    (Nelson, 18th edition)

    Takayasu's arteritis is the most common cause of reno-vascular hypertension in India.

18. **(a)** Kawasaki disease

(Nelson, 18th edition)

19. **(d)** Kawasaki's disease

(Nelson, 18th edition)

Changes in lips and oral cavity in Kawasaki's disease are erythema, cracked lips, strawberry tongue, diffuse injection of oral and pharyangeal mucosa.

20. **(a)** Thrombocytopenia

(Nelson, 18th edition)

Diagnostic Criteria of KD:

(a) Fever-lasting for at least 5 days.

(b) Presence of 4 of the following 5 conditions:

1. Bilateral non-purulent conjunctival injection.
2. Changes of mucosa of oropharynx.
3. Changes in peripheral extremities.
4. Skin rash (primarily truncal, polymorphous but non-vesicular).
5. Cervical lymphadenopathy (atleast 1 node >1.5 cm)

(c) Illness not explained by any other known disease process.

21. **(b)** AA amyloidosis

(Nelson, 18th edition)

AL amyloidosis is extremely rare in children and usually occurs in persons of middle age group. Only AA amyloidosis affects children in appreciable numbers, occurring in some persons with FMF, chronic inflammatory diseases including JRA, ankylosing spondylitis, chronic inflammation like TB, cystic fibrosis and less commonly SLE, juvenile dermatomyositis.

22. **(a)** Associated with coronary artery aneurysm in upto 25% of untreated cases

(Nelson, 18th edition)

23. **(c)** Wiskott-Aldrich syndrome

(Nelson, 18th edition)

24. **(d)** Kawasaki disease

25. **(c)** Guthrie card

(Nelson, 18th edition)

26. **(c)** Henoch-Schönlein purpura

(Nelson, 18th edition)

Leucocytoclastic Vasculitis: It is a cutaneous acute vasculitis characterized clinically by palpable purpura especially of the legs and histologically by the presence of leucoclasts. Causes of leucoclastic vasculitis are as follows:

Drug induced vasculitis, SABE, Rheumatic arthritis, Chronic active hepatitis, Primary biliary cirrhosis, H.S. purpura, Sjögren syndrome.

27. **(c)** Giant cell arthritis

(Nelson, 18th edition)

28. **(c)** IVIg

(Nelson, 18th edition)

Treatment of Kawasaki disease is ACUTE PHASE and CHRONIC PHASE.

Acute Phase: IV immunoglobins + high dose Aspirin.

Chronic Phase: Low dose Aspirin.

Corticosteroids are recommended to patients who have persistent fever despite atleast 2 doses of IVIg.

29. **(a)** Thrombocytopenia

(Nelson, 18th edition)

30. **(d)** Associated with hepatitis C

(Nelson, 18th edition)

31. **(b)** Medium and small size vessels

(Nelson, 18th edition)

32. **(c)** H.S. purpura

(Nelson, 18th edition)

33. **(c)** Mixed connective tissue disease

(Nelson, 18th edition)

34. **(a)** Common in boys

(Nelson, 18th edition)

Perthes' disease is an osteochondritis of epiphysis of femoral head. Common in boys 5-10 years.

35. **(a)** Radionuclide scan

(Nelson, 18th edition)

36. **(a)** Narrow joint space

(Nelson, 18th edition)

Radiological examination reveals collapse and sclerosis of femoral head. The hip joint space is increased.

Chapter 21

Metabolic Disorders (1)

1. **Boiled cabbage or rancid butter urine odor is found in:**
   (a) Tyrosinemia
   (b) Trimethylaminuria
   (c) Phenylketonuria
   (d) Oasthouse urine disease

2. **Classic phenylketonuria [PKU] is caused by deficiency of:**
   (a) Phenyl alanine hydroxylase
   (b) Homogentesic acid oxidase
   (c) Galactose kinase
   (d) Aldolase B

3. **Features of phenyl ketonuria are:**
   (a) The affected infant is normal at birth
   (b) Urine has mousy odor
   (c) Eczematoid rash
   (d) All of the above

4. **In phenyl ketonuria the clinical features are due to accumulation of:**
   (a) Phenyl pyruvic acid (b) Phenyl lactic acid
   (c) Phenyl acetic acid (d) All of the above

5. **Guthrie's test is a screening test for:**
   (a) Galactosemia (b) Alkaptonuria
   (c) Phenylketonuria (d) Homocystinuria

6. **Mousy odor of urine is seen in:**
   (a) Phenyl ketonuria (b) Alkaptonuria
   (c) Tyrosinemia (d) Homocystinuria

7. **Alcaptonuria is due to deficiency of:**
   (a) Homogentesic acid oxidase
   (b) Phenyl alanine hydroxylase
   (c) Galactose kinase
   (d) Aldolase B

8. **Clinical manifestations of alcaptonuria in infancy:**
   (a) Onchronosis
   (b) Arthritis
   (c) Urine turning black when exposed to air
   (d) All of the above

9. **Clinical manifestations of alcaptonuria in children:**
   (a) Onchronosis (b) Arthritis
   (c) Both (a) and (b) (d) None of the above

10. **Homocystinuria due to deficiency of:**
    (a) Cystathionine β-Synthase (CBS)
    (b) Phenyl alanine hydroxylase
    (c) Galactose kinase
    (d) Aldolase B

11. **Maximum skeletal abnormality is found in:**
    (a) Hurler disease (b) Hunter disease
    (c) Sanfilippo disease (d) Morquio disease

12. **Which of the following is vitamin B_6 dependent?**
    (a) Homocystinuria (b) Tyrosinemia
    (c) Phenylketonuria (d) Alcaptonuria

13. **Infant having ectopia lentis, elongated limbs and arachnodactyly is suffering from:**
    (a) Homocystinuria
    (b) Marfan's syndrome
    (c) Tyrosinemia
    (d) None of the above

14. **Infant having ectopia lentis, elongated limbs and arachnodactyly, mental retardation is suffering from:**
    (a) Marfan's syndrome
    (b) Homocystinuria
    (c) Tyrosinemia
    (d) None of the above

15. **Hartnup disorder causes disturbance in absorption of:**
(a) Tryptophan (b) Lysine
(c) Lucine (d) Glysine

16. **Treatment of Hartnup disorder:**
(a) Vitamin C (b) Nicotinic acid
(c) Vitamin E (d) None of the above

17. **Deficiency of which enzyme system causes MSUD (Maple Syrup Urine disease)?**
(a) Branched-chain α-ketoacid dehydrogenase
(b) Galactokinase
(c) Spingomyelinase
(d) None of the above

18. **The characteristic odor of "sweaty feet" in vomitus of an infant suggests:**
(a) Maple syrup urine disease
(b) Hartnup disorder
(c) Isovaleric acidemia
(d) All of the above

19. **In 'Galactose-1-Phosphate uridyl transferase deficiency' Galactosemia the clinical features are:**
(a) Hepatomegaly (b) Jaundice
(c) Cataract (d) All of the above

20. **Galactokinase deficiency causes:**
(a) Cataract (b) Hepatomegaly
(c) Jaundice (d) All of the above

21. **The gene for UDP-galactose-4-epimerase is located on:**
(a) Chromosome 1 (b) Chromosome 18
(c) Chromosome 17 (d) Chromosome 20

22. **GK1 [galactokinase] gene is located on:**
(a) Chromosome17q24 (b) Chromosome 15
(c) Chromosome 9 (d) None of the above

23. **GK2 gene is located on:**
(a) Chromosome 15 (b) Chromosome 20
(c) Chromosome18 (d) Chromosome 21

24. **Enzyme deficient in Canavan's disease:**
(a) UDP-galactose-4-epimerase
(b) Aspartoacylase
(c) Galactokinase
(d) None of the above

25. **True about Canavan's disease is:**
(a) Autosomal recessive disorder
(b) Spongy degeneration of the white matter of the brain
(c) Leads to a severe form of leukodystrophy
(d) All of the above

26. **Deficiency of fructokinase causes:**
(a) Essential or benign fructosuria
(b) Hereditary fructose intolerance
(c) Both of the above
(d) None

27. **Essential or benign fructosuria is characterized by:**
(a) Deficiency of fructokinase
(b) Not associated with any clinical manifestations
(c) It is an accidental finding
(d) All of the above

28. **The gene encoding fructokinase is located on chromosome:**
(a) 2p23.3 (b) 10
(c) 13 (d) 15

29. **Enzyme deficiency in hereditary fructose intolerance is:**
(a) Fructose-1,6-bisphosphate aldolase
(b) Fructokinase
(c) Spingomyelinase
(d) None

30. **Clinical manifestations of hereditary fructose intolerance are:**
(a) Clinical manifestations resemble galactosemia
(b) Jaundice
(c) Hepatomegaly
(d) All of the above

31. **The gene for aldolase B is on chromosome:**
(a) 9q22.3 (b) 2
(c) 4 (d) 7

32. **Following is an X-linked recessive disorder:**
(a) Lesch-Nyhan Disease (LND)
(b) Tay Sachs disease
(c) Hurler's disease
(d) Niemann-Pick's disease
(e) None

33. Following is an X-linked recessive disorder:
(a) Lesch-Nyhan disease (LND)
(b) Hunter's disease
(c) Fabry's disease
(d) All of the above

34. Partial deficiency in HPRT is called as:
(a) Kelley-Seegmiller syndrome
(b) Hurler's disease
(c) Hunter's disease
(d) Fabry's disease

35. Enzyme deficient in Lesch-Nyhan disease (LND):
(a) HPRT (b) Aldolase B
(c) Galactokinase (d) None

36. Highest concentration of HPRT is in:
(a) Basal ganglia (b) Liver
(c) Spleen (d) Bone

37. Self-mutilation of the mouth and fingers suggests:
(a) Lesch-Nyhan Disease (LND)
(b) Tay Sach's disease
(c) Fabry's disease
(d) None

38. Hyperuricemia is seen in:
(a) Lesch-Nyhan disease (LND)
(b) Tay Sach's disease
(c) Fabry's disease
(d) None

39. IQ is normal in:
(a) Hurler disease (b) Hunter disease
(c) Sanfilippo disease (d) Morquio disease

40. Allopurinol is used in treatment of:
(a) Lesch-Nyhan disease (LND)
(b) Tay Sach's disease
(c) Fabry's disease
(d) None

41. Action of allopurinol is:
(a) Xanthine oxidase inhibitor
(b) Uricosuric drug
(c) Auto oxidation of uric acid
(d) None

42. Enzyme deficiency in Metachromatic leuko-dystrophy:
(a) Arylsulfatase A (b) Sphingomyelinase
(c) β-Galactocerebrosidase (d) α-Galactosidase

43. Enzyme deficiency in Gaucher disease:
(a) β-.Glucocerebrosidase
(b) β-Galactocerebrosidase
(c) α-Galactosidase
(d) Sphingomyelinase

44. Gaucher disease is:
(a) Autosomal recessive (b) Autosomal dominant
(c) X-linked dominant (d) None

45. Clinical manifestations of Gaucher disease:
(a) Thrombocytopenia
(b) Anemia
(c) Bone pain or pathologic fractures
(d) All of the above

46. Most common lysosomal storage disease:
(a) Gaucher disease (b) Fabry disease
(c) Krabbe disease (d) None

47. Enzyme deficiency in Niemann-Pick disease (NPD):
(a) Sphingomyelinase (b) Fabry disease
(c) Krabbe disease (d) None

48. Clinical manifestations of Niemann-Pick disease (NPD):
(a) Cherry red spot in macula
(b) Hepatosplenomegaly
(c) Neurodevelopmental regression
(d) All of the above

49. Enzyme deficiency in Fabry disease:
(a) α-Galactosidase
(b) β-Galactocerebrosidase
(c) α-Galactosidase
(d) Sphingomyelinase

50. Angiokeratomas is seen in:
(a) Fabry disease
(b) Niemann-Pick disease (NPD)
(c) Krabbe disease
(d) None

51. Type 1 Mucopolysaccharidosis is:
(a) Hurler disease (b) Hunter disease
(c) Sanfilippo disease (d) None

52. Most common mucopolysaccharidosis is:
(a) Hurler disease (b) Hunter disease
(c) Sanfilippo disease (d) None

53. Corneal clouding is not seen in:
(a) Hurler disease (b) Hunter disease
(c) Sanfilippo disease (d) Morquio disease

Answers

1. **(a)** Tyrosinemia

(Nelson, 18th edition)

Inborn Errors of Amino Acid Metabolism Associated with Peculiar Odor

Inborn Error of Metabolism	Urine Odor
Glutaric acidemia (type II)	Sweaty feet, acrid
Hawkinsinuria	Swimming pool
Isovaleric acidemia	Sweaty feet, acrid
Maple syrup urine disease	Maple syrup
Hypermethioninemia	Boiled cabbage
Multiple carboxylase deficiency	Tomcat urine
Oasthouse urine disease	Hops-like
Phenylketonuria	Mousey or musty
Trimethylaminuria	Rotting fish
Tyrosinemia	Boiled cabbage, rancid butter

2. **(a)** Phenylalanine hydroxylase

(Nelson, 18th edition)

Phenylalanine is an essential amino acid. Dietary phenylalanine not utilized for protein synthesis is normally degraded by way of the tyrosine pathway. Deficiency of the enzyme phenylalanine hydroxylase or of its cofactor tetrahydrobiopterin causes accumulation of phenylalanine in body fluids and the central nervous system (CNS). The severity of hyperphenylalaninemia depends on the degree of enzyme deficiency and may vary from very high plasma concentrations (>20 mg/dL or >1,200 µmole/L, classic phenylketonuria [PKU]) to mildly elevated levels (2–6 mg/dL or 120–360 µmole/L). In affected infants with plasma concentrations >20 mg/dL, excess phenylalanine is metabolized to phenylketones (phenylpyruvate and phenylacetate) that are excreted in the urine, giving rise to the term *phenylketonuria* (PKU). These metabolites have no role in pathogenesis of CNS damage in patients with PKU; their presence in the body fluids simply signifies the severity of the condition. The brain is the main organ affected by hyperphenylalaninemia. The CNS damage in affected patients is caused by the elevated concentration of phenylalanine in brain tissue, which interferes with the cerebral transport of other large neutral amino acids (tyrosine, tryptophan). There are a few adults with classic PKU and normal intelligence who have never been treated with a phenylalanine-restricted diet. Phenylalanine content of the brain in these individuals was found to be close to that of normal subjects when studied by magnetic resonance spectroscopy (MRS) and imaging (MRI) techniques.

3. **(d)** All of the above

(Nelson, 18th edition)

The affected infant is normal at birth. Mental retardation may develop gradually and may not be evident for the 1st few months. It is usually severe, and most patients require institutional care if the condition remains untreated. Vomiting, sometimes severe enough to be misdiagnosed as pyloric stenosis, may be an early symptom. Older untreated children become hyperactive, with purposeless movements, rhythmic rocking and athetosis.

On physical examination, these infants are lighter in their complexion than unaffected siblings. Some may have a seborrheic or eczematoid rash, which is usually mild and disappears as the child grows older. These children have an unpleasant odor of phenylacetic acid, which has been described as musty or mousey. There are no consistent findings on neurologic examination. Most infants are hypertonic with hyperactive deep tendon reflexes. About 25% of children have seizures, and more than 50% have electroencephalographic abnormalities. Microcephaly, prominent maxilla with widely spaced teeth, enamel hypoplasia, and growth retardation are other common findings in untreated children. The clinical manifestations of classic PKU are rarely seen in those countries in which neonatal screening programs for the detection of PKU are in effect.

4. **(d)** All of the above

(Nelson, 18th edition)

The affected infant is normal at birth. Mental retardation may develop gradually and may not be evident for the 1st few months. It is usually severe, and most patients require institutional care if the condition remains untreated. Vomiting, sometimes severe enough to be misdiagnosed as pyloric stenosis, may be an early symptom. Older untreated children become hyperactive, with purposeless movements, rhythmic rocking and athetosis.

On physical examination, these infants are lighter in their complexion than unaffected siblings. Some may have a seborrheic or eczematoid rash, which is usually mild and disappears as the child grows older. These children have an unpleasant odor of phenylacetic acid, which has been described as musty or mousey. There are no consistent findings on neurologic examination. Most infants are hypertonic with hyperactive deep tendon reflexes. About 25% of children have seizures, and more than 50% have electroencephalographic abnormalities. Microcephaly, prominent maxilla with widely spaced teeth, enamel hypoplasia, and growth retardation are other common findings in untreated children. The clinical manifestations of classic PKU are rarely seen in those countries in which neonatal screening programs for the detection of PKU are in effect.

5. **(c)** Phenylketonuria

(Nelson, 18th edition)

Neonatal Screening for Hyperphenylalaninemia:

Effective and relatively inexpensive methods for mass screening of newborn infants have been developed and are used in the United States and several other countries. The bacterial inhibition assay of Guthrie, which was the 1st method for the purpose, has been replaced by more precise and quantitative methods (fluorometric and tandem mass spectrometry). All these methods require a few drops of blood, which are placed on a filter paper and mailed to a central laboratory for assay. Blood phenylalanine in affected infants with PKU may rise to diagnostic levels as early as 4 hours after birth even in the absence of protein feeding. It is recommended, however, that the blood for screening be obtained in the 1st 24–48 hours of life after feeding protein to reduce the possibility of false negative results, especially in the milder forms of the condition.

6. **(a)** Phenyl ketonuria

(Nelson, 18th edition)

Inborn Errors of Amino Acid Metabolism Associated with Peculiar Odor

Inborn error of metabolism	Urine odor
Glutaric acidemia (type II)	Sweaty feet, acrid
Hawkinsinuria	Swimming pool
Isovaleric academia	Sweaty feet, acrid
Maple syrup urine disease	Maple syrup
Hypermethioninemia	Boiled cabbage
Multiple carboxylase deficiency	Tomcat urine
Oasthouse urine disease	Hops-like
Phenylketonuria	Mousey or musty
Trimethylaminuria	Rotting fish
Tyrosinemia	Boiled cabbage, rancid butter

7. **(a)** Homogentesic acid oxidase

(Nelson, 18th edition)

Alcaptonuria

This rare (incidence ≈1/250,000) autosomal recessive disorder is due to a deficiency of homogentisic acid oxidase, which causes large amounts of homogentisic acid to accumulate in the body and then to be excreted in the urine.

8. **(c)** Urine turning black when exposed to air

(Nelson, 18th edition)

Clinical manifestations of alcaptonuria consist of ochronosis and arthritis, which occur in adulthood. The only sign of the disorder in children is a blackening of the urine on standing.

9. **(c)** Both (a) and (b)

(Nelson, 18th edition)

Clinical manifestations of alcaptonuria consist of ochronosis and arthritis, which occur in adulthood. The only sign of the disorder in children is a blackening of the urine on standing.

10. **(a)** Cystathionine β-Synthase (CBS)

(Nelson, 18th edition)

Most homocysteine, an intermediate compound of methionine degradation, is normally remethylated to methionine. This methionine-sparing reaction is catalyzed by the enzyme methionine synthase, which requires a metabolite of folic acid (5-methyltetrahydrofolate) as a methyl donor and a metabolite of vitamin B_{12} (methylcobalamin) as a cofactor. Only 20–30% of total homocysteine (and its dimer homocystine) is in free form in the plasma of normal individuals. The rest is bound to proteins as mixed disulfides. Three major forms of homocystinemia and homocystinuria have been identified.

11. **(d)** Morquio disease

(Nelson, 18th edition)

Both types of Morquio disease are characterized by short-trunk dwarfism, fine corneal deposits, a skeletal dysplasia that is distinct from other mucopolysaccharidoses, and preservation of intelligence. MPS IV-A is usually more severe than MPS IV-B, with adult heights of <125 cm in the former and >150 cm in the latter. There is considerable variability of expression in both subtypes, however. The appearance of genua valga, kyphosis, growth retardation with short trunk and neck, and waddling gait with a tendency to fall are early symptoms of MPS IV. Extra skeletal manifestations include mild corneal clouding, small teeth with abnormally thin enamel, frequent caries formation, and, occasionally, hepatomegaly and cardiac valvular lesions. Instability of the odontoid process and ligamentous laxity are regularly present and can result in life-threatening atlantoaxial instability and dislocation. Surgery to stabilize the upper cervical spine, usually by posterior spinal fusion before the development of cervical myelopathy, can be lifesaving.

12. (a) Homocystinuria

(Nelson, 18th edition)

This is the most common inborn error of methionine metabolism. About 40% of affected patients respond to high doses of vitamin B_6 and usually have milder clinical manifestations than those who are unresponsive to vitamin B_6 therapy. These patients possess some residual enzyme activity.

13. (a) Marfan syndrome

(Nelson, 18th edition)

Most homocysteine, an intermediate compound of methionine degradation, is normally remethylated to methionine. This methionine-sparing reaction is catalyzed by the enzyme methionine synthase, which requires a metabolite of folic acid (5-methyl-tetrahydrofolate) as a methyl donor and a metabolite of vitamin B_{12} (methylcobalamin) as a cofactor. Only 20–30% of total homocysteine (and its dimer homocystine) is in free form in the plasma of normal individuals. The rest is bound to proteins as mixed disulfides. Three major forms of homocystinemia and homocystinuria have been identified.

14. (b) Homocystinuria

(Nelson, 18th edition)

Most homocysteine, an intermediate compound of methionine degradation, is normally remethylated to methionine. This methionine-sparing reaction is catalyzed by the enzyme methionine synthase, which requires a metabolite of folic acid (5-methyltetra-hydrofolate) as a methyl donor and a metabolite of vitamin B_{12} (methylcobalamin) as a cofactor. Only 20–30% of total homocysteine (and its dimer homocystine) is in free form in the plasma of normal individuals. The rest is bound to proteins as mixed disulfides. Three major forms of homocystinemia and homocystinuria have been identified.

15. (a) Tryptophan

(Nelson, 18th edition)

Tryptophan is an essential amino acid and a precursor for nicotinic acid and serotonin. Presumed deficiencies of a variety of different enzymes involved in tryptophan catabolism have been reported, but no distinct clinical entity has yet emerged. Hartnup disorder causes disturbance in tryptophan absorption.

16. (b) Nicotinic acid

(Nelson, 18th edition)

Treatment with nicotinic acid or nicotinamide (50–300 mg/24 hours) and a high-protein diet results in a favorable response in symptomatic patients. Because of the intermittent nature of the clinical manifestations, the efficacy of these treatments is difficult to evaluate. The prevalence of the disorder is estimated to be 1/30,000. Normal outcome both for mother and fetus is reported in affected pregnant women. The gene for this condition has not yet been identified.

17. (a) Branched-chain α-ketoacid dehydrogenase

(Nelson, 18th edition)

Decarboxylation of leucine, isoleucine, and valine is accomplished by a complex enzyme system (branched-chain α-ketoacid dehydrogenase) using thiamine pyrophosphate (vitamin B_1) as a coenzyme. This mitochondrial enzyme consists of four subunits: $E_{1\alpha}$, $E_{1\beta}$, E_2 and E_3. The E_3 subunit is shared with two other dehydrogenases in the body, namely pyruvate dehydrogenase and α-ketoglutarate dehydrogenase. Deficiency of this enzyme system causes MSUD, named after the sweet odor of maple syrup found in body fluids, especially urine. Based on clinical findings and response to thiamine administration, five phenotypes of MSUD have been identified.

18. (c) Isovaleric acidemia

(Nelson, 18th edition)

Clinical manifestations in the *acute form* include vomiting and severe acidosis in the 1st few days of life. Lethargy, convulsions, and coma may ensue, and death may occur if proper therapy is not initiated. The vomiting may be severe enough to suggest pyloric stenosis. The characteristic odor of "sweaty feet" may be present. Infants who survive this acute episode will go on to have the chronic intermittent form later on in life. A milder form of the disease *(chronic intermittent form)* also exists; in this, the 1st clinical manifestation (vomiting, lethargy, acidosis or coma) may not appear until the child is a few months or a few years old. In both forms, acute episodes of metabolic decompensations may occur during a catabolic state such as an infection. Sensitive methods for newborn screening have identified yet a milder and potentially asymptomatic phenotype of the condition; a few older siblings of these affected newborns were found to have identical genotype and biochemical abnormalities without any clinical manifestations.

19. (d) All of the above

(Nelson, 18th edition)

The diagnosis of uridyl transferase deficiency should be considered in newborn or young infants with any of the following features: jaundice, hepatomegaly, vomiting, hypoglycemia, convulsions, lethargy, irritability, feeding difficulties, poor weight gain or failure to regain birth weight, aminoaciduria, nuclear cataracts, vitreous hemorrhage, hepatic failure, liver cirrhosis, ascites, splenomegaly, or mental retardation. Symptoms are milder and improve when milk is temporarily withdrawn and replaced by intravenous or lactose-free nutrition. Patients with galactosemia are at increased risk for *Escherichia coli* neonatal sepsis; the onset of sepsis often precedes the diagnosis of galactosemia. Death from liver and kidney failure and sepsis may follow within days. When the diagnosis is not made at birth, damage to the liver (cirrhosis) and brain (mental retardation) becomes increasingly severe and irreversible.

20. (a) Cataract

(Nelson, 18th edition)

The diagnosis of uridyl transferase deficiency should be considered in newborn or young infants with any of the following features: jaundice, hepatomegaly, vomiting, hypoglycemia, convulsions, lethargy, irritability, feeding difficulties, poor weight gain or failure to regain birth weight, aminoaciduria, nuclear cataracts, vitreous hemorrhage, hepatic failure, liver cirrhosis, ascites, splenomegaly, or mental retardation. Symptoms are milder and improve when milk is temporarily withdrawn and replaced by intravenous or lactose-free nutrition. Patients with galactosemia are at increased risk for *Escherichia coli* neonatal sepsis; the onset of sepsis often precedes the diagnosis of galactosemia. Death from liver and kidney failure and sepsis may follow within days. When the diagnosis is not made at birth, damage to the liver (cirrhosis) and brain (mental retardation) becomes increasingly severe and irreversible.

21. (a) Chromosome 1

(Nelson, 18th edition)

The gene for UDP-galactose-4-epimerase is located on chromosome 1 at 1p36. Carrier detection is possible by measurement of epimerase activity in the erythrocytes. Prenatal diagnosis for the severe form of epimerase deficiency, using an enzyme assay of cultured amniotic fluid cells, is possible

22. (a) Chromosome17q24

(Nelson, 18th edition)

The deficient enzyme is galactokinase, which normally catalyzes the phosphorylation of galactose. The principal metabolites accumulated are galactose and galactitol. Two genes have been reported to encode galactokinase: GK1 chromosome 17q24 and GK2 on chromosome 15. Cataracts are usually the sole manifestation of galactokinase deficiency; pseudotumor cerebri is a rare complication. The affected infant is otherwise asymptomatic. Heterozygote carriers may be at risk for presenile cataracts. Affected patients have an increased concentration of blood galactose levels, provided they have been fed a lactose-containing formula. The diagnosis is made by demonstrating an absence of galactokinase activity in erythrocytes or fibroblasts. Transferase activity is normal. Treatment is dietary restriction of galactose.

23. (a) Chromosome 15

(Nelson, 18th edition)

The deficient enzyme is galactokinase, which normally catalyzes the phosphorylation of galactose. The principal metabolites accumulated are galactose and galactitol. Two genes have been reported to encode galactokinase: GK1 chromosome 17q24 and GK2 on chromosome 15. Cataracts are usually the sole manifestation of galactokinase deficiency; pseudotumor cerebri is a rare complication. The affected infant is otherwise asymptomatic. Heterozygote carriers may be at risk for presenile cataracts. Affected patients have an increased concentration of blood galactose levels, provided they have been fed a lactose-containing formula. The diagnosis is made by demonstrating an absence of galactokinase activity in erythrocytes or fibroblasts. Transferase activity is normal.

24. (b) Aspartoacylase

(Nelson, 18th edition)

Canavan Disease

N-acetylaspartic acid, a derivative of aspartic acid, is synthesized in the brain and is found in a high concentration, similar to that of glutamic acid. Its function is unknown, but excessive amounts of *N*-acetylaspartic acid in urine and deficiency of the enzyme aspartoacylase that cleaves the *N*-acetyl group from *N*-acetylaspartic acid are associated with Canavan disease.

25. **(d)** All of the above

(Nelson, 18th edition)

Canavan Disease

Canavan disease, an autosomal recessive disorder characterized by spongy degeneration of the white matter of the brain, leads to a severe form of leukodystrophy. It is more prevalent in individuals of Ashkenazi Jewish descent than in other ethnic groups.

26. **(a)** Essential or benign fructosuria

(Nelson, 18th edition)

Defects in Fructose Metabolism

Deficiency of Fructokinase (Essential or benign fructosuria)

Deficiency of fructokinase is not associated with any clinical manifestations. It is an accidental finding usually made because the asymptomatic patient's urine contains a reducing substance. No treatment is necessary and the prognosis is excellent. Inheritance is autosomal recessive with an incidence of 1/120,000. The gene encoding fructokinase is located on chromosome 2p23.3.

27. **(d)** All of the above

(Nelson, 18th edition)

Deficiency of fructokinase is not associated with any clinical manifestations. It is an accidental finding usually made because the asymptomatic patient's urine contains a reducing substance. No treatment is necessary and the prognosis is excellent. Inheritance is autosomal recessive with an incidence of 1/120,000. The gene encoding fructokinase is located on chromosome 2p23.3.

28. **(a)** 2p23.3

29. **(a)** Fructose-1,6-Bisphosphate aldolase

(Nelson, 18th edition)

Deficiency of fructose-1,6-bisphosphate aldolase is a severe condition of infants that appears with the ingestion of fructose-containing food and is caused by a deficiency of fructose aldolase B activity in the liver, kidney and intestine. The enzyme catalyzes the hydrolysis of fructose-1,6-bisphosphate into triose phosphate and glyceraldehyde phosphate. The same enzyme also hydrolyzes fructose-1-phosphate. Deficiency of this enzyme activity causes a rapid accumulation of fructose-1-phosphate and initiates severe toxic symptoms when exposed to fructose.

30. **(d)** All of the above

(Nelson, 18th edition)

Patients with HFI are perfectly healthy and asymptomatic until fructose or sucrose (table sugar) is ingested (usually from fruit, fruit juice, or sweetened cereal). Symptoms may occur early in life, soon after birth if foods or formulas containing these sugars are introduced into the diet. Certain patients are very sensitive to fructose, whereas others can tolerate moderate intakes (up to 250 mg/kg/day). The average intake of fructose in Western societies is 1–2 g/kg/day. Early clinical manifestations resemble galactosemia and include jaundice, hepatomegaly, vomiting, lethargy, irritability and convulsions. Laboratory findings include a prolonged clotting time, hypoalbuminemia, elevation of bilirubin and transaminase levels, and proximal tubular dysfunction. Acute fructose ingestion produces symptomatic hypoglycemia; the higher the intake, the more severe is the clinical picture. Chronic ingestion results in failure to thrive and hepatic disease. If the intake of the fructose persists, hypoglycemic episodes recur, and liver and kidney failure progress, eventually leading to death.

31. **(a)** 9q22.3

(Nelson, 18th edition)

The true incidence of hereditary fructose intolerance (HFI) is unknown but may be as high as 1/26,000. The gene for aldolase B is on chromosome 9q22.3. Several mutations causing hereditary fructose intolerance are known. A single missense mutation, a G ≡ C transversion in exon 5 resulting in the normal alanine at position 149 being replaced by a proline, is the most common mutation identified in northern Europeans. This mutation, plus 2 other point mutations, account for 80–85% of hereditary fructose intolerance in Europe and the United States. Diagnosis of hereditary fructose intolerance can be made by direct DNA analysis.

32. **(a)** Lesch-Nyhan disease (LND)

(Nelson, 18th edition)

Lesch-Nyhan Disease (LND)

This is a rare X-linked disorder of purine metabolism that results from HPRT deficiency.

33. **(d)** All of the above

(Nelson, 18th edition)

This is a rare X-linked disorder of purine metabolism that results from HPRT deficiency. This enzyme is normally present in each cell in the body, but its highest concentration is in the brain, especially in the basal ganglia. Clinical manifestations include hyperuricemia, intellectual disability, dystonic movement disorder that may be accompanied by choreoathetosis and spasticity, dysarthric speech, and compulsive self-biting, usually beginning with the eruption of teeth.

34. **(a)** Kelley-Seegmiller syndrome

(Nelson, 18th edition)

Partial deficiency in HPRT (Kelley-Seegmiller syndrome) with >1.5–2.0% enzyme is associated with hyperuricemia and variable neurologic dysfunction (neurologic HPRT deficiency). HPRT deficiency with levels >8% leads to a severe form of gout, with apparently normal cerebral functioning (HPRT-related hyperuricemia) although cognitive deficits may occur. Qualitatively similar cognitive deficit profiles have been reported in both LND and variant cases. Variants produced scores that are intermediate between those of patients with LND and normal controls on nearly every neuropsychologic measure tested.

35. **(a)** HPRT

(Nelson, 18th edition)

This is a rare X-linked disorder of purine metabolism that results from HPRT deficiency. This enzyme is normally present in each cell in the body, but its highest concentration is in the brain, especially in the basal ganglia.

36. **(a)** Basal ganglia

This is a rare X-linked disorder of purine metabolism that results from HPRT deficiency. This enzyme is normally present in each cell in the body, but its highest concentration is in the brain, especially in the basal ganglia.

37. **(a)** Lesch-Nyhan disease (LND)

(Nelson, 18th edition)

The presence of dystonia along with self-mutilation of the mouth and fingers suggests Lesch-Nyhan disease.

38. **(a)** Lesch-Nyhan disease (LND)

(Nelson, 18th edition)

The presence of dystonia along with self-mutilation of the mouth and fingers suggests Lesch-Nyhan disease. With partial HPRT deficiency, recognition is linked to either hyperuricemia alone or hyperuricemia and a dystonic movement disorder. Serum levels of uric acid >4–5 mg uric acid/dL and a urine uric acid: creatinine ratio of 3:4 or more are highly suggestive of HPRT deficiency, particularly when associated with neurologic symptoms.

39. **(d)** Morquio disease

(Nelson, 18th edition)

Both types of Morquio disease are characterized by short-trunk dwarfism, fine corneal deposits, a skeletal dysplasia that is distinct from other muco-polysaccharidoses, and preservation of intelligence.

40. **(a)** Lesch-Nyhan disease (LND)

(Nelson, 18th edition)

Treatment

Medical management of this disorder focuses on the prevention of renal failure by pharmacologic treatment of hyperuricemia with high fluid intake along with alkali and allopurinol. Allopurinol treatment must be monitored because urinary oxypurine excretion is sensitive to allopurinol, resulting in an increased concentration of xanthine, which is extremely insoluble.

41. **(a)** Xanthine oxidase inhibitor

(Nelson, 18th edition)

Treatment of hyperuricemia involves the combination of allopurinal (a xanthine oxidase inhibitor) to decrease uric acid production, probenecid to increase uric acid clearance in those with normal renal function, alkalinization of the urine to increase the solubility of uric acid, and increased fluid intake to reduce the concentration of uric acid. A low-purine diet, weight reduction, and reduced alcohol intake are recommended.

42. **(a)** Arylsulfatase A

(Nelson, 18th edition)

Metachromatic Leukodystrophy (MLD)

This is an autosomal recessive white matter disease caused by a deficiency of arylsulfatase A (ASA), which is required for the hydrolysis of sulfated glycosphingolipids.

43. **(a)** β-Glucocerebrosidase

(Nelson, 18th edition)

Gaucher disease results from the deficient activity of the lysosomal hydrolase, acid β-glucosidase, which is encoded by a gene located on chromosome 1q21-q31.

44. **(a)** Autosomal recessive

(Nelson, 18th edition)

Gaucher Disease

This disease is a multisystemic lipidosis characterized by hematologic problems, organomegaly, and skeletal involvement, the latter usually manifesting as bone pain and pathologic fractures. It is the most common lysosomal storage disease and the most prevalent genetic defect among Ashkenazi Jews. There are three clinical subtypes delineated by the absence or presence and progression of neurologic manifestations: Type 1 or the adult, non-neuronopathic form; type 2, the infantile or acute neuronopathic form; and type 3, the juvenile or Norrbottnian form. All are autosomal recessive traits. Type 1, which accounts for 99% of cases, has a striking predilection for Ashkenazi Jews, with an incidence of about 1/1,000 and a carrier frequency of 1/18.

45. **(d)** All of the above
(Nelson, 18th edition)

Clinical manifestations of type 1 Gaucher disease have a variable age at onset, from early childhood to late adulthood, with most symptomatic patients presenting by adolescence. At presentation, patients may have bruising from thrombocytopenia, chronic fatigue secondary to anemia, hepatomegaly with or without elevated liver function test results, splenomegaly, and bone pain. Occasional patients have pulmonary involvement at the time of presentation. Patients presenting in the 1st decade frequently are not Jewish and have growth retardation and a more malignant course. Other patients may be discovered fortuitously during evaluation for other conditions or as part of routine examinations; these patients may have a milder or even a benign course. In symptomatic patients, splenomegaly is progressive and can become massive. Most patients develop radiologic evidence of skeletal involvement, including an Erlenmeyer flask deformity of the distal femur. Clinically apparent bony involvement, which occurs in >20% of patients, can present as bone pain or pathologic fractures. Lytic lesions can develop in the long bones, including the femur, ribs, and pelvis; osteosclerosis may be evident at an early age. Bone crises with severe pain and swelling can occur. Bleeding secondary to thrombocytopenia may manifest as epistaxis or bruising and is frequently overlooked until other symptoms become apparent. With the exception of the severely growth-retarded child, who may experience developmental delay secondary to the effects of chronic disease, development and intelligence are normal.

46. **(a)** Gaucher disease
(Nelson, 18th edition)

Gaucher Disease

This disease is a multisystemic lipidosis characterized by hematologic problems, organomegaly, and skeletal involvement, the latter usually manifesting as bone pain and pathologic fractures. It is the most common lysosomal storage disease and the most prevalent genetic defect among Ashkenazi Jews.

47. **(a)** Sphingomyelinase
(Nelson, 18th edition)

Neimann-Pick Disease (NPD)

The original description of NPD was what is now known as type A NPD, a fatal disorder of infancy characterized by failure to thrive, hepatosplenomegaly, and a rapidly progressive neurodegenerative course that leads to death by 2–3 years of age. Type B is a non-neuronopathic form observed in children and adults. Type C is a neuronopathic form that results from defective cholesterol transport. All the subtypes are inherited as autosomal recessive traits and display variable clinical features.

NPD types A and B result from the deficient activity of acid sphingomyelinase.

48. **(d)** All of the above
(Nelson, 18th edition)

The clinical manifestations and course of type A NPD is uniform and is characterized by a normal appearance at birth (although the newborn period is sometimes complicated by prolonged jaundice). Hepatosplenomegaly, moderate lymphadenopathy, and psychomotor retardation are evident by 6 months of age, followed by neurodevelopmental regression and death by 3 years. With advancing age, the loss of motor function and the deterioration of intellectual capabilities are progressively debilitating; and in later stages, spasticity and rigidity are evident. Affected infants lose contact with their environment. In contrast to the stereotyped type A phenotype, the clinical presentation and course of patients with type B disease are more variable. Most are diagnosed in infancy or childhood when enlargement of the liver or spleen, or both, is detected during a routine physical examination. At diagnosis, type B NPD patients usually have evidence of mild pulmonary involvement, usually detected as a diffuse reticular or finely nodular infiltration on the chest radiograph. Pulmonary symptoms usually present in adults. In most patients, hepatosplenomegaly is particularly prominent in childhood, but with increasing linear growth, the abdominal protuberance decreases and becomes less conspicuous. In mildly affected patients, the splenomegaly may not be noted until adulthood, and there may be minimal disease manifestations.

49. **(a)** α-galactosidase

(Nelson, 18th edition)

This condition is an inborn error of glycosphingolipid metabolism characterized by angiokeratomas (telangiectatic skin lesions), hypohidrosis, corneal and lenticular opacities, acroparesthesias, and vascular disease of the kidney, heart, and/or brain. The disease is an X-linked recessive trait that is manifested in affected males and has an estimated prevalence of ≈1/40,000 males. Later-onset affected males with residual α-galactosidase A activity may present with cardiac and/or renal disease including hypertrophic cardiomyopathy and renal failure. Heterozygous females for the classic phenotype can be asymptomatic or as severely affected as the males, the variability due to random X-inactivation. The disease results from the deficient activity of α-galactosidase.

50. **(a)** Fabry disease

(Nelson, 18th edition)

Fabry Disease

This condition is an inborn error of glycosphingolipid metabolism characterized by angiokeratomas (telangiectatic skin lesions), hypohidrosis, corneal and lenticular opacities, acroparesthesias, and vascular disease of the kidney, heart, and/or brain.

51. **(a)** Hurler disease

(Nelson, 18th edition)

Hurler Disease

This form of MPS I (MPS I-H) is a severe, progressive disorder with multiple organ and tissue involvement that results in premature death, usually by 10 years of age. An infant with Hurler syndrome appears normal at birth, but inguinal hernias are often present. Diagnosis is usually made between 6 and 24 months of age with evidence of hepatosplenomegaly, coarse facial features, corneal clouding, large tongue, prominent forehead, joint stiffness, short stature, and skeletal dysplasia. Acute cardiomyopathy has been found in some infants <1 year of age. Most patients have recurrent upper respiratory tract and ear infections, noisy breathing, and persistent copious nasal discharge. Valvular heart disease with incompetence, notably of the mitral and aortic valves, regularly develops, as does coronary artery narrowing. Obstructive airway disease, notably during sleep, may necessitate tracheotomy. Obstructive airway disease, respiratory infection, and cardiac complications are the common causes of death.

52. **(a)** Hurler disease

(Nelson, 18th edition)

Mucopolysaccharidosis I

MPS I is caused by mutations of the *IUA* gene on chromosome 4p16.3 encoding α-L-iduronidase. Mutation analysis reveals 2 major alleles, W402X and Q70X, that account for more than ½ the MPS-I alleles in the white population. The mutations introduce stop codons with ensuing absence of functional enzyme (null alleles); homozygosity or compound heterozygosity gives rise to Hurler disease. Other mutations occur in only 1 or a few individuals.

Deficiency of α-L-iduronidase results in a broad clinical spectrum, from severe Hurler disease to mild Scheie diseases. Homozygous nonsense mutations result in severe forms of MPS I, whereas missense mutations are more likely to preserve some residual enzyme activity associated with a milder form of the disease.

53. **(b)** Hunter disease

(Nelson, 18th edition)

Hunter Disease

Marked molecular heterogeneity explains the wide clinical spectrum of Hunter disease. Patients with severe MPS II have features similar to those of Hurler disease except for the lack of corneal clouding and the somewhat slower progression of somatic and CNS deterioration. Coarse facial features, short stature, dysostosis multiplex, joint stiffness, and mental retardation manifest between 2 and 4 years of age. Grouped skin papules are present in some patients. Extensive Mongolian spots have been observed in African and Asian patients since birth and may be an early marker of the disease. Gastrointestinal storage may produce chronic diarrhea. Communicating hydrocephalus and spastic paraplegia may develop due to thickened meninges. In severely affected patients, extensive, slowly progressive neurologic involvement precedes death, which usually occurs between 10 and 15 years of age.

Chapter 22

Metabolic Disorders (2)

1. **Hyperphenylalaninemia is inherited as:**
   (a) X linked dominant
   (b) X linked recessive
   (c) Autosomal dominant
   (d) Autosomal recessive traits

2. **Pompe disease is caused by a deficiency of:**
   (a) Acid maltase
   (b) Muscle phosphorylase
   (c) Glucose 6 phosphatase
   (d) Glycogen branching enzyme

3. **Pompe disease is inherited as:**
   (a) Autosomal dominant
   (b) Autosomal recessive
   (c) X linked dominant
   (d) X linked recessive

4. **Mucopolysaccharidosis type 1 is characterised as:**
   (a) Hepatosplenomegaly (b) Coarse facial feature
   (c) Short stature (d) All of the above

5. **Hunter disease (MPS II) is inherited as:**
   (a) X-linked disorder
   (b) Autosomal disorder
   (c) Mitochondrial inheritance
   (d) Familial

6. **Hutchinson-Gilford progeria syndrome is characterised by:**
   (a) Absent sexually maturity
   (b) Failure to thrive
   (c) Sculpted nose
   (d) All of the above

7. **Diagnostic feature of acute porphyria is:**
   (a) Gum bleeding
   (b) Coca coloured urine
   (c) Abdominal pain after puberty
   (d) All of the above

8. **Drugs regarded as safe in acute porphyrias:**
   (a) Gabapentin
   (b) Streptomycin
   (c) Acetaminophen
   (d) All of the above

9. **Drugs regarded as unsafe in acute porphyrias:**
   (a) Barbiturates (b) Phenytoin
   (c) Carbamazepine (d) All of the above

10. **Transient neonatal hyperinsulinism is present in:**
    (a) Infant of diabetic mother
    (b) Small for gestational age
    (c) Birth asphyxia
    (d) All of the above

Answers

1. **(d)** Autosomal recessive traits
2. **(a)** Acid maltase
3. **(b)** Autosomal recessive
4. **(d)** All of the above
5. **(a)** X-linked disorder
6. **(d)** All of the above
7. **(c)** Abdominal pain after puberty
8. **(d)** All of the above
9. **(d)** All of the above

Drugs Regarded as Unsafe and Safe in Acute Porphyrias

Unsafe	Safe
Barbiturates	Narcotic analgesics
Sulfonamide antibiotics	Aspirin
Meprobamate	Acetaminophen
Carisoprodol	Phenothiazines
Glutethimide	Penicillin and derivatives
Methyprylon	Streptomycin
Ethchlorvynol	Glucocorticoids
Mephenytoin	Bromides
Phenytoin	Insulin
Succinimides	Atropine
Carbamazepine	Cimetidine
Clonazepam	Ranitidine[†]
Primidone	Acetaminophen (paracetamol)
Valproic acid	Acetazolamide
Pyrazolones (aminopyrine, antipyrine)	Allopurinol
Griseofulvin	Amiloride
Ergots	Bethanidine
Metoclopramide	Bumetanide
Rifampin	Cimetidine
Pyrazinamide	Coumarins
Diclofenac	Fluoxetine
Progesterone and synthetic progestins	Gabapentin
Danazol	Gentamicin
Alcohol	Guanethidine
ACE inhibitors (especially enalapril)	Ofloxacin
Calcium channel blockers (especially nifedipine)	Propranolol
Ketoconazole	Succinylcholine
Rifampin	Tetracycline

10. **(d)** All of the above

Chapter 23

Chromosome and Genetics

1. **Which of the following is not a single gene disorder?**
(a) Sickle cell anaemia (b) Cystic fibrosis
(c) Tay Sachs disease (d) Spina bifida

2. **Treatment of lysosomal storage disorders is:**
(a) Enzyme replacement
(b) Radiotherapy
(c) Bone marrow transplant
(d) No treatment possible

3. **Prenatal diagnosis of genetic defects can be evaluated by amniocentensis at:**
(a) 24-26 weeks (b) 16-18 weeks
(c) 10-12 weeks (d) None of the above

4. **A medical geneticist is one who:**
(a) Does diagnosis and management of patients with genetic disorders
(b) Gives genetic counseling and coordination of care
(c) Supervises laboratory testing in cytogenetics, biochemical genetics, and molecular genetics
(d) Nurses and cares for patients with genetic disorders

5. **The human genome has:**
(a) 30,000 genes (b) 80,000 genes
(c) 25000 genes (d) 7500 genes

6. **The number of base pairs in the mitochondrial chromosome are:**
(a) 15 400 (b) 17800
(c) 16568 (d) 22768

7. **The most common form of chronic peripheral neuropathy of childhood is:**
(a) Charcot-Marie-Tooth disease, type 1A
(b) Peroneal muscular atrophy
(c) None of the above
(d) All of the above

8. **The most common type of short limb skeletal dysplasia is:**
(a) Marfan syndrome
(b) Ehlar Danlos
(c) Achondroplasia
(d) Fragile X syndrome

9. **In achondroplasia the basic functional defect is:**
(a) Mutation in fibrillin 1
(b) Mutation in collagen type 4
(c) Mutation in fibroblast growth factor 3
(d) None of the above

10. **Which of the following is not true about multifactorial inheritance?**
(a) The risk of recurrence is related to the incidence of the disease
(b) There is a similar rate of recurrence (typically 3-5%) among all 1st degree relatives (parents, siblings, offspring of the affected child)
(c) Disorders affect both sexes equally
(d) The risk of recurrence is increased when multiple family members are affected

11. **One of the many complications of in vitro fertilization are:**
(a) Abortions
(b) Genetic imprinting
(c) Triplet repeat expansion disorders in child
(d) It is very safe and well monitored procedure

12. **With in vitro fertilization child is at increased risk of all *except:***
(a) Beckwith Wiedemann
(b) Angelman syndrome
(c) Retinoblastoma
(d) Giant cell tumor

13. In all the following disorders the trinucleotide repeat expansion occurs in the exon *except:*

(a) Huntington disease
(b) Haw River syndrome
(c) Progressive myoclonic epilepsy type 1
(d) Cleidocranial dysplasia

14. Mitochondrial abnormalities most commonly affect:

(a) Brain
(b) Stomach
(c) Prostate
(d) Bone marrow

15. Kearns-Sayre syndrome to the maximum precision consist of:

(a) Optic neuritis, liver cirrhosis, peripheral neuropathy
(b) Dementia, convulsions, papilloedema
(c) Ophthalmoplegia, pigmentary retinopathy and cardiomyopathy
(d) Cardiomyopathy chronic pancreatitis portal hypertension

16. Which of the following is a Y linked inheritance?

(a) Leri-Weil dyschondrosteosis
(b) Wiskot Aldrich syndrome
(c) Langer mesomelic dwarfism
(d) Both (a) and (c)

17. Which of the following characteristics is not true for X-linked inheritance?

(a) Males are more commonly and more severely affected than females
(b) Affected males will have only carrier daughters. They have no chance of having an affected son
(c) Carrier women have 50% risk of having an affected son
(d) Carrier woman has 25% risk for a carrier daughter, and a 50% chance for a child that does not inherit the mutated X-linked gene

18. Hardy-Weinberg formula is used for:

(a) To calculate the atmospheric pressure
(b) To calculate the BMR in paediatric age group
(c) To calculate chemotherapeutic dose requirement in paedo oncology
(d) To calculate the frequency of the heterozygote or carrier state when the frequency of recessive disease is known

19. Which of the following is not true for autosomal dominant inheritance?

(a) The disorder is transmitted in a vertical (parent to child) pattern, appearing in multiple generations
(b) An affected individual has a 50% (1 in 2) chance of passing on the deleterious genes for each pregnancy, and therefore of having a child affected by the disorder. This is referred to as the recurrence risk for the disorder
(c) Finding of male to female transmission essentially confirms the diagnosis
(d) Unaffected individuals (family members who do not manifest the trait) do not pass the disorder to their children

20. A non-inherited disorder consisting of bizarre, patterned, hypopigmented macules arranged over the body surface in sharply demarcated whorls, streaks, and patches that follow the lines of Blaschko, having systemic manifestation is:

(a) Hypomelanosis of Ito
(b) Systematized nevus depigmentosus
(c) Incontinentia pigmenti
(d) Vogt-Koyanogi-Harada syndrome

21. Uniparental disomy is:

(a) Two chromosomes are identical
(b) Two chromosomes are different members of a pair, both of which were inherited from one parent
(c) Both of the above
(d) None of the above

22. TDT stands for:

(a) Transfer dyanamic test
(b) Temporary divident test
(c) Transmission disequilibrium test
(d) Trial dynamic test

23. What is transmission disequilibrium test?

(a) Case-control design, with a comparison of the frequency of an allele in affected people compared with unaffected people
(b) A population-based study, in which an increase in a quantitative trait or continuous measurement is correlated with genotype
(c) Family-based test, in which transmission of alleles to affected and unaffected offspring is tested
(d) All of the above

24. The interaction between genes and the environment is called:
(a) Epistasis (b) Phenocopy
(c) Variable expressivity (d) Pleiotropy effect

25. According to the hygiene hypothesis:
(a) The lack of exposure to a different set of pathogens has been shown to increase immune deregulation and asthma
(b) More the hygiene, lesser the chances of developing genetic disorders
(c) Hygiene plays no role in transmission of genetic disorders
(d) None of the above

26. A child with a family history of pancreatic cancer comes to the clinic of a medical geneticist, which of the following tests would you consider most appropriate to determine his chances of getting the disease as adult?
(a) Pharmacogenetic testing
(b) Predispositional testing
(c) Predictive testing
(d) None of the above

27. Which of the following is not true about genetic counselling?
(a) Giving family information about support groups
(b) Careful physical examination about the affected individual
(c) Documenting prenatal pregnancy delivery notes
(d) Regular follow up to motivate and give psychological support to the patient and his family
(e) None

28. Which of the following is a polygenic disorder?
(a) Diabetes mellitus (b) Hypertension
(c) Both of the above (d) None of the above

29. Which of the following is not an autosomal dominant inherited disease?
(a) Noonan syndrome
(b) Marfan's syndrome
(c) Chronic granulomatous disease
(d) Sickle cell disease

30. Jyotsna father had sickle cell anaemia. But her mother did not. Jyotsna married Ravi who also did not have sickle cell anaemia. Nor did his parents have. What is the probability of their kids being born with sickle cell anaemia?
(a) 50% (b) 25%
(c) 20% (d) None

31. Lalit married Pallavi. Both were later diagnosed with being carriers of albinism.What is the probability of their kid being born normal?
(a) 25% (b) 50%
(c) 75% (d) 0%

32. Pranavati's father has Wiskott-Aldrich disease Pranavati's maternal grandfather also had Wiskott-Aldrich disease, but her mother does not. Pranavati's mother is pregnant. What is the probability that her sibling will be born with Wiskott-Aldrich disease?
(a) 25% (b) 0%
(c) 50% (d) 75%

33. Ramu was recently diagnosed with Friedreich's ataxia. He married Sushma. Sushma was screened for genetic skeleton and was found to be normal. (Not even a carrier of Friedreich's ataxia).What is the probability that their kids be affected with Friedreich's ataxia?
(a) 25% (b) 50%
(c) 100% (d) None

34. The chances of having an unaffected baby when both parents have osteogenesis imperfecta are:
(a) 0% (b) 100%
(c) 50% (d) 25%

35.

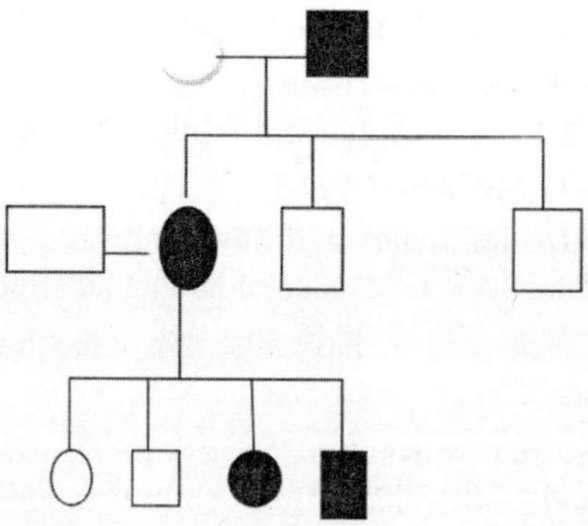

What is the type of this inheritance pattern?
(a) Autosomal recessive (b) Autosomal dominant
(c) X-linked recessive (d) X-linked dominant

36. Which of the following is not present in Down's syndrome?
(a) Short stature
(b) Hypotonia
(c) Profound mental retardation
(d) Webbed neck

37. Which of the following is not an autosomal dominant disorder?
(a) Huntington's
(b) Hereditary spherocytosis
(c) Familial hypercholesteremia
(d) Haemophilia A and B

38. The following characteristics are suggestive of which syndrome—microcephaly, mental retardation, micrognathia, rocker bottom feet?
(a) Trisomy 13 (b) Trisomy 21
(c) Trisomy 18 (d) Trisomy 22

39. The other name of Trisomy 13 is:
(a) Patau syndrome
(b) Edward syndrome
(c) Cat eye syndrome
(d) Down's syndrome

40. Match the pairs correctly:
Trisomy

1. 13	1. Down syndrome
2. 21	2. Edward syndrome
3. 22	3. Cat eye syndrome
4. 18	4. Patau syndrome

(a) 1-4, 2-3, 3-1, 4-2 (b) 1-4, 2-1, 3-3, 4-2
(c) 1-2, 2-4, 3-1, 4-3 (d) 1-3, 2-4, 3-1, 4-2

41. The most common cardiac manifestation in Noonan's syndrome is:
(a) ASD
(b) VSD
(c) Supravalvular pulmonary stenosis
(d) Coarctation of aorta

42. Noonan's syndrome is:
(a) Autosomal dominant
(b) Autosomal recessive
(c) X-linked dominant
(d) X-linked recessive

43. Autosomal dominant disease with Turner phenotype is:
(a) Achondroplasia
(b) Noonan's syndrome
(c) Wiskott-Aldrich syndrome
(d) Agammaglobulinemia

44. In which of the following diseases is anticipation phenomenon not seen?
(a) Huntington's (b) Myotonic dystrophy
(c) Fragile X syndrome (d) Marfan's disease

45. The following is not a feature of the Peirre Robin syndrome:
(a) Hearing defect
(b) Brushborder Iris
(c) Respiratory distress
(d) Mandibular hyperplasia

46. A particular genetic disorder that is passed from generations to generation only from the mother to offsprings is:
(a) Autosomal dominant
(b) Autosomal recessive
(c) X-linked recessive
(d) Mitochondrial inheritance

47. Which of the following disorders is common in advanced maternal age?
(a) Wiskott-Aldrich syndrome
(b) Vitamin D resistant rickets
(c) Down's syndrome
(d) Familial hypercholesteremia

48. Which of the following diseases have all three types of Mendelian inheritance?
(a) Chronic granulomatous diseases
(b) Ehlar Danlos syndrome
(c) Acute intermittent porphyria
(d) Friedreich's ataxia

Answers

1. **(d)** Spina bifida

(Kliegman: Nelson Textbook of Pediatrics, 18th ed.)

Sickle cell cystic fibrosis and Tay Sachs are single gene disorders while spina bifida is a multifactorial disorder.

2. **(a)** Enzyme replacement

(Kliegman: Nelson Textbook of Pediatrics, 18th ed.)

The treatment of many lysosomal storage disorders that were lethal or associated with intractable chronic illness. The basis for treatment in this case is enzyme replacement, using specially modified enzymes that are administered by intravenous infusion and are then taken up by cells and incorporated into lysosomes. Conditions such as Gaucher disease and Fabry disease are routinely treated.

3. **(b)** 16-18 weeks

(Kliegman: Nelson Textbook of Pediatrics, 18th ed.)

Prenatal diagnosis can be confirmed by amniocentesis at 16-18 weeks or chorionic villus sampling at 10-12 weeks.

4. **(a)** Does diagnosis and management of patients with genetic disorders

(Kliegman: Nelson Textbook of Pediatrics, 18th ed.)

(See the following Table)

5. **(c)** 25000 genes

(Kliegman: Nelson Textbook of Pediatrics, 18th ed.)

The human genome has approximately 25,000 genes.

6. **(c)** 16568

(Kliegman: Nelson Textbook of Pediatrics, 18th ed.)

The mitochondrial chromosome consists of a double-stranded circular piece of DNA, which contains 16,568 base pairs (bp) of DNA and is completely sequenced.

7. **(d)** All of the above

(Kliegman: Nelson Textbook of Pediatrics, 18th ed.)

Charcot-Marie-Tooth disease, type 1A, or peroneal muscular atrophy, the most common form of chronic peripheral neuropathy of childhood, results from duplication of the gene for peripheral myelin protein 22, resulting in overexpression of the gene product.

8. **(c)** Achondroplasia

(Kliegman: Nelson Textbook of Pediatrics, 18th ed.)

The gain-of-function mutation in achondroplasia, the most common of the short-limbed skeletal dysplasias, exemplifies the enhanced function of a normal protein. Achondroplasia results from a mutation in fibroblast growth receptor 3 (FGFR3), which leads to activation of the receptor, even in the absence of fibroblast growth factor (FGF).

9. **(c)** Mutation in fibroblast growth factor 3

(Kliegman: Nelson Textbook of Pediatrics, 18th ed.)

See the previous explanation.

10. **(c)** Disorders affect both sexes equally

(Kliegman: Nelson Textbook of Pediatrics, 18th ed.)

Multifactorial/Polygenic Inheritance

Multifactorial inheritance refers to traits that are caused by a combination of inherited, environmental, and stochastic factors. Multifactorial traits differ from polygenic inheritance, which refers to traits that result from the additive effects of multiple genes. Multifactorial traits segregate within families but do not exhibit a consistent or recognizable inheritance pattern. Characteristics include the following:

Ans. 4 **Types of Genetics Professionals**

Professional	Training	Certification	Role
Medical geneticist	MD and residency in medical genetics	American Board of Medical Genetics	Diagnosis and management of patients with genetic disorders
Genetic counselor	MS	American Board of Genetic Counseling	Genetic counseling and coordination of care
Laboratory geneticist	PhD or MD and 2 years fellowship	American Board of Medical Genetics	Supervision of laboratory testing in cytogenetics, biochemical genetics, and molecular genetics
Nurse-geneticist	Advanced Practice Nurse in Genetics (master's) or Genetics Clinical Nurse (baccalaureate)	Genetic Nursing Credentialing Commission	Nursing care of patients with genetic disorders

1. There is a similar rate of recurrence (typically 3-5%) among all 1st-degree relatives (parents, siblings, offspring of the affected child). It is unusual to find a substantial increase in risk for relatives related more distantly than 2nd degree to the index case.
2. The risk of recurrence is related to the incidence of the disease.
3. Some disorders have a sex predilection, as indicated by an unequal male: female incidence. Pyloric stenosis is more common in males, whereas congenital dislocation of the hips is more common in females. Where there is an altered sex ratio, the risk is higher for the relatives of an index case in the less commonly affected sex. The risk to the son of an affected female with infantile pyloric stenosis is 18% compared with the 5% risk for the son of an affected male. The female has passed on a greater genetic susceptibility to her offspring.
4. The likelihood that both identical twins will be affected with the same malformation is less than 100% but much greater than the chance that both members of a non-identical twin pair will be affected. The frequency of concordance for identical twins ranges from 21% to 63%. This distribution contrasts with that of Mendelian inheritance, in which identical twins always share a disorder due to a single mutant gene.
5. The risk of recurrence is increased when multiple family members are affected; these instances are often the most problematic for distinguishing multifactorial from Mendelian etiology. A simple example is that the risk of recurrence for unilateral cleft lip and palate is 4% for a couple with one affected child and increases to 9% with two affected children.
6. The risk of recurrence may be greater when the disorder is more severe. The infant who has long-segment Hirschsprung disease has a greater chance of having an affected sibling than the infant who has short-segment Hirschsprung disease.

11. **(b)** Genetic imprinting

(Kliegman: Nelson Textbook of Pediatrics, 18th ed.)

There is an increased incidence of imprinting disorders associated with in vitro fertilization or intracytoplasmic sperm injection (Beckwith-Wiedemann and Angelman syndrome). Retinoblastoma has also been reported in association with assisted reproductive technologies.

12. **(d)** Giant cell tumor

(Kliegman: Nelson Textbook of Pediatrics, 18th ed.)

See the previous explanation.

13. **(c)** Progressive myoclonic epilepsy type 1

(Kliegman: Nelson Textbook of Pediatrics, 18th ed.)

Ans. 12 **Diseases Associated with Repeat Expansions**

Disease	Description	Repeat sequence	Normal range, Abnormal range	Parent in whom expansion usually occurs	Location of expansion
Category 1					
Huntington disease	Loss of motor control, dementia, affective disorder	CAG	6–34;36–100 or more	More often through father	Exon
Spinal and bulbar muscular atrophy	Adult-onset motor-neuron disease associated with androgen insensitivity	CAG	11–34;40–62	More often through father	Exon
Spinocerebellar ataxia type 1	Progressive ataxia, dysarthria, dysmetria	CAG	6–39;41–81	More often through father	Exon
Spinocerebellar ataxia type 2	Progressive ataxia, dysarthria	CAG	15–29;35–59	—	Exon
Spinocerebellar ataxia type 3 (Machado-Joseph disease)	Dystonia, distal muscular atrophy, ataxia, external ophthalmoplegia	CAG	13–36;68–79	More often through father	Exon
Spinocerebellar ataxia type 6	Progressive ataxia, dysarthria, nystagmus	CAG	4–16;21–27	—	Exon
Spinocerebellar ataxia type 7	Progressive ataxia, dysarthria, retinal degeneration	CAG	7–35;38–200	More often through father	—

Contd.

Contd.

Disease	Description	Repeat sequence	Normal range, abnormal range	Parent in whom expansion usually occurs	Location of expansion
Spinocerebellar ataxia type 17	Progressive ataxia, dementia, bradykinesia, dysmetria	CAG	29–42;47–55	—	Exon
Dentatorubral-pallidoluysian atrophy/Haw River syndrome	Cerebellar atrophy, ataxia, myoclonic epilepsy, choreoathetosis, dementia	CAG	7–25;49–88	More often through father	Exon
Category 2					
Pseudoachondroplasia/ multiple epiphyseal dysplasia	Short stature, joint laxity, degenerative joint disease	GAC	5;6–7	—	Exon
Oculopharyngeal muscular dystrophy	Proximal limb weakness, dysphagia, ptosis	GCG	6;7–13	—	Exon
Cleidocranial dysplasia	Short stature, open skull sutures with bulging calvaria, clavicular hypoplasia, shortened fingers, dental anomalies	GCG, GCT, GCA	17;27 (expansion observed in one family)	—	Exon
Synpolydactyly	Polydactyly and syndactyly	GCG, GCT, GCA	15;22–25	—	Exon
Category 3					
Myotonic dystrophy (DMI; chromosome 19)	Muscle loss, cardiac arrhythmia, cataracts, frontal balding	CTG	5–37;100 to several thousand	Either parent, but expansion to congenital form through mother	3' untranslated region
Myotonic dystrophy (DM2; chromosome 3)	Muscle loss, cardiac arrhythmia, cataracts, frontal balding	CCTG	<75; 75–11,000	—	3' untranslated region
Friedreich ataxia	Progressive limb ataxia, dysarthria, hypertrophic cardiomyopathy, pyramidal weakness in legs	GAA	7–2; 200–900 or more	Autosomal recessive inheritance, so disease alleles are inherited from both parents	Intron
Fragile X syndrome (FRAXA)	Mental retardation, large ears and jaws, macroorchidism in males	CGG	6–52; 200–2,000 or more	Exclusively through mother	5' untranslated region
Fragile site (FRAXE)	Mild mental retardation	GCC	6–35; >200	More often through mother	3' untranslated region
Spinocerebellar ataxia type 8	Adult-onset ataxia, dysarthria, nystagmus	CTG	16–37; 107–127	More often through mother	3' untranslated region
Spinocerebellar ataxia type 10	Ataxia and seizures	ATTCT	12–16; 800–4,500	More often through father	Intron
Spinocerebellar ataxia type 12	Ataxia, eye movement disorders; variable age at onset	CAG	7–28; 66–78	—	5' untranslated region
Progressive myoclonic epilepsy type 1	Juvenile-onset convulsions, myoclonus, dementia	12-bp repeat motif	2–3; 30–75	Autosomal recessive inheritance, so transmitted by both parents	5' untranslated region

14. **(a)** Brain

(Kliegman: Nelson Textbook of Pediatrics, 18th ed.)

The mitochondria are the cell's suppliers of energy, so that the organs that are most affected by the presence of abnormal mitochondria are those that have the greatest energy requirements, such as the brain, muscle, heart and liver.

15. **(c)** Ophthalmoplegia, pigmentary retinopathy and cardiomyopathy

(Kliegman: Nelson Textbook of Pediatrics, 18th ed.)

The criteria for KSS include a triad of (1) onset before age 20 years, (2) progressive external ophthalmoplegia (PEO) with ptosis, and (3) pigmentary retinopathy. There must also be at least one of the following: heart block, cerebellar syndrome, or cerebrospinal fluid protein >100 mg/dL. Other nonspecific but common features include dementia, sensorineural hearing loss, and multiple endocrine abnormalities, including short stature, diabetes mellitus, and hypoparathyroidism. There is no treatment for KSS. The prognosis is poor, despite placement of a pacemaker, and progressively downhill, with death resulting by the 3rd or 4th decade. Unusual clinical presentations can include renal tubular acidosis and Lowe syndrome. There are also a few overlap cases of children with KSS and strokelike episodes. Muscle biopsy shows RRF and variable cytochrome oxidase (COX)-negative fibers. Most patients have mtDNA deletions, and some have duplications. These may be new mutations accounting for the generally sporadic nature of KSS. A few pedigrees have shown autosomal dominant transmission.

16. **(d)** Both (a) and (c)

(Kliegman: Nelson Textbook of Pediatrics, 18th ed.)

There are few Y-linked traits. These demonstrate only male-to-male transmission, and only males are affected. Most Y-linked genes are related to male sex determination and reproduction, and are associated with infertility. Therefore, it is rare to see familial transmission of a Y-linked disorder. Advances in assisted reproductive technologies may make possible familial transmission of male infertility. Of special note is the pseudoautosomal region on the Y chromosome, the small region of homology that is shared by both Xp and Yp. Very few genes reside in this region. One of the few is SHOX. Heterozygous SHOX mutations cause Leri-Weil dyschondrosteosis, a rare skeletal dysplasia that involves bilateral bowing of the forearms with dislocations of the ulna at the wrist and generalized short stature. Homozygous mutations cause the much more severe Langer mesomelic dwarfism.

17. **(c)** Carrier women have 50% risk of having an affected son

(Kliegman: Nelson Textbook of Pediatrics, 18th ed.)

X-linked Inheritance

Characteristics of X-linked inheritance include the following: (1) Males are more commonly and more severely affected than females. (2) Female carriers are generally unaffected, or if affected, they are affected more mildly than males. (3) Affected males will have only carrier daughters. They have no chance of having an affected son (male-to-male transmission excludes X-linkage and is seen with autosomal dominant and Y-linked inheritance). (4) Carrier women have a 25% risk for having an affected son, a 25% risk for a carrier daughter, and a 50% chance for a child that does not inherit the mutated X-linked gene.

18. **(d)** To calculate the frequency of the heterozygote or carrier state when the frequency of recessive disease is known

(Kliegman: Nelson Textbook of Pediatrics, 18th ed.)

If the frequency of an autosomal recessive disease is known, the frequency of the heterozygote or carrier state can be calculated from the Hardy-Weinberg formula: (p*p)+2pq+(q*q)=1

where is the frequency of one of a pair of alleles and q is the frequency of the other. For example, if the frequency of cystic fibrosis among white Americans is 1 in 2,500 (p^2), then the frequency of the heterozygote (2pq) can be calculated: if p^2 = ½,500, then p = 1/50 and q = 49/50; 2pq = 2 × 1/50 × 49/50, or approximately 1/25 (or 3.92%).

19. **(c)** Finding of male to female transmission essentially confirms the diagnosis

(Kliegman: Nelson Textbook of Pediatrics, 18th ed.)

The pedigree for an autosomal dominant disorder demonstrates certain characteristics. (1) The disorder is transmitted in a vertical (parent to child) pattern, appearing in multiple generations. This is illustrated by individual I.1 passing on the changed gene to II.2 and II.5. (2) An affected individual has a 50% (1 in 2) chance of passing on the deleterious genes for each pregnancy, and therefore of having a child affected by the disorder. This is referred to as the recurrence risk for the disorder. (3) Unaffected individuals (family members who do not manifest the trait) do not pass the disorder to their children. (4) Males and females are equally affected. Although not a characteristic per se. (5) The finding of male-to-male transmission essentially confirms autosomal dominant inheritance. Vertical transmission can also be seen with X-linked traits. However, since a father passes on his Y chromosome to a son, male-to-male transmission cannot be seen with an X-linked trait. Therefore, male-to-male transmission eliminates X-linked inheritance as a possible explanation. While male-to-male transmission can occur with Y-linked genes as well, there are very few Y-linked disorders compared with thousands having the autosomal dominant inheritance pattern.

20. **(a)** Hypomelanosis of Ito

(Kliegman: Nelson Textbook of Pediatrics, 18th ed.)

Hypomelanosis of Ito

This congenital skin disorder affects children of both sexes and is frequently associated with defects in several organ systems. There is no evidence for genetic transmission; chromosomal mosaicism and chromosomal translocations have been reported. Hypomelanosis of Ito is currently a descriptive rather than definitive diagnosis.

The skin lesions of hypomelanosis of Ito are generally present at birth but may be acquired in the 1st 2 years of life. The lesions are similar to a negative image of that present in incontinentia pigmenti, consisting of bizarre, patterned, hypopigmented macules arranged over the body surface in sharply demarcated whorls, streaks, and patches that follow the lines of Blaschko. The palms, soles and mucous membranes are spared. The hypopigmentation remains unchanged throughout childhood but fades during adulthood. The degree of depigmentation varies from hypopigmented to achromic. Neither inflammatory nor vesicular lesions precede the development of the pigmentary changes as in incontinentia pigmenti. The hypopigmented areas demonstrate fewer and smaller melanocytes and a decreased number of melanin granules in the basal cell layer than normal. Inflammatory cells and pigment incontinence are lacking.

The most commonly associated abnormalities involve the nervous system, including mental retardation (70%), seizures (40%), microcephaly (25%), and muscular hypotonia (15%). The musculoskeletal system is the 2nd most frequently involved system, affected by scoliosis and thoracic and limb deformities. Minor ophthalmologic defects (strabismus, nystagmus) are present in 25% of patients, and 10% have cardiac defects. The differential diagnosis includes systematized nevus depigmentosus, which is a stable leukoderma not associated with systemic manifestations. Differentiation from incontinentia pigmenti, particularly the hypopigmented 4th stage, is critical for genetic counseling because incontinentia pigmenti, unlike hypomelanosis of Ito, is inherited.

21. **(a)** Two chromosomes are identical

(Kliegman: Nelson Textbook of Pediatrics, 18th ed.)

Uniparental isodisomy means that the two chromosomes are identical, whereas uniparental heterodisomy means that the two chromosomes are different members of a pair, both of which were inherited from one parent. The phenotypical result of UPD varies according to the chromosome involved, the parent who contributed the chromosomes, and whether it is isodisomy or heterodisomy. Three types of phenotypic effects are seen in UPD: (1) those related to imprinted genes, that is, the absence of a gene that is expressed only when inherited from a parent of a specific gender, (2) those related to autosomal recessive disorders, and (3) those related to a vestigial aneuploid producing mosaicism.

22. **(c)** Transmission disequilibrium test

(Kliegman: Nelson Textbook of Pediatrics, 18th ed.)

Three basic designs are used: (1) A case-control design, with a comparison of the frequency of an allele in affected people compared with unaffected people, (2) A population-based study, in which an increase in a quantitative trait or continuous measurement is correlated with genotype, and (3) A family-based test, in which transmission of alleles to affected and unaffected offspring is tested. This last type of analysis, known as a transmission disequilibrium test (TDT), looks for an allele that is transmitted to an affected person more often than the other allele.

23. **(d)** All of the above

(Kliegman: Nelson Textbook of Pediatrics, 18th ed.)

Refer to the explanation above.

24. **(a)** Epistasis

(Kliegman: Nelson Textbook of Pediatrics, 18th ed.)
The interaction between genes and the environment is called epistasis. Epistatic effects could affect the expressivity of a trait as well as the penetrance. An example of this is G6PD deficiency. An individual could carry the altered gene and be deficient in the enzyme, yet would never have a hemolytic crisis unless exposed to an oxidative stress. People with inherited propensity for malignant melanoma who live in darker geographic regions or limit their sun exposure may never express the phenotype of cancer. Asthma in some susceptible people may develop only after exposure to certain antigens or pollutants.

25. **(a)** The lack of exposure to a different set of pathogens has been shown to increase immune deregulation and asthma

The lack of exposure to a different set of pathogens has been shown to increase immune deregulation and asthma, as proposed in the hygiene hypothesis. Exposure to parasites in early childhood has been correlated with protection against asthma and atopy.

26. **(c)** Predictive testing

(Kliegman: Nelson Textbook of Pediatrics, 18th ed.

Predictive genetic testing involves performance of a test in an individual who is at risk of developing a genetic disorder (presymptomatic), usually on the basis of family history, yet does not manifest signs or symptoms. This is usually done for disorders that display age-dependent penetrance; the likelihood of manifesting signs and symptoms increases with age, as in cancer or Huntington disease.

27. **(e)** None

Genetic Counseling

Providing accurate information to families requires (1) Taking a careful family history and constructing a pedigree that lists the patient's relatives (including abortions, stillbirths, deceased individuals) with their sex, age, and state of health, up to and including third-degree relatives; (2) Gathering information from hospital records about the affected individual (in some cases, about other family members); (3) Documenting prenatal, pregnancy, and delivery histories; (4) Reviewing the latest available medical, laboratory, and genetic information concerning the disorder; (5) Careful physical examination of the affected individual (photographs, measurements) and of apparently unaffected individuals in the family; (6) Establishing or confirming the diagnosis by the diagnostic tests available; (7) Giving the family information about support groups; (8) Providing new information to the family as it becomes available (a mechanism for updating needs to be established).

28. **(c)** Both of the above

A trait is called polygenic if multiple genes are thought to contribute to the phenotype of an individual.

29. **(d)** Sickle cell disease

(Kliegman: Nelson Textbook of Pediatrics, 18th ed.)

Sickle cell disorder is an autosomal recessive disorder.

30. **(d)** None

(Kliegman: Nelson Textbook of Pediatrics, 18th ed.)

As Jyotsna is a carrier and Ravi is normal, 50% of their kids will be carrier but none with have profound complete sickle cell anaemia as it is a autosomal recessive disorder.

31. **(a)** 25%

(Kliegman: Nelson Textbook of Pediatrics, 18th ed.)

Albinism is an autosomal recessive disorder. And it will be manifestated in homozygous state only. Hence there is only 25% chance of a child born with normal genetic framework. 50% will be carrier and 25% will be affected.

32. **(a)** 25%

(Kliegman: Nelson Textbook of Pediatrics, 18th ed.)

Wiskott-Aldrich is an X linked recessive disorder. Occurs only in homozygous state. Pranavati's father has Wiskott-Aldrich disease. And her mother is a carrier as her maternal grandfather had the disease. In such a situation there is 25% probability of the child being born with the disease.

33. **(d)** None

(Kliegman: Nelson Textbook of Pediatrics, 18th ed.)

Friedreich's ataxia is an autosomal recessive disease. Ramu is affected and Sushma is normal. As one is affected and the other is normal, all the children will be born as carriers. But none of them will be affected.

34. **(d)** 25%

(Kliegman: Nelson Textbook of Pediatrics, 18th ed.)

Osteogenesis imperfecta is an autosomal dominant condition. Both parents are affected. So obviously, 50% will be affected. 25% will be dead as they are incompatible with life and 25% will be unaffected.

35. **(d)** X linked dominant

(Kliegman: Nelson Textbook of Pediatrics, 18th ed.)

As the disease is transmitted only from father to daughter, it is a X linked disease. And it is dominant because the other X inherited from mother in spite being normal is subdued by this defective X.

36. **(c)** Profound mental retardation

(Kliegman: Nelson Textbook of Pediatrics, 18th ed.)

Down syndrome is characterized by mild to moderate mental retardation.

Characteristics	Percentage	Characteristics	Percentage
Stunted growth	100%	Flattened nose	60%
Mental retardation	99.8%	Small teeth	60%
Atypical fingerprints	90%	Clinodactyly	52%
Separation of the abdominal muscles	80%	Umbilical hernia	51%
Flexible ligaments	80%	Short neck	50%
Hypotonia	80%	Shortened hands	50%
Brachycephaly	75%	Congenital heart disease	45%
Smaller genitalia	75%	Single transverse palmar crease	45%
Eyelid crease	75%	Macroglossia (larger tongue)	43%
Shortened extremities	70%	Epicanthic fold	42%
Oval palate	69%	Strabismus	40%
Low-set and rounded ear	60%	Brushfield spots (iris)	35%

37. **(d)** Haemophilia A and B

(Kliegman: Nelson Textbook of Pediatrics, 18th ed.)

Haemophilia A and B is X linked recessive syndrome.The others are autosomal dominant disorder.

38. **(c)** Trisomy 18

(Kliegman: Nelson Textbook of Pediatrics, 18th ed.)

Microcephaly, mental retardation and micrognathia may be present in many syndromes. But rocker bottom feet is characteristic of Trisomy 18 (Edwards syndrome).

Children born with Edwards syndrome may have some or all of the following characteristics: kidney malformations, structural heart defects at birth (i.e., ventricular septal defect, atrial septal defect, patent ductus arteriosus), intestines protruding outside the body (omphalocele), esophageal atresia, mental retardation, developmental delays, growth deficiency, feeding diff iculties, breathing difficulties, and arthrogryposis (a muscle disorder that causes multiple joint contractures at birth).

Some physical malformations associated with Edwards syndrome include small head (microcephaly) accompanied by a prominent back portion of the head (occiput); low-set, malformed ears; abnormally small jaw (micrognathia); cleft lip/cleft palate; upturned nose; narrow eyelid folds (palpebral fissures); widely spaced eyes (ocular hypertelorism); drooping of the upper eyelids (ptosis); a short breast bone; clenched hands; choroid plexus cysts; underdeveloped thumbs and or nails, absent radius, webbing of the second and third toes; clubfoot or Rocker bottom feet; and in males, undescended testicles.

Clenched hand and overlapping fingers: index finger overlaps third finger and fifth finger overlaps fourth finger, characteristically seen in Trisomy 18.

In utero, the most common characteristic is cardiac anomalies, followed by central nervous system anomalies such as head shape abnormalities. The most common intracranial anomaly is the presence of choroid plexus cysts, which are pockets of fluid on the brain. These are not problematic in themselves, but their presence may be a marker for trisomy 18. Sometimes excess amniotic fluid or polyhydramnios is exhibited.

39. **(a)** Patau syndrome

(Kliegman: Nelson Textbook of Pediatrics, 18th ed.)

Patau syndrome is Trisomy 13.

Trisomy 18 is Edwards syndrome.

Partial Trisomy 22 is cat eye syndrome.

Down's syndrome is Trisomy 21.

40. **(b)** 1-4, 2-1, 3-3, 4-2

(Kliegman: Nelson Textbook of Pediatrics, 18th ed.)

Refer to the previous answer.

41. **(c)** Supravalvular pulmonary stenosis

(Kliegman: Nelson Textbook of Pediatrics, 18th ed.)

Coarctation of aorta is most common characteristic feature in Turner's syndrome, whereas Noonan's is characterized by supravalvular pulmonary stenosis.

42. **(a)** Autosomal dominant

(Kliegman: Nelson Textbook of Pediatrics, 18th ed.)

Noonan's syndrome is autosomal dominant syndrome. It is characterised by Turner like phenotype.

43. **(b)** Noonan's syndrome

(Kliegman: Nelson Textbook of Pediatrics, 18th ed.)

Noonan syndrome is characteristically Turner phenotype with normal karyotype.

44. **(d)** Marfan's disease

(Kliegman: Nelson Textbook of Pediatrics, 18th ed.)

Hungtintons, Myotonic dystrophy, Fragile X syndrome, Friedreich's ataxia are certain tri nucleotide repeat disorders in which anticipation phenomenon is seen.

45. **(b)** Brushborder iris

(Kliegman: Nelson Textbook of Pediatrics, 18th ed.)

Pierre Robin syndrome is a congenital condition of facial abnormalities in humans. PRS is a sequence, i.e., a chain of certain developmental malformations, one entailing the next. The 3 main features are cleft palate, micrognathia (a small jaw) and glossoptosis (airway obstruction caused by backwards displacement of the tongue base). A genetic cause to PRS was recently identified. Pierre Robin sequence may be caused by genetic anomalies at chromosomes 2, 11,17.

PRS is characterized by an unusually small mandible, posterior displacement or retraction of the tongue (glossoptosis), and upper airway obstruction. Incomplete closure of the roof of the mouth (cleft palate) is present in the majority of patients, and is commonly U-shaped.

46. **(d)** Mitochondrial inheritance

(Kliegman: Nelson Textbook of Pediatrics, 18th ed.)

In most multicellular organisms, mtDNA is inherited from the mother (maternally inherited). Mechanisms for this include simple dilution (an egg contains 100,000 to 1,000,000 mtDNA molecules, whereas a sperm contains only 100 to 1000), degradation of sperm mtDNA in the fertilized egg, and, at least in a few organisms, failure of sperm mtDNA to enter the egg. Whatever the mechanism, this single parent (uniparental) pattern of mtDNA inheritance is found in most animals, most plants and in fungi as well.

In short, during fertilization the mitochondria of the zygote is derived from mother. So if a disease is being passed from mother to offspring then the pattern of inheritance is considered mitochondrial.

47. **(c)** Down's syndrome

(Kliegman: Nelson Textbook of Pediatrics, 18th ed.)

Elderly females in pregnancy have the most likelihood of giving birth to Down's syndrome babies.

48. **(b)** Ehlar Danlos syndrome

(Kliegman: Nelson Textbook of Pediatrics, 18th ed.)

Ehlar Danlos has all three types of Mendelian inheritance unlike chronic granulomatous disease, acute intermittent porphyria, Friedreich's ataxia.

Chapter 24

Bone and Joint Disorders

1. **What is degree of hip and knee flexion in normal full-term newborn?**
(a) 10-20 degree (b) 20-30 degree
(c) 30-45 degree (d) 90 degree

2. **What is degree of hip extension in normal full-term newborn?**
(a) 80-90 degrees (b) 60-50 degree
(c) 45 degree (d) 10-20 degree

3. **What is ratio of head height to total height at birth?**
(a) 1 : 1 (b) 1 : 2
(c) 1 : 3 (d) 1 : 4

4. **At what age wide gait diminishes?**
(a) 1 year (b) 2 years
(c) 3 years (d) 4 years

5. **At what age fully mature gait pattern develops?**
(a) 7 years (b) 5 years
(c) 3 years (d) 2 years

6. **Macrodactyly is seen in:**
(a) Proteus syndrome
(b) Neurofibromatosis
(c) Klippel-Trenaunay-Weber syndrome
(d) All of the above

7. **At what intrauterine age the hip joint forms?**
(a) 11 weeks (b) 9 weeks
(c) 5 weeks (d) 4 weeks

8. **What is normal tibiofemoral angle at birth?**
(a) Less than 10 degree (b) 10-15 degree
(c) 20-25 degree (d) 30-45 degree

9. **At what age physiologic bowleg disappears?**
(a) 6 months (b) 1 year
(c) 2 years (d) 4 years

10. **Which is cause of pathologic bowleg?**
(a) Vitamin D deficiency (b) Rickets
(c) Hypophosphatasia (d) All of the above

11. **Pathologic condition leading to knock-knees:**
(a) Ricket
(b) Renal osteodystrophy
(c) Skeletal dysplasia
(d) All of the above

12. **At what intrauterine age knee joint develops?**
(a) 2-3 months (b) 3- 4 months
(c) 5-6 months (d) 8 months

13. **At what intrauterine age patellar ossification center appears in girls?**
(a) 1-1.5 year (b) 1.5-2 years
(c) 2nd - 4th year (d) 6 years

14. **At what intrauterine age patellar ossification center appears in boys?**
(a) 3rd -5th year (b) 5-7th year
(c) 8-9th year (d) Above 10 years

15. **Which is the largest joint in the body?**
(a) Hip (b) Ankle
(c) Knee (d) Patella

16. **At what intrauterine age the hip joint begins to develop?**
(a) 4th week (b) 7th week
(c) 10th week (d) 12th week

17. **Klippel-Feil syndrome is characterized by:**
(a) Short neck
(b) Low hairline
(c) Restriction of neck motion
(d) All of the above

18. Which syndrome is commonly associated with radial deficiency?
(a) Holt-Oram (b) Fanconi anemia
(c) VACTERL (d) All of the above

19. Syndrome associated with polydactyly:
(a) Carpenter syndrome
(b) Meckel-Gruber syndrome
(c) Ellis-van Creveld syndrome
(d) All of the above

20. Syndrome associated with syndactyly:
(a) Apert syndrome
(b) Carpenter syndrome
(c) Holt-Oram syndrome
(d) All of the above

21. Which systemic diseases mimic of child abuse?
(a) Osteogenesis imperfecta (b) Osteomyelitis
(c) Caffey disease (d) All of the above

22. Which is the most common infecting organism in all age groups for osteomyelitis?
(a) Staphylococcus aureus
(b) Staphylococcus epidermidis
(c) Streptococcus viridans
(d) H. influenza

23. Which is the component of female athlete triad?
(a) Disordered eating (b) Amenorrhea
(c) Osteoporosis (d) All of the above

24. Ellis-van Creveld syndrome constitutes:
(a) Short limbs
(b) Postaxial polydactyly
(c) Nail dysplasia
(d) All of the above

25. Jeune syndrome is composed of:
(a) Autosomal recessive (b) Long, narrow thorax
(c) Postaxial polydactyly (d) All of the above

26. Osteogenesis imperfecta has component of:
(a) Fragile bones (b) Blue sclerae
(c) Early deafness (d) All of the above

27. Marfan syndrome is inherited as:
(a) Autosomal dominant (b) Autosomal recessive
(c) X linked recessive (d) X linked dominant

28. Marfan syndrome is characterized by:
(a) Tall stature (b) Dental crowding
(c) Long, thin face (d) All of the above

29. Which drug commonly causes osteoporosis?
(a) Glucocorticosteroids (b) Anticonvulsants
(c) Chemotherapy (d) All of the above

Answers

1. **(b)** 20–30 degree
2. **(a)** 80–90 degree
3. **(d)** 1 : 4
4. **(b)** 2 years
5. **(a)** 7 years
6. **(d)** All of the above
7. **(a)** 11 weeks
8. **(b)** 10– 5 degrees
9. **(c)** 2 years
10. **(d)** All of the above
11. **(d)** All of the above
12. **(b)** 3-4 months
13. **(c)** 2nd-4th year
14. **(a)** 3rd-5th year
15. **(c)** Knee
16. **(b)** 7th week
17. **(d)** All of the above
18. **(d)** All of the above
19. **(d)** All of the above
20. **(d)** All of the above
21. **(d)** All of the above
22. **(a)** Staphylococcus aureus
23. **(d)** All of the above
24. **(d)** All of the above
25. **(d)** All of the above
26. **(d)** All of the above
27. **(a)** Autosomal dominant
28. **(d)** All of the above
29. **(d)** All of the above

Chapter 25

Immunology

1. **If an infant's neutrophil count is persistently elevated to extreme levels in the absence of any signs of infection, condition is known as:**
   (a) Congenital neutropenia
   (b) Acquired neutropenia
   (c) Leukocyte adhesion deficiency
   (d) None of the above

2. **Severe combined immunodeficiency (SCID) could be detected at birth by:**
   (a) Direct Coomb test
   (b) Indirect Coomb test
   (c) ELISA
   (d) CBC and differential counts of cord blood

3. **Which of the following is not present in DiGeorge anomaly?**
   (a) Hypocalcemia (b) Unusual facies
   (c) Heart disease (d) Bloody stool

4. **Which of the following is not present in Wiskott-Aldrich syndrome?**
   (a) Bloody stool (b) Draining ears
   (c) Mouth ulcer (d) Eczema

5. **Chédiak-Higashi syndrome is:**
   (a) Oculocutaneous albinism, recurrent infection
   (b) Bloody stools, draining ears, eczema
   (c) Mouth ulcers, neutropenia, recurrent infections
   (d) Maculopapular rash, alopecia, lymphadenopathy

6. **Recurrent neisserial meningitis is due to:**
   (a) Hyper-IgE syndrome
   (b) C6, C7, or C8 deficiency
   (c) Severe combined immunodeficiency
   (d) Biotin-dependent cocarboxylase deficiency

7. **Omenn syndrome is:**
   (a) Autosomal recessive (b) Autosomal dominant
   (c) X-linked recessive (d) X-linked dominant

8. **Screening test for B-cell defects is:**
   (a) Serum IgA
   (b) WBC count
   (c) Titre of isohemagglutinins
   (d) Serum IgG

9. **To evaluate a patient's ability to respond to polysaccharide antigens, anti-pneumococcal antibodies can be measured:**
   (a) Before and after 2 weeks
   (b) Before and after 3 weeks
   (c) After 4 weeks
   (d) After 1 year

10. **Antibodies seen in serum after vaccination is:**
    (a) IgG (b) IgA
    (c) IgM (d) IgD

11. **All of the following are secondary lymphatic organs *except:***
    (a) Thymus (b) Spleen
    (c) Lymph nodes (d) Tonsils

12. **______ is primary lymphatic organ.**
    (a) Thymus (b) Peyer patches
    (c) Spleen (d) Tonsils

13. **'CD' in immunology stands for:**
    (a) Common of differentiate
    (b) Clusters of differentiation
    (c) Compact differentiation
    (d) Cells of differentiation

14. T cells migrate to thymus from liver in _____ intrauterine life.
(a) 3rd week (b) 5th week
(c) 6th week (d) 8th week

15. B cells migrate to long bones from liver in _____ of intrauterine life.
(a) 4th week (b) 6th week
(c) 8th week (d) 10th week

16. CD 2, CD 3, CD 4 are related to:
(a) Monocytes
(b) T lymphocytes
(c) B lymphocytes
(d) NK cells

17. CD 19, CD 20, CD 21 are related to:
(a) B lymphocyte (b) T lymphocyte
(c) Macrophage (d) NK cells

18. Following is T helper cell receptor:
(a) CD 2 (b) CD 4
(c) CD 6 (d) CD 8

19. _____ act as receptor for HLA 1.
(a) CD 2 (b) CD 4
(c) CD 6 (d) CD 8

20. CD 34 is marker present on:
(a) T lymphocytes
(b) B lymphocytes
(c) Haemopoetic stem cells
(d) Macrophages

21. _____ CD marker is present on all lymphocyte.
(a) CD 20 (b) CD 1
(c) CD 34 (d) CD 45

22. Average half-life in the circulation of neutrophil:
(a) 6 hours (b) 12 hours
(c) 24 hours (d) 48 hours

23. Average half-life in the circulation of monocyte is:
(a) 36-104 hours (b) 48-72 hours
(c) 72-96 hours (d) 12-24 hours

24. The proliferation, differentiation, and survival of immature hematopoietic progenitor cells are governed by:
(a) IL (b) CSF
(c) Both (d) GF

25. Immature committed progenitors bear receptors for:
(a) IL-3 (b) IL-4
(c) IL-5 (d) IL-6

26. Osteoclast is type of:
(a) Bone forming cell
(b) Cartilage forming cell
(c) Bone eating macrophage
(d) Cartilage eating macrophage

27. _____are circulating precursor of macrophages.
(a) Neutrophils (b) Monocytes
(c) Basophils (d) Eosinophils

28. Classical activation of macrophages occurs by:
(a) IL-4 (b) IL-5
(c) INF-gamma (d) TNF-alfa

29. Autosomal recessive gene responsible for FMF (Familial Mediterranean fever) on:
(a) Chromosome 12 (b) Chromosome 14
(c) Chromosome 16 (d) Chromosome 18

30. All of the following are causes of eosinophilia *except:*
(a) Wiskott-Aldrich syndrome
(b) Eosinophilic leukemia
(c) Toxoplasmosis
(d) Pneumonia

Answers

1. **(c)** Leukocyte adhesion deficiency

(Nelson Textbook of Pediatrics, 18th ed.)

If an infant's neutrophil count is persistently elevated to extreme levels in the absence of any signs of infection, a leukocyte adhesion deficiency should be suspected. If the absolute neutrophil count is normal, congenital and acquired neutropenias and leukocyte adhesion defects are excluded.

2. **(d)** CBC and differential counts of cord blood

(Nelson Textbook of Pediatrics, 18th ed.)

If a CBC and a manual differential were performed on the cord blood of all infants, severe combined immunodeficiency (SCID) could be detected at birth by the identification of lymphopenia, and life saving immunologic reconstitution could then be provided to all affected infants.

3. **(d)** Bloody stool

(Nelson Textbook of Pediatrics, 18th ed.)

Features	**Diagnosis**
In newborns and young infants (0 to 6 months)	
Hypocalcemia, heart disease, unusual facies	DiGeorge anomaly
Delayed umbilical cord detachment, leukocytosis, recurrent infections	Leukocyte adhesion defect–Autosomal recessive
Diarrhea, pneumonia, thrush, failure to thrive	Severe combined immunodeficiency
Maculopapular rash, alopecia, lymphadenopathy	Severe combined immunodeficiency with graft-versus-host disease
Bloody stools, draining ears, eczema	Wiskott-Aldrich syndrome
Mouth ulcers, neutropenia, recurrent infections	XL-Hyper IgM syndrome

4. **(c)** Mouth ulcer

(Nelson Textbook of Pediatrics, 18th ed.)

Refer above table.

5. **(a)** Oculocutaneous albinism, recurrent infection

(Nelson Textbook of Pediatrics, 18th ed.)

Chédiak-Higashi syndrome–Oculocutaneous albinism, recurrent infection.

6. **(b)** C6, C7, or C8 deficiency

(Nelson Textbook of Pediatrics, 18th ed.)

In older children (older than 5 years) and adults	
Progressive dermatomyositis with chronic enterovirus encephalitis	X-linked agammaglobulinemia
Sinopulmonary infections, neurologic deterioration, telangiectasia	Ataxia-telangiectasia
Recurrent neisserial meningitis	C6, C7, or C8 deficiency
Sinopulmonary infections, malabsorption, splenomegaly, autoimmunity	Common variable immunodeficiency
Candidiasis with raw egg ingestion	Biotin-dependent cocarboxylase deficiency

7. **(a)** Autosomal recessive

(Nelson Textbook of Pediatrics, 18th ed.)

Omen syndrome is T + B Severe combined immunodeficiency–AR.

8. **(a)** Serum IgA

(Nelson Textbook of Pediatrics, 18th ed.)

- A simple screening test for B-cell defects is the measurement of serum IgA. If the IgA level is normal, selective IgA deficiency, which is the most common B-cell defect, is excluded, as are most of the permanent types of hypogammaglobulinemia since IgA is usually very low or absent in those conditions. If IgA is low, IgG and IgM should also be measured.
- One of the most useful tests for B-cell function is to determine the presence and titer of isohemagglutinins, or antibodies to type A and B red blood cell polysaccharide antigens. This test measures predominantly IgM antibodies. Isohemagglutinins may be absent normally in the 1st 2 years of life and are always absent if the patient is blood type AB.

9. **(b)** Before and after 3 weeks

(Nelson Textbook of Pediatrics, 18th ed.)

To evaluate a patient's ability to respond to polysaccharide antigens, anti-pneumococcal antibodies can be measured before and 3 weeks after immunization with pneumococcal polysaccharide vaccine (PPV23) in patients >2–3 years. Antibodies detected in these tests are of the IgGiso type.

10. **(a)** IgG

(Nelson Textbook of Pediatrics, 18th ed.)

Refer above question.

In children >2 years of age with low anti-pneumococcal antibody titers, it is useful to boost with conjugate pneumococcal vaccine twice, 1 month apart, before giving a polysaccharide pneumococcal vaccine 1 month later and then measuring antibody titers 3 weeks later.

11. **(a)** Thymus

(Nelson Textbook of Pediatrics, 18th ed.)

Development of the primary lymphoid organs—thymus and bone marrow—begins during the middle of the 1st trimester of gestation and proceeds rapidly. Development of the secondary lymphoid organs—spleen, lymph nodes, tonsils, Peyer patches, and lamina propria—soon follows.

12. **(a)** Thymus

(Nelson Textbook of Pediatrics, 18th ed.)

Development of the primary lymphoid organs—thymus and bone marrow—begins during the middle of the 1st trimester of gestation and proceeds rapidly. Development of the secondary lymphoid organs—spleen, lymph nodes, tonsils, Peyer patches, and lamina propria—soon follows.

13. **(b)** Clusters of differentiation

(Nelson Textbook of Pediatrics, 18th ed.)

The complexity and number of lymphoid cell surface molecules led to the development of an international nomenclature for clusters of differentiation (CD).

14. **(d)** 8th week

(Nelson Textbook of Pediatrics, 18th ed.)

15. **(d)** 10th week

(Nelson Textbook of Pediatrics, 18th ed.)

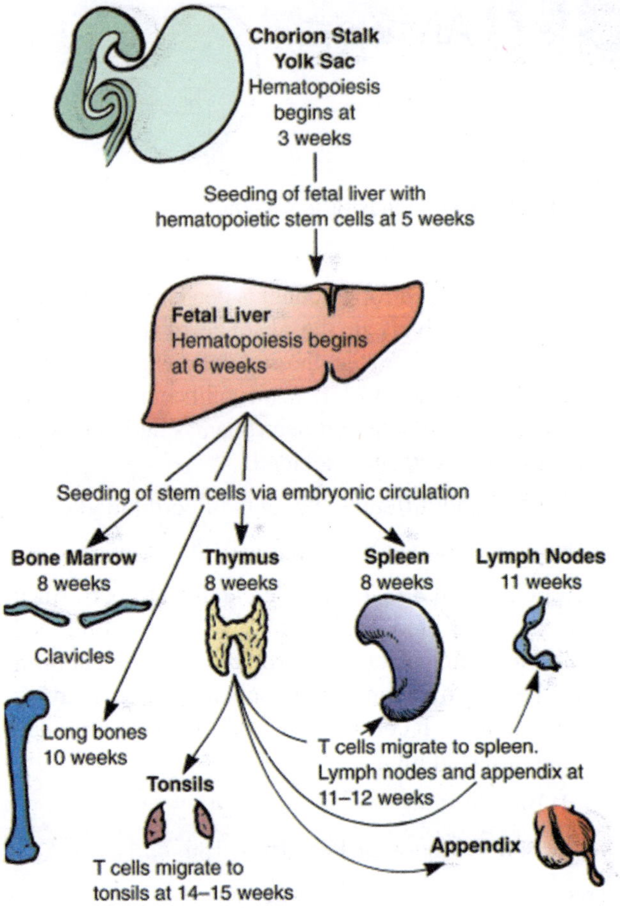

16. **(b)** T lymphocytes

(Nelson Textbook of Pediatrics, 18th ed.)

17. **(a)** B lymphocyte

(Nelson Textbook of Pediatrics, 18th ed.)

18. **(b)** CD 4

(Nelson Textbook of Pediatrics, 18th ed.)

19. **(d)** CD 8

(Nelson Textbook of Pediatrics, 18th ed.)

20. **(c)** Haemopoetic stem cells

(Nelson Textbook of Pediatrics, 18th ed.)

21. **(d)** CD 45

(Nelson Textbook of Pediatrics, 18th ed.)

CD Number[*]	Other Names	Tissue/Lineage	Function
CD1	T6	Cortical thymocytes; Langerhans cells	Antigen presentation to TCRää cells
CD2	SRBC receptor	T and NK cells	Binds LFA-3 (CD58); alternative pathway of T-cell activation
CD3	T3, Leu 4	T cells	TCR-associated; transduces signals from TCR
CD4	T4, Leu 3a	Helper T-cell subset	Receptor for HLA Class II antigens; associated with p56 Ick tyrosine kinase
CD7	3A1, Leu 9	T and NK cells and their precursors	Co-mitogenic for T lymphocytes
CD8	T8, Leu 2a	Cytotoxic T-cell subset; also on 30% of NK cells	Receptor for HLA Class I antigens; associated with p56 Ick tyrosine kinase
CD10	cALLA	B-cell progenitors	Peptide cleavage
CD11a	LFA-1a ∀ chain	T, B and NK cells	With CD18, ligand for ICAMS 1, 2 and 3
CD11b, c	MAC-1, CR3; CR4	NK cells	With CD18, receptors for C3bi
CD16	FcRIII	NK cells	FcR for IgG
CD19	B4	B cells	Regulates B-cell activation
CD20	B1	B cells	Mediates B-cell activation
CD21	B2	B cells	C3d, also the receptor for EBV; CR2
CD25	IL-2Rα	T, B and NK cells	Mediates signaling by IL-2
CD34	My10	Precursor cells	Binds to L-selectin
CD38	T10	T, B and NK cells and monocytes	Associates with hyaluronic acid
CD40	CD40	B cells and monocytes	Initiates isotype switching when ligated
CD45	Leukocyte common antigen, T200	All leukocytes	Tyrosine phosphatase that regulates lymphocyte activation; CD45R0 isoform on memory T cells, CD45RA isoform on naive T cells
CD56	NCAM; NKH-1	NK cells	Mediates NK homotypic adhesion
CD73	Ecto-5′-nucleotidase	T and B cells	Associates with AMP
CD127	IL-7Rα	T cells	Mediates IL-7 signaling
CD132	Common γ chain (γc)	T, B and NK cells	Mediates signaling by IL-2, IL-4, IL-7, IL-9, IL-15 and IL-21
CD154	CD40 ligand, gp39	Activated CD4+ T cells	Ligates CD40 on B cells and initiates isotype switching
CD278	ICOS	T cells	Interacts with B7-H2

22. **(a)** 6 hours

(Nelson Textbook of Pediatrics, 18th ed.)

Neutrophils	
Average time in mitosis (myeloblast to myelocyte)	7-9 days
Average time in postmitosis and storage (metamyelocyte to neutrophil)	3-7 days
Average half-life in the circulation	6 hours
Average total body pool	6.5 × 108 cells/kg
Average circulating pool	3.2 × 108 cells/kg
Average marginating pool	3.3 × 108 cells/kg
Average daily turnover rate	1.8 × 108 cells/kg

23. **(a)** 36–104 hours

(Nelson Textbook of Pediatrics, 18th ed.)

Mononuclear Phagocytes	
Average time in mitosis	30–48 hours
Average half-life in the circulation	36–104 hours
Average circulating pool (monocytes)	1.8 × 107 cells/kg
Average daily turnover rate	1.8 × 109 cells/kg
Average survival in tissues (macrophages)	Months

24. **(c)** Both

(Nelson Textbook of Pediatrics, 18th ed.)

The proliferation, differentiation, and survival of immature hematopoietic progenitor cells are governed by hematopoietic growth factors (HGFs), a family of glycoproteins. Besides regulating proliferation and differentiation of progenitors, these factors influence the survival and function of mature blood cells. The HGFs include the interleukins and the colony-stimulating factors (CSFs), which are named for their ability to stimulate progenitor cells to form colonies of recognizable mature cells in vitro.

25. **(a)** IL-3

(Nelson Textbook of Pediatrics, 18th ed.)

The majority of lineage-specific progenitors require the presence of additional growth factors such as interleukin 3 (IL-3) or granulocyte-macrophage CSF (GM-CSF) in addition to a lineage-specific HGF to generate the colonies for which they are programmed. Hence, immature committed progenitors bear receptors for IL-3, stem cell factor (SCF), GM-CSF, and IL-6.

26. **(c)** Bone eating macrophage

(Nelson Textbook of Pediatrics, 18th ed.)

Principal Sites of Macrophages in Tissues

- Liver (Kupffer cells)
- Lung (interstitial and alveolar macrophages)
- Connective tissue
- Serous cavities (pleural and peritoneal macrophages)
- Synovial membrane (type A synoviocytes)
- Bone (osteoclasts)
- Brain and retina (microglial cells)
- Spleen, lymph nodes, bone marrow
- Intestinal wall
- Breast milk
- Placenta
- Granuloma (multinucleated giant cells)

27. **(b)** Monocytes

(Nelson Textbook of Pediatrics, 18th ed.)

Monocytes, the circulating precursors of tissue macrophages, develop more rapidly in the bone marrow and remain longer in the circulation than do neutrophils.

28. **(c)** INF-gamma

(Nelson Textbook of Pediatrics, 18th ed.)

Classical activation is driven by specifically activated T-helper 1 (Th1)–type lymphocytes and natural killer cells through their release of interferon-γ (IFN-γ). Tumor necrosis factor–α (TNF-α) secreted by activated macrophages amplifies their activation, as does bacterial cell wall protein or endotoxin. Alternative activation is driven by T-helper 2 (Th2)–type lymphocytes through release of interleukin (IL)-4 and IL-13. These cytokines regulate antibody responses, allergy, and resistance to parasites. They can upregulate macrophage endocytosis, antigen presentation, and expression of certain chemo-attractant cytokines (chemokines) and intracellular enzymes.

29. **(c)** Chromosome 16

(Nelson Textbook of Pediatrics, 18th ed.)

Familial Mediterranean fever (FMF)	Autosomal recessive gene responsible for FMF on Chromosome 16, which encodes for a protein, called pyrin, that may modify neutrophil activation	Excessive accumulation of neutrophils at inflamed	Recurrent fever, peritonitis, pleuritis, sites arthritis, and amyloidosis

30. **(a)** Wiskott-Aldrich syndrome

(Nelson Textbook of Pediatrics, 18th ed.)

Causes of Eosinophilia

Allergic Disorders

- Allergic rhinitis
- Acute and chronic urticaria
- Hypersensitivity drug reactions
- Asthma
- Pemphigoid

Infectious Diseases

- Tissue-Invasive Helminth Infections
  - Trichinosis
  - Strongyloidosis
  - Filariasis
  - Echinococcosis
  - Toxocariasis
  - Ascariasis
  - Schistosomiasis
- Pneumocystis carinii
- Toxoplasmosis
- Amebiasis
- Malaria
- Bronchopulmonaryaspergillosis
- Coccidioidomycosis
- Scabies

Malignant Disorders

- Brain tumors
- Hodgkin disease and T-cell lymphoma
- Acute myelogenousleukemia
- Myeloproliferative disorders

Gastrointestinal Disorders

- Inflammatory bowel disease
- Eosinophilic gastroenteritis
- Chronic active hepatitis
- Peritoneal dialysis
- Milk precipitin disease

Rheumatologic Disease

- Rheumatoid arthritis
- Eosinophilic fascitis

Immunodeficiency Disease

- Hyper-IgE syndrome
- Wiskott-Aldrich syndrome
- Graft vs host reaction
- Omenn syndrome
- Pulmonary disease
- Löffler syndrome
- Eosinophilicleukemia Hypersensitivity pneumonia

Miscellaneous

- Thrombocytopenia with absent radii
- Vasculitis
- Postirradiation of abdomen
- Histiocytosis with cutaneous involvement

Chapter 26

Skin

1. **What is monthly scalp hair growth?**
   (a) 0.2 cm (b) 0.5 cm
   (c) 1 cm (d) 2 cm

2. **Type of hairs:**
   (a) Terminal (b) Lanugo
   (c) Vellus (d) All of the above

3. **At what intrauterine life lanugo hairs are replaced by vellus hairs?**
   (a) 32-34 weeks (b) 34-36 weeks
   (c) 36-40 weeks (d) 40-42 weeks

4. **Which is site for terminal hairs?**
   (a) Beard (b) Eyebrows
   (c) Pubic areas (d) All of the above

5. **What is name of hairs which are unpigmented and distributed all over body?**
   (a) Vellus hair (b) Terminal
   (c) Lanugo (d) None

6. **What is site of apocrine gland?**
   (a) Axillae (b) Areolae
   (c) Genital area (d) All of the above

7. **What is growth rate of the nail plate?**
   (a) 0.2 cm/3 months (b) 1cm/month
   (c) 1 cm/3 months (d) 0.5 cm/month

8. **What is a minimum Sun Protection factor required for most fair-skinned individuals to prevent sunburn?**
   (a) 5 (b) 10
   (c) 12 (d) 15

9. **Harlequin color change is commonly seen in:**
   (a) Low birth weight infants
   (b) Post term infants
   (c) Term infants
   (d) All neonates

10. **Sacral dimple is commonly seen in:**
    (a) Bloom syndrome
    (b) Smith-Lemli-Opitz syndrome
    (c) Spina bifida occulta
    (d) All of the above

11. **The limb-body wall complex involves:**
    (a) Exencephaly (b) Facial clefts
    (c) Limb defects (d) All of the above

12. **Branchio-otorenal dysplasia consists of:**
    (a) External ear malformations
    (b) Branchial fistulas
    (c) Renal anomalies
    (d) All of the above

13. **Setleis syndrome consists of:**
    (a) Leonine facies
    (b) Nasal bridge abnormalities
    (c) Low frontal hairline
    (d) All of the above

14. **Goltz syndrome consists of:**
    (a) Reticulated hypopigmentation
    (b) Congenital absence of skin
    (c) Syndactyly
    (d) All of the above

15. **Child syndrome consists of:**
    (a) Congenital hemidysplasia
    (b) Ichthyosiform erythroderma
    (c) Limb defects
    (d) All of the above

16. **Ephelid a light or dark brown macules having size:**
    (a) > 3 mm in diameter
    (b) < 3 mm in diameter
    (c) < 1 mm in diameter
    (d) > 1 mm in diameter

17. Lamb syndrome is characterised by:
(a) Lentigines of the face and vulva
(b) Atrial myxoma
(c) Blue nevi
(d) All of the above

18. Leopard syndrome is characterised by:
(a) Autosomal dominant
(b) Generalized, symmetric distribution of lentigines
(c) Sensorineural deafness
(d) All of the above

19. The Peutz-Jeghers syndrome is characterized by:
(a) Melanotic macules on the lips
(b) Gastrointestinal polyposis
(c) Autosomal dominant trait
(d) All of the above

20. What is most familiar cutaneous hallmark of neurofibromatosis Type 1 -Von Recklinghausen disease?
(a) Café-au-lait spot
(b) Xeroderma pigmentosa
(c) Shagreen patch
(d) All of the above

21. What are disorders associated with Café-au-Lait spots?
(a) McCune-Albright syndrome
(b) Fanconi anemia
(c) Gaucher disease
(d) All of the above

22. Hermansky-Pudlak syndrome is characterised by:
(a) Autosomal recessive
(b) Oculocutaneous albinism,
(c) Prolonged bleeding
(d) All of the above

23. Chédiak-Higashi syndrome is characterised by:
(a) Hypopigmentation of the skin
(b) Prolonged bleeding time
(c) Peripheral neuropathy
(d) All of the above

24. What is the hallmark of Waardenburg type 1?
(a) Vitiligo (b) Albinism
(c) White forelock (d) Leukoderma

25. Vogt-Koyanogi-Harada syndrome is associated with:
(a) Vitiligo (b) Uveitis
(c) Dysacusia (d) All of the above

26. What is the most common cause of sunburn?
(a) Infra red light (b) White light
(c) Ultraviolet B radiation (d) All of above

27. Cockayne syndrome is characterised by:
(a) Facial erythema in a butterfly distribution after sun exposure
(b) Dwarfism
(c) Mental retardation
(d) All of the above

28. Rothmund-Thomson syndrome is characterised by:
(a) Poikiloderma
(b) Autosomal recessive trait
(c) Hypogenitalism
(d) All of the above

29. What is inheritance pattern in Harlequin fetus?
(a) Autosomal recessive (b) Autosomal dominant
(c) X linked recessive (d) X linked dominant

30. Sjögren-Larsson syndrome is characterised by:
(a) Ichthyosis (b) Mental retardation
(c) Spasticity (d) All of the above

31. What is inheritance pattern of Netherton Syndrome?
(a) Autosomal recessive (b) Autosomal dominant
(c) X linked recessive (d) X linked dominant

32. Netherton syndrome is characterised by:
(a) Ichthyosis
(b) Trichorrhexis invaginata
(c) Atopic diathesis
(d) All of the above

33. What is inheritance pattern of Mal de Meleda?
(a) Autosomal dominant (b) Autosomal recessive
(c) X linked recessive (d) X linked dominant

34. Which drug causes of hyperhidrosis (increased production of eccrine sweat)?
(a) Meperidine (b) Emetics
(c) Antipyretics (d) All of the above

35. Wart is commonly caused by:
(a) Human papilloma virus (b) Herpes simplex virus
(c) H. ducrei (d) Syphilis

36. Acrodermatitis enteropathica is characterised by:
(a) Autosomal recessive
(b) Inability to absorb sufficient zinc from the diet
(c) Cutaneous eruption
(d) All of the above

Answers

1. **(c)** 1 cm
2. **(d)** All of the above
3. **(c)** 36–40 weeks
4. **(d)** All of the above
5. **(a)** Vellus hair
6. **(d)** All of the above
7. **(c)** 1 cm/3 months
8. **(d)** 15
9. **(a)** Low birth weight infants
10. **(d)** All of the above
11. **(d)** All of the above
12. **(d)** All of the above
13. **(d)** All of the above
14. **(d)** All of the above
15. **(d)** All of the above
16. **(b)** < 3 mm in diameter
17. **(d)** All of the above
18. **(d)** All of the above
19. **(d)** All of the above
20. **(a)** Café-au-lait spot
21. **(d)** All of the above
22. **(d)** All of the above
23. **(d)** All of the above
24. **(c)** White forelock
25. **(d)** All of the above
26. **(d)** All of the above
27. **(d)** All of the above
28. **(d)** All of the above
29. **(a)** Autosomal recessive
30. **(d)** All of the above
31. **(a)** Autosomal recessive
32. **(d)** All of the above
33. **(b)** Autosomal recessive
34. **(d)** All of the above
35. **(a)** Human papilloma virus
36. **(d)** All of the above

Chapter 27

Eye

1. **What is average size of cornea in newborn?**
   (a) 10 mm (b) 12mm
   (c) 14mm (d) 16mm

2. **At what age neonate achieves adult corneal size (12 mm)?**
   (a) 1 year (b) 2 years
   (c) 3 years (d) 4 years

3. **At what age chidren having eye with hyperopia?**
   (a) 7-9 years (b) Birth upto 7 years
   (c) 10-13 years (d) Above 13 years

4. **Upto what age the level of hyperopia tends to decreases?**
   (a) 14 years (b) 10 years
   (c) 9 years (d) 7 years

5. **What is approximate visual acuity in newborns?**
   (a) 6/6 (b) 20/400
   (c) 20/20 (d) 20/6

6. **Which is one of the earliest responses to a formed visual stimulus in an infant?**
   (a) Head turning towards light
   (b) Eye blinking
   (c) Infant's regard for the mother's face
   (d) None

7. **At what age normal infant can follow an object through an arc of 180 degrees?**
   (a) 8-10 weeks (b) 10-12 weeks
   (c) 14-16 weeks (d) 18-20 weeks

8. **At what age the visual acuity improves reaches 20/30-20/20?**
   (a) 6 months (b) 15 months
   (c) 18 months (d) 2-3 years

9. **At what age tears appears in babies eyes?**
   (a) 1 month (b) 1-3 months
   (c) 5-7 months (d) 7-9 months

10. **Which is a type of ametropia?**
    (a) Hyperopia (b) Myopia
    (c) Astigmatism (d) All of the above

11. **Cause of childhood severe visual impairment:**
    (a) Optic coloboma (b) Porencephaly
    (c) Optic glioma (d) All of the above

12. **Diplopia is seen in condition like:**
    (a) Increased intracranial pressure
    (b) Brain tumor
    (c) Orbital mass
    (d) All of the above

13. **Monocular diplopia is seen:**
    (a) Dislocation of the lens (b) Cataract
    (c) Defect in macula (d) All of the above

14. **Duane syndrome is characterized by:**
    (a) Retraction of the globe on adduction
    (b) Absence of the 6th nerve nucleus
    (c) Impairment of abduction
    (d) All of the above

15. **Mobius syndrome is characterized by:**
    (a) Congenital facial paresis
    (b) Abduction weakness
    (c) Bilateral
    (d) All of the above

16. **Parinaud syndrome is characterized by:**
    (a) Palsy of vertical gaze
    (b) 3rd cranial nerve paresis
    (c) Lesion of mesencephalic tegmentum
    (d) All of the above

17. Spasmus nutans is characterized by:
(a) Pendular nystagmus
(b) Head nodding
(c) Torticollis
(d) All of the above

18. Which is the first sign of neuroblastoma?
(a) Opsoclonus
(b) Headache
(c) Hearing defect
(d) Tingling

19. Allgrove syndrome is characterized by:
(a) Adrenocorticotropic hormone-resistant adrenal insufficiency
(b) Achalasia of the esophageal cardia
(c) Alacrima
(d) All of the above

20. Peters anomaly is characterized by:
(a) Leukoma
(b) Iridocorneal adhesions
(c) Microcornea
(d) All of the above

21. Cogan syndrome is characterized by:
(a) A nonluetic interstitial keratitis
(b) Hearing loss
(c) Vestibular symptoms
(d) All of the above

22. At what intrauterine age retinal angiogenesis normally proceeds from the optic disc to the outer rim of the retina nasally?
(a) 12 weeks (b) 40 weeks
(c) 36 weeks (d) 48 weeks

23. At what intrauterine age retinal angiogenesis normally proceeds from the optic disc to the outer rim of the retina to temporally?
(a) 12 weeks (b) 40 weeks
(c) 36 weeks (d) 48 weeks

24. Retinoblastoma manifests with:
(a) Leukocoria (b) Pseudohypopyon
(c) Hyphema (d) All of the above

25. Cherry red spot is observed in:
(a) Tay-Sachs disease
(b) Sandhoff variant (GM_2 type 2)
(c) Generalized gangliosidosis (GM_1 type 1)
(d) All of the above

26. Coats disease is characterized by:
(a) Telangiectasia of retinal vessels
(b) Leakage of plasma to form intraretinal and subretinal exudates
(c) Retinal hemorrhages and detachment
(d) All of the above

27. Infantile glaucoma is characterized by:
(a) Epiphora (b) Photophobia
(c) Blepharospasm (d) All of the above

Answers

1. **(a)** 10 mm
2. **(b)** 2 years
3. **(b)** Birth upto 7 years
4. **(a)** 14 years
5. **(b)** 20/400
6. **(c)** Infant's regard for the mother's face
7. **(a)** 8–10 weeks
8. **(d)** 2–3 years
9. **(b)** 1–3 months
10. **(d)** All of the above
11. **(d)** All of the above
12. **(d)** All of the above
13. **(d)** All of the above
14. **(d)** All of the above
15. **(d)** All of the above
16. **(d)** All of the above
17. **(d)** All of the above
18. **(a)** Opsoclonus
19. **(d)** All of the above
20. **(d)** All of the above
21. **(d)** All of the above
22. **(c)** 36 weeks
23. **(b)** 40 weeks
24. **(d)** All of the above
25. **(d)** All of the above
26. **(d)** All of the above
27. **(d)** All of the above

Chapter 28

Ear

1. **Purulent otorrhea is seen in conditions like:**
   (a) Otitis externa
   (b) Otitis media with perforation of the tympanic membrane
   (c) Drainage from a branchial cleft sinus
   (d) All of the above

2. **Bloody otorrhea is seen in conditions like:**
   (a) Trauma (b) Neoplasm
   (c) Blood dyscrasia (d) All of the above

3. **Clear otorrhea is seen in conditions like:**
   (a) Pyogenic meningitis
   (b) Cerebrospinal fluid leak from the middle ear
   (c) Head trauma
   (d) None

4. **Cause of congenital infectious pathogens implicated in sensorineural hearing loss in children:**
   (a) Cytomegalovirus
   (b) Rubella virus
   (c) Toxoplasma gondii
   (d) All of the above

5. **Cause of autosomal recessive genetic sensory neural hearing loss is:**
   (a) Usher syndrome
   (b) Pendred syndrome
   (c) Jervell and Lange-Nielsen syndrome
   (d) All of the above

6. **Condition associated with craniofacial abnormalities, conductive hearing loss and sensory neural hearing loss:**
   (a) Pierre Robin syndrome
   (b) Treacher Collins syndrome
   (c) Osteogenesis imperfecta
   (d) All of the above

7. **Drug causing sensory neural hearing loss includes:**
   (a) Aminoglycosides
   (b) Loop diuretics
   (c) Chemotherapeutic agents
   (d) All of the above

8. **Ramsay Hunt syndrome is characterized by:**
   (a) Herpes vesicles in the ear canal
   (b) Facial paralysis
   (c) Pain
   (d) All of the above

9. **Which is the preferred drug for uncomplicated acute otitis media?**
   (a) Azithromycin (b) Amoxicillin
   (c) Doxycycline (d) Cefixime

10. **Gradenigo syndrome is characterized by:**
    (a) Suppurative otitis media
    (b) Paralysis of the external rectus muscle
    (c) Pain in the ipsilateral orbit
    (d) All of the above

Answers

1. **(d)** All of the above
2. **(d)** All of the above
3. **(b)** Cerebrospinal fluid leak from the middle ear
4. **(d)** All of the above
5. **(d)** All of the above
6. **(d)** All of the above
7. **(d)** All of the above
8. **(d)** All of the above
9. **(b)** Amoxicillin
10. **(d)** All of the above

Chapter 29

Cancer and Benign Tumors

1. **Chromosome 11p-(deletion) with sporadic aniridia is associated with:**
(a) Wilm's tumor (b) Retinoblastoma
(c) Osteosarcoma (d) MEN I

2. **Chromosomal 13q-(deletion) is associated with:**
(a) Wilm's tumor (b) Retinoblastoma
(c) Osteosarcoma (d) MEN I

3. **Trisomy 21 is associated with:**
(a) Down's syndrome
(b) Turner's syndrome
(c) Noonan's syndrome
(d) Megakaryocytic leukemia

4. **Klinefelter syndrome (47, XXY) is associated with malignancy of:**
(a) Neck (b) Breast
(c) Thorax (d) Liver

5. **Noonan's syndrome is associated with malignancy of:**
(a) Atrial myxoma
(b) Carotid angioma
(c) Juvenile myelomonocytic leukemia
(d) Hepatoma

6. **Rothmund-Thompson syndrome is associated with malignancy of:**
(a) Osteosarcoma (b) Wilm's tumour
(c) Retinoblastoma (d) Pinealoblastoma

7. **Viruses have been implicated in the pathogenesis of malignancy:**
(a) Epstein-Barr virus
(b) Human papillomavirus
(c) Human herpesvirus 8
(d) All of the above

8. **Adverse reaction of methotrexate:**
(a) Myelosuppression (b) Stomatitis
(c) Hepatitis (d) All of the above

9. **Adverse reaction of 6-Mercaptopurine:**
(a) Myelosuppression (b) Hepatic necrosis
(c) Mucositis (d) All of the above

10. **Adverse reaction of cytarabine on intrathecal administration:**
(a) Arachnoiditis
(b) Leukoencephalopathy
(c) Leukomyelopathy
(d) All of the above

11. **Indication of cyclophosphamide (Cytoxan):**
(a) Non-Hodgkin lymphoma
(b) Hodgkin lymphoma
(c) Ewing sarcoma
(d) All of the above

12. **Indication of doxorubicin:**
(a) Osteosarcoma (b) Ewing sarcoma
(c) Neuroblastoma (d) All of the above

13. **Which is the most common malignant neoplasms in childhood?**
(a) Nervous tumours
(b) Haematological tumours
(c) Cardiovasular system
(d) None

14. **Which is the most common childhood leukemia?**
(a) Acute myeloblastic leukemia
(b) Neuroblastoma
(c) Acute lymphoblastic leukemia
(d) None

15. **Which is the hallmark of Hodgkin lymphoma?**
(a) Warthin cells
(b) Reed-Sternberg cell
(c) Lymphocytes
(d) Giant cells

16. **What is the characteristic feature of lymphadenopathy of Hodgkin lymphoma?**
(a) Painless (b) Non-tender
(c) Firm and rubbery (d) All of the above

17. **Which condition have an increased risk of Wilm's tumor?**
(a) Pearlman syndrome (b) Sotos syndrome
(c) von Willebrand disease (d) All of the above

18. **Beckwith-Wiedemann syndrome consists of:**
(a) Macroglossia (b) Omphalocele
(c) Hemihypertrophy (d) All of the above

19. **Most common age of occurrence of hepatoblastoma in children:**
(a) 1 year (b) < 3 years of age
(c) 5 years (d) 15 years

20. **Which is a valuable serum tumor marker in the diagnosis and monitoring of hepatic tumors?**
(a) LDH levels
(b) Alkaline phosphatase
(c) α-fetoprotein
(d) Thyroglobulin

Answers

1. **(a)** Wilm's tumor
2. **(b)** Retinoblastoma
3. **(d)** Megakaryocytic leukemia
4. **(b)** Breast
5. **(c)** Juvenile myelomonocytic leukemia
6. **(a)** Osteosarcoma
7. **(d)** All of the above
8. **(d)** All of the above
9. **(d)** All of the above
10. **(d)** All of the above
11. **(d)** All of the above
12. **(d)** All of the above
13. **(a)** Nervous tumours
14. **(c)** Acute lymphoblastic leukemia
15. **(b)** Reed-Sternberg cell
16. **(d)** All of the above
17. **(d)** All of the above
18. **(d)** All of the above
19. **(b)** $<$ 3 years of age
20. **(c)** α-fetoprotein

Chapter 30

National Programmes Related to Pediatrics

1. **Should one restart with 1st dose of a vaccine, if child is brought late for a dose?**
   (a) Yes, start the schedule again
   (b) Do not start the schedule again; pick up where schedule was left off
   (c) Don't give the vaccination at all if once missed
   (d) None of these

2. **Why is it not advisable to clean the injection site with spirit swab before vaccination?**
   (a) Child/baby may be allergic to it
   (b) Late immune reaction will occur
   (c) Live components of vaccine are killed in contact
   (d) All of the above

3. **Why should there be minimum gap of 4 weeks between 2 doses of DPT?**
   (a) Child may suffer from cold, fever etc
   (b) It may cause diarrhoea
   (c) Due to antibody products and protection
   (d) Due to pain at injection site

4. **Why 2nd dose of measles in national immunization programme is given?**
   (a) 1st dose is not so effective
   (b) Measles is highly infective disease
   (c) 1st dose is less in amount
   (d) None of the above

5. **Why give DPT vaccine in anterolateral mid thigh and not gluteal region?**
   (a) Prevent damage to sciatic nerve
   (b) Not effective in other region
   (c) Not invoke immune reponse on arm
   (d) Causes infection if given on other sites

6. **Why give measles vaccine only on right upper arm?**
   (a) Left arm will not evoke immune response
   (b) To maintain unifomity
   (c) To help surveyors in verifying the reciept of vaccine
   (d) Both (b) and (c)

7. **Why do we give 0.05 ml of dose of BCG to newborns?**
   (a) Large dose may be inflective
   (b) Skin of newborn is thin
   (c) More dose cause local abscess
   (d) Both (b) and (c)

8. **Which is the 1st country in the world to introduce ORS?**
   (a) America (b) Japan
   (c) India (d) Russia

9. **In which year RCH camps started?**
   (a) January 2001 (b) March 2005
   (c) June 2010 (d) May 2013

10. **Aim of RCH camp scheme:**
    (a) To provide medicines
    (b) To administer PHC's
    (c) To make available services of gynaeclogists and pediatrics available
    (d) None of these

11. **Which of the following is UNICEF assisted activity?**
    (a) NRHM (b) BDCS
    (c) RCH (d) CSSM

12. **DPT not give on gluteal region:**
    (a) Do not invoke immune response
    (b) Not given I.M.
    (c) Will cause reaction
    (d) None

13. If no scar appears affect administering BCG, should one revaccinate child?
(a) Yes, child may suffer from infections
(b) No there is no need
(c) Yes, child may suffer TB
(d) None of these

14. Birth of Hep. B vaccine is given within ________ hours of birth.
(a) 12 hours (b) 72 hours
(c) 48 hours (d) 24 hours

15. Why birth dose of Hep. B vaccine only within 24 hours of birth?
(a) To prevent perinatal transmission
(b) Later it may not be effective
(c) May not invoke immune response later
(d) None

16. Enlist minor reactions following vaccination:
(a) Mild fever (b) Redness
(c) Pain (d) All of these

17. In which year child survival and safe motherhood programme was launched?
(a) 1992 (b) 1990
(c) 2000 (d) 2005

18. RCH programme launched on:
(a) 15th October 1997 (b) 22nd August 1990
(c) 26 January 1998 (d) 2nd February 2000

19. RCH programme phase II began from:
(a) 2000 (b) 2005
(c) 1990 (d) None

20. Triage of sick newborns:
(a) Sorting of sick neonates
(b) Screening of sick neonates
(c) Sorting of sick neonates for management
(d) All of these

21. National worshop on pediatric TB under RNTCP held in:
(a) 2000 (b) 1990
(c) 2003 (d) 1999

22. Under national workshop on pediatrics TB, treatment is based on:
(a) Child's height
(b) Child's mid arm circumference
(c) Child's weight
(d) None

23. Pediatric PWBs (patient wise boxes) to treat TB is global 1st for RNTCP because:
(a) It was the national programme
(b) There was no such treatment earliest
(c) Has PWBs for pediatric TB
(d) None

24. National policy on pediatric ART (antiretroviral treatment) formed in:
(a) 2005 (b) 2006
(c) 2000 (d) 1998

25. "Learning for life" module is prepared for:
(a) Learning to know what is life
(b) Art of living
(c) School AIDS education programme
(d) None

26. Prevention of parent to child transmission (PPTCT) programme invokes:
(a) Testing of pregnant women
(b) Detection of positive pregnant women
(c) Administration of prophylactic neurapine to mother and infants
(d) All of them

27. PPTCT programme was started in:
(a) 2000 (b) 2005
(c) 2013 (d) 2001

28. NACO launched national pediatric initiatives on:
(a) 30th November 2006 (b) 21 February 2007
(c) 1st December 1998 (d) None of these

29. HIV exposed infant should be given:
(a) ARV prophylaxis (b) Early infant diagnosis
(c) PCP prohylaxis (d) All of these

30. Under school eye screening programme:
(a) Children are 1st screened by trained teacher
(b) Suspected children are seen by ophthalmic assistants
(c) Connective spectacles are prescribed
(d) All of these

31. EPI (expanded programme of immunization) renamed as universal child immunization in:
(a) 1985 (b) 1990
(c) 1974 (d) 2000

32. Government of India launched EPI in:
(a) 1978 (b) 1985
(c) 1974 (d) 2000

33. Universal immunization programme started in India in:
(a) 1978 (b) 1974
(c) 1985 (d) 1990

34. Pulse polio immunization programme started in:
(a) 1985 (b) 1978
(c) 1974 (d) 1995

35. Hepatitis B vaccine was introduced in national imunization schedule in:
(a) March 2000 (b) June 2002
(c) August 1998 (d) September 1999

36. Components of RCH programme includes:
(a) Child survival and safe motherhood
(b) Family planning
(c) Health care
(d) All of these

37. Major inerventions of RCH programme are:
(a) Essential obstetric care
(b) 24 hours delivery services
(c) Emergency obstetric care
(d) All of them

38. Major interventions under RCH II/ NRHM is:
(a) IMNCI (b) BDCS
(c) CSSM (d) None

39. Child's welfare ICDS scheme was prepared in:
(a) 1975 (b) 1977
(c) 1978 (d) 2000

40. Objectives of ICDS scheme are:
(a) To improve nutritional and health status of children
(b) To reduce mortality, morbidity, malnutritional and school drop out
(c) Child development
(d) All of these

41. National policy for children adopted in ________ by Government of India.
(a) 1978 (b) 1974
(c) 1998 (d) 2000

42. Integrated child protection scheme (ICPS) launched to all *except:*
(a) Safe and secure environment in country
(b) For children of migrant, prisoners, prostitutes, drug abusers
(c) For child beggers
(d) For reducing mortality rate

43. Emergency outreach services "child line" dedicated number is __________ under ICPS scheme.
(a) 2000 (b) 1098
(c) 1094 (d) None

Answers

1. **(b)** Do not start the schedule again; pick up where schedule was left off

   (Park, 22nd edition)

   For example: If child has received BCG, Hep B-1, DPT-1 and OPV-1 at 5 months and returns at 11 months, vaccinate the child with DPT-2, Hep B-2, OPV-2 and measles, do not start from DPT-1, Hep B-1 again.

2. **(c)** Live components of vaccine are killed in contact (Park, 22nd edition)

3. **(c)** Due to antibody products and protection

   (Park, 22nd edition)

   Bz reducing interval between 2 doses may not obtain antibody production for protection.

4. **(b)** Measles is highly infective disease

   (Park, 22nd edition)

   One dose of measles vaccine at 9 months of age protects 85% of infants, 2nd dose protects all children, measles highly infectious disease.

5. **(a)** Prevent damage to sciatic nerve

   (Park, 22nd edition)

   To prevent damage to sciatic nerve DPT, is given in anterolateral mid thigh.

6. **(d)** Both (b) and (c)

   (Park, 22nd edition)

   To maintain uniformity and due to this surveyors can also verify vaccine given.

7. **(d)** Both (b) and (c)

   (Park, 22nd edition)

8. **(c)** India

   (Park, 22nd edition)

   India is the 1st country to introduce low osmolality oral rehydration solution.

9. **(a)** January 2001

   (Park, 22nd edition)

   Scheme for holding camps have been initiated in 102 districts covering 17 states from January 2001.

10. **(c)** To make available services of gynaecologists and pediatrics available

    (Park, 22nd edition)

    In order to make services of specialists like gynaecologists and pediatrics available to people in remote areas, scheme for holding camps initiated.

11. **(b)** BDCS

    (Park, 22nd edition)

    Border district cluster, strategy (BDCS), selected for reducing infant mortality and maternal mortality, it is UNICEF assisted activity.

12. **(a)** Do not invoke immune response

    (Park, 22nd edition)

    DPT given in anterolateral midthigh to prevent damage to sciatic nerve and not on gluteal region Bz not invoke immune response.

13. **(b)** No there is no need

    There is no need to revaccinate even if no scar appears. (Park, 22nd edition)

14. **(d)** 24 hours

    (Park, 22nd edition)

    Birth dose of Hep B+ve vaccine is effective in preventing perinatal transmission of Hep B, if given within 24 hours.

15. **(a)** To prevent perinatal transmission

    (Park, 22nd edition)

    Birth dose of Hep B+ve vaccine is effective in preventing perinatal transmission of Hep B, if given within 24 hours.

16. **(d)** All of these

    (Park, 22nd edition)

    Mild fever of 3 days, redness, pain are minor reactions may occur following vaccinations.

17. **(a)** 1992

    (Park, 22nd edition)

18. **(a)** 15th October 1997

    (Park, 22nd edition)

19. **(b)** 2005

(Park, 22nd edition)

20. **(d)** All of these

(Park, 22nd edition)

Triage of sick newborn is sorting and screening neonates for management of them.

21. **(c)** 2003

Treatment under national workshop on pediatrics TB is based on child's body weight and this is to be global 1st for RNCTP as the world has such PWB's for treatment of children TB.

22. **(c)** Child's weight

Treatment under national workshop on pediatrics TB is based on child's body weight and this is to be global 1st for RNCTP as the world has such PWB's for treatment of children TB.

23. **(c)** Has PWBs for pediatric TB

Treatment under national workshop on pediatrics TB is based on child's body weight and this is to be global 1st for RNCTP as no other dots programme in world has such PWB's for treatment of children TB.

24. **(b)** 2006

(Park, 22nd edition)

25. **(c)** School AIDS education programme

26. **(b)** Detection of positive pregnant women

(Park, 22nd edition)

27. **(d)** 2001

(Park, 22nd edition)

28. **(a)** 30th November 2006

(Park, 22nd edition, Pg 405)

29. **(d)** All of these

(Park, 22nd edition)

30. **(d)** All of these

(Park, 22nd edition, Pg 407)

31. **(a)** 1985

(Park, 22nd edition, Pg 408)

32. **(a)** 1978

(Park, 22nd edition, Pg 408)

33. **(c)** 1985

34. **(d)** 1995

(Park, 22nd edition, Pg 409)

35. **(b)** June 2002

(Park, 22nd edition, Pg 109)

36. **(d)** All of these

(Park, 22nd edition, Pg 415)

37. **(a)** All of them

(Park, 22nd edition, Pg 416)

38. **(a)** IMNCI

(Park, 22nd edition, Pg 424)

39. **(a)** 1975

(Park, 22nd edition, Pg 546)

40. **(a)** All of these

(Park, 22nd edition, Pg 546)

41. **(b)** 1974

(Park, 22nd edition, Pg 546)

42. **(d)** For reducing mortality rate

(Park, 22nd edition, Pg 546)

43. **(b)** 1098

It is 24 hours toll free telephone service is available to all children in distress.

Chapter 31

Infestations in Children

1. **Growing pain is common in children between _________ of age:**
   (a) 1and 2 years (b) 2 and 4 years
   (c) 4 and 8 years (d) 10 and 12 years

2. **Erythema nodosum is the first manifestation of:**
   (a) Inflammatory bowel disease
   (b) Sarcoidosis
   (c) Spondyloarthropathy
   (d) All of the above

3. **Erythema nodosum develop after exposure to:**
   (a) Sulfonamides (b) Phenytoin
   (c) Oral contraceptive agent (d) All of the above

4. **Virus associated with arthritis:**
   (a) Rubella (b) Parvovirus
   (c) Cytomegalovirus (d) All of the above

5. **Crest syndrome refers to the manifestations of:**
   (a) Calcinosis
   (b) Raynaud phenomenon
   (c) Sclerodactyly
   (d) All of the above

6. **Papa syndrome consists of:**
   (a) Pyogenic arthritis
   (b) Pyoderma gangrenosum
   (c) Acne
   (d) All of the above

7. **Blau syndrome is characterized by:**
   (a) Granulomatous arthritis
   (b) Uveitis
   (c) Flexion contractures at the fingers
   (d) All of the above

8. **What is a hallmark of all mycobacteria?**
   (a) Acid fastness (b) Rod shape
   (c) Gram staining (d) Droplet infection

9. **Newborns tuberculin skin test become positive at:**
   (a) 1-3 months (b) 3-6 months
   (c) 6-8 months (d) 8-12 months

10. **What is adverse reaction of ethambutol?**
    (a) Optic neuritis (b) Liver failure
    (c) Nephritis (d) CCF

11. **Manifestations of congenital syphilis:**
    (a) Olympian brow (b) Saber shins
    (c) Hutchinson teeth (d) All of the above

12. **Drug of choice for congenital syphilis:**
    (a) Tetracycline
    (b) Gentamycin
    (c) Cefixime
    (d) Crystalline penicillin G

13. **Which is the natural hosts, reservoirs and vectors of R. rickettsii?**
    (a) Mice (b) Mosquitos
    (c) Ticks (d) Lice

14. **Complications of amebic colitis includes:**
    (a) Necrotizing colitis
    (b) Ameboma
    (c) Toxic megacolon
    (d) All of the above

15. **Drug of choice treatment for amebiasis:**
    (a) Chloramphenicol (b) Metronidazole
    (c) Erythromycin (d) Ceftriaxone

Answers

1. **(c)** 4 and 8 years
2. **(d)** All of the above
3. **(d)** All of the above
4. **(d)** All of the above

Viruses Associated with Arthritis

• Togaviruses
• Rubivirus
• Rubella
• Alphaviruses
• Ross River
• Chikungunya
• O'nyong-nyong
• Mayaro
• Sindbis
• Ockelbo
• Pogosta
• Parvovirus
• B_{19}
• Hepadnavirus
• Hepatitis B
• Adenoviruses
• Adenovirus 7
• Herpesviruses
• Herpes simplex
• Cytomegalovirus
• Epstein-Barr
• Varicella-zoster
• Paramyxoviruses
• Mumps
• Enteroviruses
• Echovirus
• Coxsackievirus B
• Orthopoxviruses
• Variola virus (smallpox)
• Vaccinia virus

5. **(d)** All of the above
6. **(d)** All of the above
7. **(d)** All of the above
8. **(a)** Acid fastness
9. **(a)** 1–3 months
10. **(a)** Optic neuritis
11. **(d)** All of the above
12. **(d)** Crystalline penicillin G
13. **(c)** Ticks
14. **(d)** All of the above
15. **(b)** Metronidazole

Chapter 32

Anatomy and Embryology

1. **Adenohypophysis develops from:**
   (a) Endoderm (b) Mesoderm
   (c) Neural crest cell (d) Oral ectoderm

2. **Craniopharyngiomas arise from remnant of:**
   (a) Connection between oropharynx and Rathke's pouch
   (b) From hypothalamus
   (c) From median eminence
   (d) From neurohypophysis

3. **Which factor is necessary for the differentiation into testis?**
   (a) SRY factor (b) DAX1
   (c) WNT4 (d) FOXL2

4. **The central tendon of the diaphragm develops from:**
   (a) Pleura-peritoneal membranes
   (b) Septum transversum
   (c) Oesophageal mesentery
   (d) Intercostal muscles

5. **The major bronchi and terminal bronchi are formed in which of the following phases of lung development?**
   (a) Canalicular phase
   (b) Pseudoglandular phase
   (c) Saccular phase
   (d) Alveolar phase

6. **The umbilical cord contains all *except:***
   (a) 2 arteries, 1 vein (b) Allantois
   (c) 2 veins, 1 artery (d) Wharton jelly

7. **The anatomical closure of the umbilical vessels occurs at:**
   (a) 2-3 days (b) 5-7 days
   (c) 8-10 days (d) 10-15 days

8. **A persistent urachus is due to the failure of closure of:**
   (a) Vitelline duct
   (b) Mullerian duct
   (c) Allantoic duct
   (d) Omphalomesenteric duct

9. **Gut rotation and attachment is completed by:**
   (a) 2 months of gestation
   (b) 3 months of gestation
   (c) 4 months of gestation
   (d) 5 months of gestation

10. **During intestinal rotation, the caecum rotates**
    (a) Clockwise (b) Counterclockwise
    (c) Towards right (d) Towards left

11. **Which of the following acts an axis for the bowel rotation?**
    (a) Celiac trunk
    (b) Superior mesenteric artery
    (c) Inferior mesenteric artery
    (d) Abdominal aorta

12. **In the most common type of malrotation the caecum is found at:**
    (a) Subhepatic area
    (b) Subphrenic area
    (c) Right lower quadrant
    (d) Left lower quadrant

13. **The most common form of duodenal atresia is:**
    (a) Fibrous cord connecting 2 blind duodenal pouches
    (b) Gap between non connecting ends of the duodenum
    (c) Intact membrane obstructing the lumen
    (d) Windsock web variety

14. Duodenal atresia is most commonly associated with:
(a) Congenital heart diseases
(b) Malrotaion
(c) Anorectal and renal anomalies
(d) Oesophageal atresia

15. Which one among the following statements is true regarding gastric duplications?
(a) Extrinsic defect along the greater curvature of stomach
(b) Usually communicate with the lumen
(c) Usually do not communicate with the lumen
(d) Result due to the failure of solid stage of development of intestine

16. The calcification of primary teeth begins at:
(a) 1-2 months (b) 2-3 months
(c) 3-4 months (d) 4-5 months

17. The enamel of the teeth is derived from:
(a) Ectoderm (b) Endoderm
(c) Mesoderm (d) Neural crest cells

18. Twinning phenomenon is most commonly noticed in:
(a) Maxillary incisors (b) Mandibular incisors
(c) Maxillary molars (d) Mandibular molars

19. Concrescence, seen as an anomaly of dentition is:
(a) Joining of incompletely formed teeth
(b) Bifid crown with a single tooth
(c) Attachment of roots of adjacent teeth
(d) Absence of teeth

20. The first evidence of primary dentition in the maxilla and the mandible is seen by:
(a) 8 weeks of intrauterine life
(b) 10 weeks of intrauterine life
(c) 12 weeks of intrauterine life
(d) 14 weeks of intrauterine life

21. The hepatic lobules are identifiable by:
(a) 6th week of gestation (b) 7th week of gestation
(c) 8th week of gestation (d) 10th week of gestation

22. The canalization of the cystic duct is fully completed by:
(a) 2-3 weeks of gestation
(b) 4-5 weeks of gestation
(c) 6-7 weeks of gestation
(d) 7-8 weeks of gestation

23. The paired cardiac tubes are formed by:
(a) 10 days of gestation
(b) 12 days of gestation
(c) 14 days of gestation
(d) 18 days of gestation

24. The developing left ventricle expresses which of the following transcription molecules?
(a) dHAND (b) eHAND
(c) hHAND (d) fHAND

25. The embryonic sinus venosus represents the future:
(a) Right atria (b) Left atria
(c) Both (d) None

26. The septation of the atria begin at:
(a) 10 days (b) 22 days
(c) 26 days (d) 30 days

27. The dorsal aortae in the embryo fuse to form:
(a) Aortic arch (b) Ascending aorta
(c) Descending aorta (d) Brachiocephalic trunk

28. The 3rd aortic arch participates in the formation of:
(a) Maxillary artery
(b) Hyoid artery
(c) Common and external carotid arteries
(d) Common and internal carotid arteries

29. Atrial natriuretic peptide and is expressed by all *except:*
(a) Mature ventricular myocytes
(b) Immature ventricular myocytes
(c) Mature atrial myocytes
(d) Immature atrial myocytes

30. All the following molecules play a role in cardiac differentiation *except:*
(a) MLC (b) GATA-4
(c) MEF2 (d) Nkx

31. Holt Oram syndrome is characterized by all *except:*
(a) Absent radii (b) ASD
(c) VSD (d) 1st degree heart block

32. Mesoblastic haematopoeisis begins by:
(a) 4 days of intrauterine life
(b) 10 days of intrauterine life
(c) 20 days of intrauterine life
(d) 30 days of intrauterine life

33. The liver replaces the yolk sac as the primary site of blood cell production by:
(a) 2-4 weeks of gestation
(b) 4-6 weeks of gestation
(c) 6-8 weeks of gestation
(d) 8-10 weeks of gestation

34. The mean corpuscular volume in the embryo is:
(a) > 100 fl (b) > 140 fl
(c) > 160 fl (d) > 180 fl

35. The splenic precursor is first identifiable at:
(a) 5th week of gestation (b) 6th week of gestation
(c) 7th week of gestation (d) 8th week of gestation

36. At birth the spleen weighs:
(a) 10 grams (b) 20 grams
(c) 30 grams (d) 40 grams

37. The red pulp of the spleen consists of all the following components *except:*
(a) Cords of billroth (b) B cells
(c) Macrophages (d) Reticular cells

38. Congenital absence of spleen is associated with all *except:*
(a) Cyanotic heart disease (b) Malrotation of gut
(c) Dextrocardia (d) Trilobed lungs

39. The protein content of lymph is same as:
(a) Transudate
(b) Exudates
(c) Plasma
(d) Between transudate and exudates

40. The kidney is derived from:
(a) Only mesonephros
(b) Only metanephros
(c) Only ureteral bud
(d) Both ureteral bud and metanephros

41. The collecting system of the kidney is formed by:
(a) 20 weeks of gestation (b) 30 weeks of gestation
(c) 40 weeks of gestation (d) 45 weeks of gestation

42. The nephron differentiation begins by:
(a) 5th week of gestation (b) 6th week of gestation
(c) 7th week of gestation (d) 8th week of gestation

43. Defect of the Wolffian duct development leads to:
(a) Renal agenesis (b) Renal aplasia
(c) Renal dysplasia (d) Renal cystic disease

44. The Mayer-Rokitansky-Hauser-Kuster syndrome is characterized by all *except:*
(a) Unilateral renal ectopia
(b) Unilateral renal dysplasia
(c) Mullerian duct abnormalities
(d) Vaginal agenesis

45. The testis develop by:
(a) 4-5 weeks of gestation
(b) 5-6 weeks of gestation
(c) 7-8 weeks of gestation
(d) 9-10 weeks of gestation

46. The testicular descent is regulated by all the following factors *except:*
(a) Mullerian inhibiting factor
(b) Gubernaculum
(c) Abdominal pressure
(d) Processes vaginalis

47. Histologically, the undescended testis are:
(a) Normal at birth
(b) Show hyalinization of seminiferous tubules
(c) Reduced germ cell number
(d) Reduced number of leydig cells

48. T3 and T4 synthesis and secretion begins at:
(a) 10th week of gestation
(b) 12th week of gestation
(c) 14th week of gestation
(d) 16th week of gestation

49. Anatomically the pituitary is:
(a) Intradural
(b) Extradural
(c) Subdural
(d) Subarachnoidal and in contact with CSF

50. The pituitary is supplied by:
(a) Internal carotid artery
(b) External carotid artery
(c) Ophthalmic artery
(d) Middle meningeal artery

Answers

1. **(d)** Oral ectoderm

(Nelson, Textbook of Pediatrics, 18th ed.)

The anterior pituitary gland originates from the Rathke's pouch as an invagination of the oral ectoderm. It then detaches from the oral epithelium and becomes an individual structure of rapidly proliferating cells. By 6 weeks gestation, the connection between the Rathke's pouch and the oropharynx is completely obliterated and the pouch establishes a direct connection with the downward extension of the hypothalamus, which gives rise to the pituitary stalk.

2. **(a)** Connection between oropharynx and Rathke's pouch

(Nelson, Textbook of Pediatrics, 18th ed.)

Persistent remnants of the original connection between the Rathke's pouch and the oral cavity can develop into **craniopharyngiomas,** the most common type of tumor in this area.

3. **(a)** SRY factor

(Nelson, 18th ed.)

The undifferentiated, bipotential fetal gonad arises from a thickening of the urogenital ridge, close to the region that forms the kidney and adrenal cortex. At 6 weeks of gestation, the gonad contains germ cells—stromal cells that will become Leydig cells in testes, or theca, interstitial or hilar cells in the ovary, and supporting cells that will develop into Sertoli cells in testes or granulosa cells in ovaries. In the absence of a testis-determining factor, thought to be the SRY (sex-determining region on the Y chromosome), the gonad develops into an ovary. SRY is thought to normally suppress a putative factor 2 (not yet identified) that functions as repressor of male development.

4. **(b)** Septum transversum

(Nelson, 18th ed.)

The septum transversum gives rise to the central tendon and separates the pericardial and peritoneal cavities. The central tendon constitutes 30% of the diaphragm and is the largest portion. The pleuroperitoneal membranes give rise to the dorsal lateral portions of the diaphragm; this separates the paired pleural cavities and the "fetal diaphragm" at approximately 8 weeks gestation. The esophageal mesentery forms the dorsal crura and the intercostal muscle groups give rise to the muscular portion of the diaphragm. CDH may be due to defective formation of the pleuroperitoneal membrane. When the abdominal contents return to the abdomen from the umbilical sac at 10 weeks gestation, herniation of the abdominal contents may occur.

5. **(b)** Pseudoglandular phase

(Nelson, 18th ed.)

The *pseudoglandular* phase begins at the 5th week with lung bud formation and ends at the 16–17th week of gestation. During this stage, the major bronchi and terminal bronchi are formed. The next stage is the *canalicular* stage, characterized by the development of the respiratory bronchioles, alveolar ducts, and pulmonary vessels from week 16 to 24–25. Initial alveolar or terminal sac development occurs during the *saccular* phase (24 week term). Gas exchange is now possible. After delivery, alveoli continue to develop until approximately 8 years of life. The stage is appropriately termed the *alveolar* stage. Lung hypoplasia was initially thought to be solely due to the compression of the lung from the herniated abdominal contents, which impaired lung growth. Pulmonary hypoplasia may occur, however, early in embryonic development, before the defect.

6. **(c)** 2 veins, 1 artery

(Nelson, 18th ed.)

The cord contains the two umbilical arteries, the vein, the rudimentary allantois, the remnant of the omphalomesenteric duct, and a gelatinous substance called Wharton jelly. The sheath of the umbilical cord is derived from the amnion. The muscular umbilical arteries contract readily, but the vein does not. The vein retains a fairly large lumen after birth. The normal cord at term is 55 cm long.

7. **(d)** 10-15 days

(Nelson, 18th ed.)

The blood vessels are functionally closed, but anatomically patent for 10–20 days.

8. **(c)** Allantoic duct

(Nelson, 18th ed.)

A persistent urachus (urachal cyst, sinus, patent urachus, or diverticulum) is due to failure of closure of the allantoic duct and is associated with bladder outlet obstruction.

9. **(b)** 3 months of gestation

(Nelson, 18th ed.)

Malrotation is incomplete rotation of the intestine during fetal development. The gut starts as a straight tube from stomach to rectum. The mid bowel (distal duodenum to mid-transverse colon) begins to elongate and progressively protrudes into the umbilical cord until it lies totally outside the confines of the abdominal cavity. As the developing bowel rotates in and out of the abdominal cavity, the superior mesenteric artery, which supplies blood to this section of gut, acts as an axis. The duodenum, on re-entering the abdominal cavity, moves to the region of the ligament of Treitz, and the colon that follows is directed to the left upper quadrant. The cecum subsequently rotates counterclockwise within the abdominal cavity and comes to lie in the right lower quadrant. The duodenum becomes fixed to the posterior abdominal wall before the colon is completely rotated. After rotation, the right and left colon and the mesenteric root become fixed to the posterior abdomen. These attachments provide a broad base of support to the mesentery and the superior mesenteric artery, thus preventing twisting of the mesenteric root and kinking of the vascular supply. Abdominal rotation and attachment are completed by 3 months of gestation.

10. **(b)** Counterclockwise

(Nelson, 18th ed.)

Malrotation is incomplete rotation of the intestine during fetal development. The gut starts as a straight tube from stomach to rectum. The mid bowel (distal duodenum to mid-transverse colon) begins to elongate and progressively protrudes into the umbilical cord until it lies totally outside the confines of the abdominal cavity. As the developing bowel rotates in and out of the abdominal cavity, the superior mesenteric artery, which supplies blood to this section of gut, acts as an axis. The duodenum, on re-entering the abdominal cavity, moves to the region of the ligament of Treitz, and the colon that follows is directed to the left upper quadrant. The cecum subsequently rotates counterclockwise within the abdominal cavity and comes to lie in the right lower quadrant. The duodenum becomes fixed to the posterior abdominal wall before the colon is completely rotated. After rotation, the right and left colon and the mesenteric root become fixed to the posterior abdomen. These attachments provide a broad base of support to the mesentery and the superior mesenteric artery, thus preventing twisting of the mesenteric root and kinking of the vascular supply. Abdominal rotation and attachment are completed by 3 months of gestation.

11. **(c)** Inferior mesenteric artery

(Nelson, 18th ed.)

Malrotation is incomplete rotation of the intestine during fetal development. The gut starts as a straight tube from stomach to rectum. The mid bowel (distal duodenum to mid-transverse colon) begins to elongate and progressively protrudes into the umbilical cord until it lies totally outside the confines of the abdominal cavity. As the developing bowel rotates in and out of the abdominal cavity, the superior mesenteric artery, which supplies blood to this section of gut, acts as an axis. The duodenum, on re-entering the abdominal cavity, moves to the region of the ligament of Treitz, and the colon that follows is directed to the left upper quadrant. The cecum subsequently rotates counterclockwise within the abdominal cavity and comes to lie in the right lower quadrant. The duodenum becomes fixed to the posterior abdominal wall before the colon is completely rotated. After rotation, the right and left colon and the mesenteric root become fixed to the posterior abdomen. These attachments provide a broad base of support to the mesentery and the superior mesenteric artery, thus preventing twisting of the mesenteric root and kinking of the vascular supply. Abdominal rotation and attachment are completed by 3 months of gestation.

12. **(a)** Subhepatic area

(Nelson, 18th ed.)

The most common type of malrotation involves failure of the cecum to move into the right lower quadrant. The usual location of the cecum is in the subhepatic area. Failure of the cecum to rotate properly is associated with failure to form the normal broad-based adherence to the posterior abdominal wall.

13. **(c)** Intact membrane obstructing the lumen

(Nelson, 18th ed.)

Duodenal atresia is thought to arise from failure to recanalize the lumen after the solid phase of intestinal development in the 4th and 5th week of gestation. The incidence of duodenal atresia is 1/10,000 births and accounts for 25–40% of all intestinal atresias. Half the patients are born prematurely. Duodenal atresia can take several forms, including an intact membrane obstructing the lumen, a short fibrous cord connecting two blind duodenal pouches, or a gap between the nonconnecting ends of the duodenum.

An unusual cause of obstruction is a "windsock" web, which is a distensible flap of tissue associated with anomalies of the biliary tract. The membranous form of atresia is most common, with obstruction occurring distal to the ampulla of Vater in the majority of patients

14. **(b)** Malrotaion

(Nelson, 18th ed.)

Congenital anomalies that are associated with duodenal atresia include malrotation (20%), esophageal atresia (10–20%), congenital heart disease (10–15%), and anorectal and renal anomalies (5%).

15. **(c)** Usually do not communicate with the lumen

(Nelson, 18th ed.)

Gastric duplications are uncommon cystic or tubular structures that usually occur within the wall of the stomach. Most are smaller than 12 cm in diameter and do not usually communicate with the stomach lumen. Associated anomalies occur in as many as 35% of patients. Duplications have been attributed to a failure of recanalization after the solid stage of intestinal development.

The most common clinical manifestations are associated with partial or complete gastric outlet obstruction. In 33% of patients, the cyst may be palpable. Communicating duplications may cause gastric ulceration and be associated with hematemesis or melena.

Gastric duplications are visualized on upper gastrointestinal series as an extrinsic defect usually located along the lesser curve of the stomach. CT or ultrasonography may be helpful in defining a cystic structure. Surgical excision is the treatment for symptomatic gastric duplications.

16. **(c)** 3-4 months

(Nelson, 18th ed.)

Calcification of primary teeth begins at 3–4 months in utero and concludes postnatally at ≈ 12 months with mineralization of the 2nd primary molars.

17. **(a)** Ectoderm

(Nelson, 18th ed.)

As the epithelial bud proliferates, the deeper surface invaginates and a mass of mesenchyme becomes partially enclosed. The epithelial cells differentiate into the ameloblasts that lay down an organic matrix that forms enamel; the mesenchyme forms the dentin and dental pulp.

18. **(b)** Mandibular incisors

Twinning, in which two teeth are joined together, is most often observed in the mandibular incisors of the primary dentition. It can result from gemination, fusion, or concrescence. **Gemination** is the result of the division of one tooth germ to form a bifid crown on a single root with a common pulp canal; an extra tooth appears to be present in the dental arch. **Fusion** is the joining of incompletely developed teeth that, owing to pressure, trauma, or crowding, continue to develop as one tooth. Fused teeth are sometimes joined along their entire length; in other cases, a single wide crown is supported on two roots. **Concrescence** is the attachment of the roots of closely approximated adjacent teeth by an excessive deposit of cementum. This type of twinning, unlike the others, is found most often in the maxillary molar region.

19. **(c)** Attachment of roots of adjacent teeth

(Nelson, 18th ed.)

Twinning, in which two teeth are joined together, is most often observed in the mandibular incisors of the primary dentition. It can result from gemination, fusion, or concrescence. **Gemination** is the result of the division of one tooth germ to form a bifid crown on a single root with a common pulp canal; an extra tooth appears to be present in the dental arch. **Fusion** is the joining of incompletely developed teeth that, owing to pressure, trauma, or crowding, continue to develop as one tooth. Fused teeth are sometimes joined along their entire length; in other cases, a single wide crown is supported on two roots. **Concrescence** is the attachment of the roots of closely approximated adjacent teeth by an excessive deposit of cementum. This type of twinning, unlike the others, is found most often in the maxillary molar region.

20. **(c)** 12 weeks of intrauterine life

(Nelson, 18th ed.)

The primary teeth form in dental crypts that arise from a band of epithelial cells incorporated into each developing jaw. By 12 weeks of fetal life, each of these epithelial bands **(dental laminae)** has five areas of rapid growth on each side of the maxilla and the mandible, seen as rounded, budlike enlargements. Organization of adjacent mesenchyme takes place in each area of epithelial growth, and the two elements together are the beginning of a tooth.

21. **(a)** 6th week of gestation

(Nelson, 18th ed.)

Within the ventral mesentery, proliferation of migrating cells forms anastomosing hepatic cords, with the network of primitive liver cells, sinusoids, and septal mesenchyme establishing the basic architectural pattern of liver lobule. The solid *cranial* portion of the hepatic diverticulum (pars hepatis) eventually forms the hepatic parenchyma and the intrahepatic bile ducts; the *caudal* portion (pars cystica) becomes the gallbladder, cystic duct, and common bile duct. The hepatic lobules are identifiable in the 6th human gestational week. The bile canalicular structures that include microvilli and junctional complexes are specialized loci of the liver cell membrane; these appear very early in gestation, and by 6–7 weeks, large canaliculi bounded by several hepatocytes are seen. The intrahepatic bile ducts are derived through branching and remodeling of the hepatic duct; formation is complete by the 3rd mo. The cystic duct and the gallbladder are fully recanalized by the 7th–8th week.

22. **(d)** 7-8 weeks of gestation

(Nelson, 18th ed.)

The cystic duct and the gallbladder are fully recanalized by the 7th–8th week.

23. **(d)** 18 days of gestation

(Nelson, 18th ed.)

In the early presomite embryo, the 1st identifiable cardiac precursors are angiogenetic cell clusters arranged on both sides of the embryo's central axis; these clusters form paired cardiac tubes by 18 days of gestation.

24. **(b)** eHAND

(Nelson, 18th ed.)

Chamber-specific transcription factors participate in the differentiation of the right and left ventricles. The basic helix-loop-helix transcription factor dHAND is expressed in the developing right ventricle; disruption of this gene or of other transcriptional factors such as myocyte enhancer factors 2C (MEF2C) in mice leads to hypoplasia of the right ventricle. The transcription factor eHAND is expressed in the developing left ventricle and conotruncus and is also critical to their development.

25. **(c)** Both

(Nelson, 18th ed.)

As early as 20–22 days, before cardiac looping, the embryonic heart begins to contract and exhibit phases of the cardiac cycle that are surprisingly similar to those in a mature heart. Morphologists have identified segments of the heart tube that were believed to correspond to structures in a mature heart: the sinus venosus and atrium (right and left atria), the primitive ventricle (left ventricle), the bulbus cordis (right ventricle), and the truncus arteriosus (aorta and pulmonary artery).

26. **(d)** 30 days

(Nelson, 18th ed.)

Septation of the atria begins at ≈ 30 days with growth of the septum primum downward toward the endocardial cushions. The orifice that remains is the ostium primum. The endocardial cushions then fuse and, together with the completed septum primum, divide the atrioventricular canal into right and left segments. A 2nd opening appears in the posterior portion of the septum primum, the ostium secundum, and it allows a portion of the fetal venous return to the right atrium to pass across to the left atrium. Finally, the septum secundum grows downward, just to the right of the septum primum. Together with a flap of the septum primum, the ostium secundum forms the foramen ovale, through which fetal blood passes from the inferior vena cava to the left atrium.

27. **(c)** Descending aorta

(Nelson, 18th ed.)

The aortic arch, head and neck vessels, proximal pulmonary arteries, and ductus arteriosus develop from the aortic sac, arterial arches, and dorsal aortae. When the straight heart tube develops, the distal outflow portion bifurcates into the right and left 1st aortic arches, which join the paired dorsal aortae. The dorsal aortae will fuse to form the descending aorta.

28. **(d)** Common and internal carotid arteries

(Nelson, 18th ed.)

1st aortic arch giving rise to the maxillary artery and the 2nd to the stapedial and hyoid arteries. The 3rd arches participate in the formation of the innominate artery and the common and internal carotid arteries. The right 4th arch gives rise to the innominate and right subclavian arteries, and the left 4th arch participates in formation of the segment of the aortic arch between the left carotid artery and the ductus arteriosus. The 5th arch does not persist as a major structure in the mature circulation. The 6th arches join the more distal pulmonary arteries, with the right 6th arch giving rise to a portion of the proximal right pulmonary artery and the left 6th arch giving rise to the ductus arteriosus.

29. **(a)** Mature ventricular myocytes

(Nelson, 18th ed.)

Developmental processes are chamber specific. Early in development, ventricular myocytes express both ventricular and atrial isoforms of several proteins, such as atrial natriuretic peptide (ANP) and myosin light chain (MLC). Mature ventricular myocytes do not express ANP and express only a ventricular-specific MLC 2v isoform, whereas mature atrial myocytes express ANP and an atrial-specific MLC 2a isoform.

30. **(a)** MLC

(Nelson, 18th ed.)

Signaling molecules interact with receptors on the cell surface; these receptors activate 2nd messengers, which, in turn, activate specific nuclear transcription factors (GATA-4, MEF2, Nkx, bHLH, and the retinoic acid receptor family) that induce the expression of specific gene products to regulate cardiac differentiation. Some of the primary disorders of cardiac muscle, the **cardiomyopathies,** may be related to defects in some of these signaling molecules.

31. **(c)** VSD

(Nelson, 18th ed.)

1st degree heart block

The majority of cases of ASD are sporadic; autosomal dominant inheritance does occur as part of the Holt-Oram syndrome (hypoplastic or absent radii, 1st degree heart block, ASD) or in families with secundum ASD and heart block.

32. **(b)** 10 days of intrauterine life

(Nelson, 18th ed.)

Mesoblastic hematopoiesis occurs in extraembryonic structures, principally in the yolk sac, and begins between the 10th and 14th days of gestation. By 6–8 weeks of gestation the liver replaces the yolk sac as the primary site of blood cell production, and by 10–12 weeks extraembryonic hematopoiesis has essentially ceased. **Hepatic hematopoiesis** occurs in the liver throughout the remainder of gestation, although production begins to diminish during the second trimester as bone marrow **(myeloid) hematopoiesis** increases. The liver remains the predominant hematopoietic organ through 20–24 weeks of gestation.

33. **(c)** 6-8 weeks of gestation

(Nelson, 18th ed.)

Mesoblastic hematopoiesis occurs in extraembryonic structures, principally in the yolk sac, and begins between the 10th and 14th days of gestation. By 6–8 weeks of gestation the liver replaces the yolk sac as the primary site of blood cell production, and by 10–12 weeks extraembryonic hematopoiesis has essentially ceased. **Hepatic hematopoiesis** occurs in the liver throughout the remainder of gestation, although production begins to diminish during the second trimester as bone marrow **(myeloid) hematopoiesis** increases. The liver remains the predominant hematopoietic organ through 20–24 weeks of gestation.

34. **(d)** >180 fl

(Nelson, 18th ed.)

Mean cell volumes usually are inversely proportional to gestation and to the life span of the cell. The *mean cell volume* (MCV) of erythrocytes is >180 fL in the embryo, falls to ≈ 130 by midgestation, then decreases to 110 fL by 40 weeks of gestation. *Mean platelet volumes* (MPV) range from 8–10 fL at birth and sometimes can be helpful in determining whether diminished platelet counts are caused primarily by decreased production (normal MPV) or increased destruction (large MPV).

35. **(a)** 5th week of gestation

(Nelson, 18th ed.)

The splenic precursor is recognizable by 5 weeks of gestation. At birth, the spleen weighs approximately 11 g. Thereafter, it enlarges until puberty, reaching an average weight of 135 g before diminishing in size during adulthood.

36. **(a)** 10 grams

(Nelson, 18th ed.)

The splenic precursor is recognizable by 5 weeks of gestation. At birth, the spleen weighs approximately 11 g. Thereafter, it enlarges until puberty, reaching an average weight of 135 g before diminishing in size during adulthood.

37. **(b)** B cells

(Nelson, 18th ed.)

The white pulp consists of periarterial lymphatic sheaths of T cells with embedded germinal centers containing B cells. The red pulp has a skeleton of fixed reticular cells, mobile macrophages, partially collapsed endothelial passages (cords of Billroth), and splenic sinuses. A *marginal zone* rich in dendritic (antigen-presenting) cells separates the red pulp from the white pulp.

38. **(b)** Malrotation of gut

(Nelson, 18th ed.)

Congenital absence of the spleen is associated with complex cyanotic heart defects, dextrocardia, bilateral trilobed lungs, and heterotopic abdominal organs (**Ivemark syndrome**).

39. **(d)** Between transudate and exudates

(Nelson, 18th ed.)

The composition of lymph can vary with the site of lymph drainage. It is usually clear, but lymph drained from the intestinal tract may be milky (chylous) because of the presence of fats. The protein content is intermediate between that of an exudate and that of a transudate. The protein level may be increased with inflammation and in lymph drained from the liver or intestines. Lymph also contains variable numbers of lymphocytes.

40. **(d)** Both ureteral bud and metanephros

(Nelson 18th ed.)

The kidney is derived from the ureteral bud and the metanephric blastema. During the 5th week of gestation, the ureteral bud arises from the mesonephric (wolffian) duct and penetrates the metanephric blastema, which is an area of undifferentiated mesenchyme on the nephrogenic ridge.

41. **(a)** 20 weeks of gestation

(Nelson, 18th ed.)

The kidney is derived from the ureteral bud and the metanephric blastema. During the 5th week of gestation, the ureteral bud arises from the mesonephric (wolffian) duct and penetrates the metanephric blastema, which is an area of undifferentiated mesenchyme on the nephrogenic ridge. The ureteral bud undergoes a series of approximately 15 generations of divisions and by the 20th week of gestation forms the entire collecting system: the ureter, renal pelvis, calyces, papillary ducts, and collecting tubules.

42. **(c)** 7th week of gestation

(Nelson, 18th ed.)

The kidney is derived from the ureteral bud and the metanephric blastema. During the 5th weeks of gestation, the ureteral bud arises from the mesonephric (wolffian) duct and penetrates the metanephric blastema, which is an area of undifferentiated mesenchyme on the nephrogenic ridge. The ureteral bud undergoes a series of approximately 15 generations of divisions and by the 20th week of gestation forms the entire collecting system: the ureter, renal pelvis, calyces, papillary ducts, and collecting tubules. Signals from the mesenchymal cells induce ureteric bud formation from the wolffian duct as well as ureteric bud branching. Reciprocal signals from the ureteric bud and, later, from its branching tips induce mesenchymal cells to condense, proliferate, and convert into epithelial cells. Under the inductive influence of the ureteral bud, nephron differentiation begins during the 7th week of gestation.

43. **(a)** Renal agenesis

(Nelson, 18th ed.)

Renal agenesis, or absent kidney development, can occur secondary to a defect of the wolffian duct, ureteric bud, or metanephric blastema. Unilateral renal agenesis has an incidence of 1 in 450 to 1,000 births.

44. **(b)** Unilateral renal dysplasia

(Nelson, 18th ed.)

The **Mayer-Rokitansky-Kuster-Hauser** syndrome refers to a group of associated findings that includes unilateral renal agenesis or ectopia, ipsilateral müllerian defects, and vaginal agenesis.

45. **(c)** 7-8 weeks of gestation

(Nelson, 18th ed.)

The testis develops at 7–8 weeks of gestation.

46. **(d)** Processes vaginalis

(Nelson, 18th ed.)

The process of testicular descent is regulated by an interaction between hormonal and mechanical factors, including testosterone, dihydrotestosterone, müllerian-inhibiting factor, the gubernaculum, intra-abdominal pressure, and the genitofemoral nerve. The testis develops at 7–8 weeks of gestation. At 10–11 weeks, the Leydig cells produce testosterone, which stimulates differentiation of the wolffian (mesonephric) duct into the epididymis, vas deferens, seminal vesicle, and ejaculatory duct. At 32–36 weeks, the testis, which is anchored at the internal inguinal ring by the gubernaculum, begins its process of descent. The gubernaculum distends the inguinal canal and guides the testis into the scrotum. Following testicular descent, the patent processus vaginalis (hernia sac) normally involutes.

47. **(a)** Normal at birth

(Nelson, 18th ed.)

The **consequences of cryptorchidism** include infertility, testicular malignancy, associated hernia, torsion of the cryptorchid testis, and the possible psychologic effects of an empty scrotum.

The undescended testis is normal at birth histologically, but pathologic changes can be demonstrated by 6–12 months. Delayed germ cell maturation, reduction in germ cell number, hyalinization of the seminiferous tubules, and reduced Leydig cell number are typical; these changes are progressive over time if the testis remains undescended. Similar, although less severe, changes are found in the contralateral descended testis after 4–7 years.

48. **(b)** 12th week of gestation

(Nelson, 18th ed.)

The fetal thyroid bilobed shape is recognized by 7 weeks of gestation, and characteristic thyroid follicle cell and colloid formation is seen by 10 weeks. Thyroglobulin synthesis occurs from 4 weeks, iodine trapping occurs by 8–10 weeks and thyroxine (T_4) and, to a lesser extent, triiodothyronine (T_3) synthesis and secretion occur from 12 weeks of gestation.

49. **(b)** Extradural

(Nelson, 18th ed.)

The pituitary gland is located at the base of the skull in a saddle-shaped cavity of the sphenoid bone: the sella turcica. The bony structure protects and surrounds the pituitary bilaterally and inferiorly. The dura, a dense layer of connective tissue, forms the roof of the sella. An external layer of the dura continues into the sella to form its lining. The pituitary is extradural and is not normally in contact with cerebrospinal fluid. The pituitary gland is connected to the hypothalamus by the pituitary stalk. The pituitary gland is composed of an anterior **(adenohypophysis)** and a posterior **(neurohypophysis)** lobe. The anterior lobe constitutes about 80% of the gland.

50. **(a)** Internal carotid artery

(Nelson, 18th ed.)

The arterial blood supply of the pituitary gland originates from the internal carotid via the inferior, middle, and superior hypophyseal arteries. This network of vessels forms a unique portal circulation connecting the hypothalamus and pituitary. The branches of the superior hypophyseal arteries penetrate the stalk and form a network of vessels that traverse the pituitary stalk and terminate in a network of capillaries within the anterior lobe. It is through this portal venous system that hypothalamic hormones are delivered to the anterior pituitary gland. Anterior pituitary hormones, in turn, are secreted into a secondary plexus of portal veins that drain into the dural venous sinuses.

Chapter 33

Pediatric Microbiology

1. **Coagulase negative bacteria are all *except:***
(a) S. epidermidis (b) S. saprophyticus
(c) S. hemolyticus (d) S. aureus

2. **All of the following virulence factors of S. aureus result in epidemic furunculosis *except:***
(a) Collagen-adhesin protein (CAN)
(b) Bacteriocin
(c) Enterotoxins
(d) LukE+LukD

3. **Staphylococcal enterotoxins are all *except:***
(a) A (b) B
(c) C1 (d) F

4. **All the following skin infections are caused by staph *except:***
(a) Impetigo contagiosum (b) Ecthyma
(c) Erysipelas (d) Folliculitis

5. **The most common cause of osteomyelitis and suppurative arthritis in children is ________.**
(a) S. aureus (b) Group A streptococci
(c) Group B streptococci (d) S. epidermidis

6. **The principal cause of toxic shock syndrome is________.**
(a) S. aureus (b) S. epidermidis
(c) Group A streptococci (d) Group B streptococci

7. **Quellung reaction is given by ________.**
(a) S. aureus (b) N. meningitidis
(c) S. pyogenes (d) None of the above

8. **All of the following are major criteria of staphylococcal toxic shock *except:***
(a) Acute fever
(b) Mucous membrane inflammation
(c) Rash
(d) Hypotension

9. **The most frequent cause of bacteremia and otitis media in children is:**
(a) S. aureus (b) S. pneumoniae
(c) S. pyogenes (d) S. agalactiae

10. **Children with high risk of developing invasive pneumococcal disease are all *except*:**
(a) Children with sickle cell disease
(b) With chronic cardiac disease
(c) With cochlear implants
(d) With HIV infection

11. **The cause of 2 potentially serious nonsuppurative complications: rheumatic fever and acute glomerulonephritis is:**
(a) S. pneumonie
(b) S. pyogenes
(c) S. agalactiae
(d) None of the above

12. **Group A streptococci can be identified by:**
(a) Latex agglutination
(b) Coagglutination
(c) Enzyme immunoassay
(d) All of the above

13. **Virulence of GAS depend on ______. (GAS-group A streptococci)**
(a) M protein (b) N protein
(c) Both (d) None of the above

14. **The rash of scarlet fever is caused by following pyrogenic exotoxins *except* ________.**
(a) Exotoxin A (b) Exotoxin B
(c) Exotoxin C (d) Exotoxin D

15. **Clinical criteria for Streptococcal toxic shock syndrome involves all of the following *except* ___.**
(a) Hypotension (b) Myositis
(c) Coagulopathy (d) Renal impairment

16. The only common cause of acute pharyngitis for which antibiotic therapy is definitely indicated is _______.

(a) S. pyogenes (Group A streptococci)
(b) N. gonorrhoea
(c) S. aureus
(d) All of the above

17. The organism which is identified by Lancefield's group B carbohydrate antigen is _______.

(a) S. agalactiae (b) S. pyogenes
(c) S. pneumoniae (d) None of the above

18. The common serotypes of group B Strepyococci which are involved in the early onset disease are all *except*____.

(a) 1a (b) 3
(c) 5 (d) All of the above

19. The diagnosis of invasive group B streptococci disease is done by isolation from sites *except* _____.

(a) Blood (b) Urine
(c) Csf (d) Gastric aspirate

20. Out of the non group A beta haemolytic streptococci, the most frequent cause of disease in children is_____.

(a) Group C (b) Group G
(c) Both (d) None of the above

21 M. tuberculosis grows on which media?

(a) Lowenstein Jenson media
(b) Venkatraman media
(c) BHI media
(d) None of these

22. The Mantoux tuberculin skin test is the intradermal injection of 0.1 mL containing __________units of purified protein derivative (PPD).

(a) 5 (b) 7
(c) 10 (d) 12

23. All of the following children should be given immediate tuberculin sensitivity test *except:*

(a) Contacts of people with confirmed contagious TB
(b) Childern with clinical or radiographic signs suggestive of TB
(c) Children immigrating from endemic areas (e.g. Asia)
(d) Children infected with HIV

24. Enterococci have mostly ____ type of haemolytic activity in children.

(a) Alpha haemolytic (b) Beta haemolytic
(c) Y-hemolytic (d) None of these

25. Enterococci are able to grow on:

(a) 6.5% NaCl (b) Bile
(c) Blood (d) Both (a) and (b)

26. _______enterococcus colonization predominantly occurs in 1st week of life.

(a) Enterococcus faecalis
(b) Enterococcus faecium
(c) Enterococcus gallinarium
(d) Enterococcus classiliflavus

27. True about corynebacterium is:

(a) C. diphtheriae is urease-negative
(b) C. ulcerans is urease-positive
(c) Both
(d) None

28. The remote sites affected by C. diphtheriae apart from nasopharynx are:

(a) Heart
(b) Nervous system
(c) Both
(d) None

29. Presumptive identification of L. monocytogenes can be done by all ____.

(a) Tumbling motility
(b) Umbrella formation in semisolid medium
(c) Typical cAMP test
(d) All of these

30. Characteristic features of early onset listeriosis are all *except*_____.

(a) Obstetric complications
(b) Neonatal sepsis
(c) Normal birth weight
(d) Premature delivery

31. ______________ species predominantly causes actinomycosis in children is:

(a) A. israelii (b) Aturicensis
(c) A. odontolyticus (d) None

32. "Beaded pattern" is seen in _____.

(a) Actinomyces (b) Nocardia
(c) Listeria (d) Enterococci

33. In a 7-month-old child suffering from meningo-ccocemia, the clinical feature which is seen most commonly is:

(a) Leg pain (b) Thirst
(c) Diarrhoea (d) Cold hand and feet

34. In a 4-year-old child suffering from meningo-coccemia, following classical features are seen *except*:

(a) Hemorrhagic rash (b) Neck pain
(c) Bulging fontanelle (d) Photophobia

35. The following clinical manifestations are typically seen in meningococcal meningitis:

(a) Headache (b) Photophobia
(c) Lethargy (d) All of the above

36. The features of meningococcal meningitis can overlap with:

(a) S. aureus (b) S. pneumoniae
(c) Group a streptococci (d) All of the above

37. Earliest IgG to appear in fetus is:

(a) IgA (b) IgM
(c) IgG (d) IgE

38. Every year vaccination is done on fixed dates for which vaccine:

(a) Malaria (b) Polio
(c) Diphtheria (d) Tetanus

39. _____is the most commonly STD found in sexually abused children.

(a) Syphilis
(b) Gonorrhoea
(c) Lympho granuloma venerum
(d) Herpes

40. Ophthalmia neonatorum due to N. gonorrhoeae usually appears from 1 to 4 days after birth:

(a) 1 to 4 days
(b) 4 to 8 days
(c) 1 week
(d) None of these

41. In children, the diarrhoea which doesn't produce pain is:

(a) V. cholerae (b) C. jejuni
(c) Shigella (d) Salmonella

42. Fetal loss is caused most frequently by:

(a) Measles (b) Rubella
(c) Syphilis (d) Herpes genitalis

43. When a newborn receives antibodies from its immunised mother it is example of:

(a) Natural active immunity
(b) Natural passive immunity
(c) Acquired active immunity
(d) Acquired passive immunity

44. Ion deficiency anemia in children is caused by infestation of:

(a) Hookworm (b) Roundworm
(c) Necator americanus (d) Strongyloides

45. The following lab indicator is earliest and best for used for monitoring healing rickets:

(a) Serum ca level (b) Seum vitamin D level
(c) Urinary ca level (d) None of these

46. In early childhood the most important cause of severe dehydrating diarrhoea is:

(a) Rotavirus (b) Calcivirus
(c) Coronavirus (d) Astrovirus

47. Rotavirus infection typically begins after an incubation period of:

(a) < 24 hours (b) < 48 hours
(c) < 72 hours (d) None of these

48. The most common finding in children with severe viral enteritis:

(a) Isotonic dehydration with acidosis
(b) Isotonic dehydration with alkalosis
(c) Hypotonic dehydration with acidosis
(d) None of these

49. Koplik's spots are pathognomic of:

(a) Measles (b) Mumps
(c) Rubella (d) Polio

50. The hallmarks of common HSV infections in children are:

(a) Skin vesicles (b) Shallow ulcers
(c) Both (a) and (b) (d) None

51. Most common micro-organism causing pneumonia in neonates:

(a) Group B streptococci
(b) Streptococcus pneumonia
(c) Haemophilus influenzae type B
(d) Moraxella catarrhalis

52. Most common organism responsible for acute suppurative thyroiditis is:

(a) Streptococcus viridans (b) Staphylococcus aureus
(c) Pneumococcus (d) H. influenza

Answers

1. **(d)** S. aureus

   (Nelson's Textbook of Pediatrics, 18th edition)

   Strains are classified as Staphylococcus aureus if they are coagulase positive or as 1 of the many species of coagulase-negative staphylococci (S. epidermidis, S. saprophyticus, S. haemolyticus).

2. **(d)** Luk E+Luk D

   (Nelson's Textbook of Pediatrics, 18th edition)

   (See the following Table)

3. **(d)** F

   (Nelson's Textbook of Pediatrics, 18th edition)

   One or more staphylococcal enterotoxins (types A, B, C_1, C_2, D, E) are elaborated by most strains of S. aureus. Ingestion of preformed enterotoxin A or B is associated with food poisoning resulting in vomiting and diarrhea and, in some cases, with the development of profound hypotension. By 10 years of age, almost all individuals have antibodies to at least 1 enterotoxin.

Virulence Factor	Characteristic	Clinical Syndrome
Resistance Determinants		
SCC mec type IV	Resistance to methicillin	
SCC_{476}	Resistance to fusidic acid	
Adherence		
Collagen-adhesin protein (CNA)	Greater adherence to host tissues	EF, NP, arthritis, osteomyelitis
Colonization		
Bacteriocin of SA (bsa)	Intraspecies and interspecies competition	EF
Unknown	Greater tolerance to salt	EF
Superantigens		
Enterotoxins	Activation of T cells	EF, NP, TSS-like illness
Staphylococcal enterotoxin A (sea, sak)		
Staphylococcal enterotoxin B		
Staphylococcal enterotoxin C (sec4)		
Staphylococcal enterotoxin G (seg2)		
Staphylococcal enterotoxin H	Extremely potent superantigen	
Staphylococcal enterotoxin K (sek2)		
Staphylococcal enterotoxin L (sel2)		
Staphylococcal enterotoxin O2 (seo2)		
Exotoxins		
Staphylococcal exotoxin T (set16–26)	Possible defence against immunity	
Pore-Forming Toxins		
PVL (LukSPV+LukPFV)	Necrosis, edema	EF, NP
LukE+LukD	Destruction of intestinal microvilli	Postantibiotic diarrhea
LukEv+LukDv	Necrosis	EF
α-Haemolysin	Necrosis, vascular leakage, shock	EF, NP Bullous impetigo

4. **(c)** Erysipelas

(Nelson's Textbook of Pediatrics, 18th edition)

Staphylococcus is an important cause of pyogenic skin infections, including impetigo contagiosa, ecthyma, bullous impetigo, folliculitis, hydradenitis, furuncles, carbuncles, staphylococcal scalded skin syndrome, and a syndrome resembling the rash of scarlet fever. Infection may also complicate wounds or occur as superinfection of other noninfectious skin disease (eczema). Recurrent furunculosis is a disorder of unknown cause and is associated with repeated episodes of pyoderma over months to years. Recurrent skin and soft tissue abscesses is noted with community-associated methicillin resistant S. aureus (MRSA). Staphylococcus is also an important cause of nosocomial skin infections.

Erysipelas is a relatively rare acute GAS infection involving the deeper layers of the skin and the underlying connective tissue. The skin in the affected area is swollen, red, and very tender. Superficial blebs may be present. The most characteristic finding is the sharply defined, slightly elevated border. At times, reddish streaks of lymphangitis project out from the margins of the lesion. The onset is abrupt, and signs and symptoms of a systemic infection, such as high fever, are often present. Cultures obtained by needle aspirate of the inflamed area often reveal the causative agent.

5. **(a)** S. aureus

(Nelson's Textbook of Pediatrics, 18th edition)

S. aureus is the most common cause of osteomyelitis and suppurative arthritis in children.

Most common clinical association	Microorganism
Frequent microorganism in any type of osteomyelitis	Staphylococcus aureus (susceptible or resistant to methicillin)
Foreign body–associated infection	Coagulase-negative staphylococci or Propionibacterium spp.
Common in nosocomial infections	Enterobacteriaceae, Pseudomonas aeruginosa, Candida spp.
Associated with bites, diabetic foot lesions, and decubitus ulcers	Streptococci and/or anaerobic bacteria
Sickle cell disease	Salmonella spp., S. aureus, or Streptococcus pneumonia
HIV infection	Bartonella Henselae or Bartonella Quintana
Human or animal bites	Pasteurella multocida or Eikenella corrodens
Immunocompromised patients	Aspergillus spp., Candida albicans, or Mycobacteria spp.
Populations in which tuberculosis is prevalent	Mycobacterium tuberculosis

The microbial spectrum is diverse in suppurative arthritis, but staphylococcus aureus infection is most common.

6. **(a)** S. aureus

(Nelson's Textbook of Pediatrics, 18th edition)

TSS is an acute multisystem disease characterized by high fever, hypotension, vomiting, diarrhea, myalgias, nonfocal neurologic abnormalities, conjunctival hyperemia, strawberry tongue, and an erythematous rash with subsequent desquamation on the hands and feet.

Etiology

TSS is caused by TSST-1-producing strains of S. aureus, which may colonize the vagina or cause focal sites of staphylococcal infection.

7. **(d)** None of the above

(Nelson's Textbook of Pediatrics, 18th edition)

S. pneumoniae is a gram-positive, lancet-shaped, polysaccharide-encapsulated diplococcus, occurring occasionally as individual cocci or in chains. Antisera to some pneumococcal polysaccharides cross react with other pneumococcal types defining serogroups (6A and 6B), or other bacteria (Escherichia coli, group B streptococcus, H. influenzae type B). Smooth or encapsulated strains cause most serious disease in humans. Capsular polysaccharides impede phagocytosis. Virulence is related in part to capsular size, but pneumococcal types with capsules of the same size can vary widely in virulence.

On solid media, S. pneumoniae forms unpigmented, umbilicated colonies surrounded by a zone of incomplete (α) hemolysis. S. pneumoniae is bile soluble (10% deoxycholate) and Optochin sensitive. S. pneumoniae is closely related to the viridans groups of Streptococcus mitus, which phenotypically overlap with pneumococci. Pneumococcal capsules can be microscopically visualized and typed by exposing organisms to type-specific antisera that combine with their unique capsular polysaccharide, rendering the capsule refractile (Quellung reaction).

8. **(b)** Mucous membrane inflammation
(Nelson's Textbook of Pediatrics, 18th edition)

Diagnostic Criteria of Staphylococcal Toxic Shock Syndrome

Major Criteria (All Required)
• Acute fever; temperature >38.8°C • Hypotension (orthostatic, shock; below age-appropriate norms) • Rash (erythroderma with late desquamation)

Contd.

Contd.

Minor Criteria (Any 3)
• Mucous membrane inflammation • Vomiting, diarrhea • Liver abnormalities • Renal abnormalities • Muscle abnormalities • Central nervous system abnormalities • Thrombocytopenia
Exclusionary Criteria
• Absence of another explanation • Negative blood cultures (except occasionally for S. aureus)

9. **(b)** S. pneumoniae

(Nelson's Textbook of Pediatrics, 18th edition)

S. pneumoniae is the most frequent cause of bacteremia, bacterial pneumonia, and otitis media, and the second most common cause of meningitis in children.

10. **(b)** With chronic cardiac disease

(Nelson's Textbook of Pediatrics, 18th edition)

High risk (incidence of invasive pneumococcal disease =150 cases/ 100,000 people per year)
Children with: • Sickle cell disease, congenital or acquired asplenia, or splenic dysfunction • Human immunodeficiency virus infection • Cochlear implants
Presumed high risk (insufficient data to calculate rates)
Children with: • Congenital immune deficiency; some B-(humoral) or T-lymphocyte deficiencies, complement deficiencies (particularly C1, C2, C3 and C4), or phagocytic disorders (excluding chronic granulomatous disease) • Chronic cardiac disease (particularly cyanotic congenital heart disease and cardiac failure) • Chronic pulmonary disease (including asthma treated with high-dose oral corticosteroid therapy) • Cerebrospinal leaks from a congenital malformation, skull fracture, or neurologic procedure • Chronic renal insufficiency, including nephrotic syndrome • Diseases associated with immunosuppressive therapy or radiation therapy (including malignant neoplasms, leukemias, lymphomas, and Hodgkin disease) and solid organ transplantation • Diabetes mellitus

11. **(b)** S. pyogenes

(Nelson's Textbook of Pediatrics, 18th edition)

GAS is also the cause of 2 potentially serious nonsuppurative complications: rheumatic fever and acute glomerulonephritis.

Group A streptococcus (GAS), also known as Streptococcus pyogenes, is a common cause of infections of the upper respiratory tract (pharyngitis) and the skin (impetigo, pyoderma) in children.

12. **(d)** All of the above

(Nelson's Textbook of Pediatrics, 18th edition)

Group A organisms can be identified more readily by any 1 of a number of latex agglutination, coagglutination, or enzyme immunoassay procedures. Group A strains can also be distinguished from other groups by differences in sensitivity to bacitracin.

13. **(a)** M protein

(Nelson's Textbook of Pediatrics, 18th edition)

Virulence of GAS depends primarily on the M protein, and strains rich in M protein resist phagocytosis in fresh human blood, whereas M-negative strains do not. GAS isolated from chronic pharyngeal carriers contain little or no M protein and are relatively avirulent. The M protein antigen stimulates the production of protective antibodies. These antibodies are type specific. They protect against infection with a homologous M type but confer no immunity against other M types.

14. **(d)** Exotoxin D

(Nelson's Textbook of Pediatrics, 18th edition)

GAS produces a large variety of enzymes and toxins, including erythrogenic toxins (known as streptococcal pyrogenic exotoxins). Streptococcal pyrogenic exotoxins A, B and C are responsible for the rash of scarlet fever and are elaborated by streptococci that are infected with a particular bacteriophage.

15. **(b)** Myositis

(Nelson's Textbook of Pediatrics, 18th edition)

Definition of Streptococcal Toxic Shock Syndrome
• Clinical criteria
• Hypotension plus 2 or more of the following:
• Renal impairment
• Coagulopathy
• Hepatic involvement
• Adult respiratory distress syndrome
• Generalized erythematous macular rash
• Soft tissue necrosis
• Definite case
• Clinical criteria plus group A streptococcus from a normally sterile site

16. **(a)** S. pyogenes (Group A streptococci)

(Nelson's Textbook of Pediatrics, 18th edition)

GAS pharyngitis is the only common cause of acute pharyngitis for which antibiotic therapy is definitely indicated.

17. **(a)** S. agalactiae

(Nelson's Textbook of Pediatrics, 18th edition)

Group B streptococci are facultative anaerobic gram-positive cocci that form chains or diplococci in broth and small gray-white colonies on solid medium. GBS is definitively identified by demonstration of the Lancefield group B carbohydrate antigen, such as with latex agglutination techniques widely used in clinical laboratories.

18. **(d)** All of the above

(Nelson's Textbook of Pediatrics, 18th edition)

Characteristics of Early- and Late-Onset GBS Disease

	Early-onset disease	**Late-onset disease**
Age at onset	0–6 days	7–90 days
Increased risk after obstetric complications	Yes	No
Common clinical manifestations	Sepsis, pneumonia, meningitis	Bacteremia, meningitis, other focal infections
Common serotypes	Ia, III, V, II Ib	III predominates
Case fatality rate	4.7%	2.8%

19. **(d)** Gastric aspirate

(Nelson's Textbook of Pediatrics, 18th edition)

The diagnosis of invasive GBS disease is established by isolation and identification of the organism from a normally sterile site, such as blood, urine, or cerebrospinal fluid (CSF). Isolation of GBS from gastric or tracheal aspirates or from skin or mucous membranes indicates colonization and is not diagnostic of invasive disease.

20. **(c)** Both

(Nelson's Textbook of Pediatrics, 18th edition)

Of the non-group A β-hemolytic streptococci, groups C and G streptococcus are the most frequent cause of human disease.

Group C streptococcus is a much more common cause of infection in animals than in humans. Humans infected with this organism often have had some animal contact. Both group C and group G streptococcus often can be part of the normal human flora of the nasopharynx, skin, and genital tract. Group C streptococcus can be cultured from the umbilicus of asymptomatic newborns and from routine puerperal vaginal cultures. Group G streptococcus also can be cultured from the gastrointestinal tract. Because of the relatively low virulence of group C and group G streptococci, most humans infected with either of these organisms have some underlying medical disorder (diabetes mellitus, malignancy, alcohol abuse, immunosuppression.

21. **(c)** Lowenstein-Jenson media

(Nelson's Textbook of Pediatrics, 18th edition)

M. tuberculosis is the most important cause of tuberculosis disease in humans. The tubercle bacilli are non-spore-forming, nonmotile, pleomorphic, weakly gram-positive curved rods 2–4 µm long. They may appear beaded or clumped in stained clinical specimens or culture media. They are obligate aerobes that grow in synthetic media containing glycerol as the carbon source and ammonium salts as the nitrogen source (Loewenstein-Jensen culture media). These mycobacteria grow best at 37–41°C, produce niacin, and lack pigmentation.

22. **(a)** 5

(Nelson's Textbook of Pediatrics, 18th edition)

The Mantoux tuberculin skin test is the intradermal injection of 0.1 mL containing 5 tuberculin units of purified protein derivative (PPD) stabilized with Tween 80.

23. **(d)** Children infected with HIV

(Nelson's Textbook of Pediatrics, 18th edition)

Tuberculin Skin Test (TST) Recommendations for Infants, Children and Adolescents[*]

Children for whom immediate TST is indicated:

- Contacts of people with confirmed or suspected contagious tuberculosis (contact investigation)
- Children with radiographic or clinical findings suggesting tuberculosis disease
- Children immigrating from countries with endemic infection (e.g., Asia, Middle East, Africa, Latin America, countries of the former Soviet Union) including international adoptees
- Children with travel histories to countries with endemic infection and substantial contact with indigenous people from such countries[‡]

Children who should have annual TST:

- Children infected with HIV
- Incarcerated adolescents

24. **(c)** Y-hemolytic

(Nelson's Textbook of Pediatrics, 18th edition)

Enterococci are gram-positive, catalase-negative facultative anaerobes that grow in pairs or short chains. Most are nonhemolytic (also called γ-hemolytic) on sheep blood agar, although some isolates have α- or β-hemolytic activity.

25. **(d)** Both (a) and (b)

(Nelson's Textbook of Pediatrics, 18th edition)

Enterococci are gram-positive, catalase-negative facultative anaerobes that grow in pairs or short chains. Most are nonhemolytic (also called γ-hemolytic) on sheep blood agar, although some isolates have α- or β-hemolytic activity. Enterococci are distinguished from most Lancefield groupable streptococci by their ability to grow in bile and hydrolyze esculin. Enterococci are able to grow in 6.5% NaCl and hydrolyze L-pyrrolidonyl-β-naphthylamide (PYR), features used by clinical laboratories to distinguish Enterococcus from group D streptococcus. Identification at the species level is enabled by differing patterns of carbohydrate fermentation.

26. **(a)** Enterococcus faecalis

(Nelson's Textbook of Pediatrics, 18th edition)

Enterococci are normal inhabitants of the gastrointestinal tract of humans and animals. Oral secretions and dental plaque, the upper respiratory tract, skin and vagina may also be colonized by Enterococcus. Enterococcus faecalis is the predominant organism, with colonization commonly occurring in the 1st week of life. By the time of adulthood, E. faecalis colonization is nearly ubiquitous.

27. **(c)** Both

(Nelson's Textbook of Pediatrics, 18th edition)

Corynebacteria are aerobic, nonencapsulated, non-spore-forming, mostly nonmotile, pleomorphic, gram-positive bacilli. C. diphtheriae is by far the most commonly isolated agent of diphtheria. C. ulcerans is more commonly isolated from cattle and can cause similar disease. As corynebacteria are not fastidious in growth requirements, their isolation is enhanced by use of a selective medium (i.e., cystine-tellurite blood agar) that inhibits growth of competing organisms and, when reduced by C. diphtheriae, renders colonies gray-black. Differentiation of C. diphtheriae from C. ulcerans is based on urease activity, as C. ulcerans is urease-positive.

28. **(c)** Both

(Nelson's Textbook of Pediatrics, 18th edition)

Respiratory tract obstruction by pseudomembranes may require bronchoscopy or intubation and mechanical ventilation. Two other tissues usually remote from sites of C. diphtheriae infection can be significantly affected by diphtheritic toxin: the heart and the nervous system.

29. **(d)** All of these

(Nelson's Textbook of Pediatrics, 18th edition)

Selected biochemical tests together with the demonstration of tumbling motility, umbrella-type formation below the surface in semisolid medium, hemolysis, and a typical cyclic adenosine monophosphate (cAMP) test are usually sufficient to establish a presumptive identification of L. monocytogenes.

30. **(c)** Normal birth weight

(Nelson's Textbook of Pediatrics, 18th edition)

Characteristic Features of Early- and Late-Onset Neonatal Listeriosis

Early onset (<5 days)	Late onset (≥5 days)
Positive maternal Listeria culture	Negative maternal Listeria culture
Obstetric complications	Uncomplicated pregnancy
Premature delivery	Term delivery
Low birthweight	Normal birthweight
Neonatal sepsis	Neonatal meningitis
Mean age at onset 1.5 days	Mean age at onset 14.2 days
Mortality rate >30%	Mortality rate <10%
	Nosocomial outbreaks

31. **(a)** A. israelii

(Nelson's Textbook of Pediatrics, 18th edition)

Actinomyces is a member of the order Actinomycetales, which includes gram-positive filamentous bacteria such as Nocardia, Streptomyces, and mycobacteria. Actinomyces israelii is the predominant species causing human actinomycosis. Other implicated species, in order of importance, include Propionibacterium propionicum (formerly Arachnia propionicum), A. turicensis, A. odontolyticus, A. meyeri, A. naeslundii, A. viscosus, A. europaeus, and A. radingae. Arcanobacterium pyogenes (previously in the Actinomyces genus) also causes human actinomycosis.

32. **(b)** Nocardia

(Nelson's Textbook of Pediatrics, 18th edition)

Nocardia is a member of the order Actinomycetales, which includes gram-positive filamentous bacteria such as Actinomyces, Streptomyces and mycobacteria. Nocardia organisms are environmental saprophytes that are ubiquitous in soil and decaying vegetable matter. These organisms are obligate aerobes and grow on ordinary culture media. Growth is achieved best at 37°C, although many isolates of Nocardia are thermophilic and grow at temperatures up to 50°C. At 25°C, the organisms grow very slowly. Colonies appear within 1–2 weeks on brain-heart infusion agar and Lowenstein-Jensen media, usually as waxy, folded, or heaped colonies at the edges. With further incubation, these colonies develop aerial hyphae that tend to give them a white, chalky appearance. Using the modified Kinyoun acid-fast staining of biopsy specimens or body fluids, Nocardia demonstrates fragmented bacilli with stain concentrated in a beaded pattern along portions of the branching filaments.

33. **(d)** Cold hand and feet

(Nelson's Textbook of Pediatrics, 18th edition)

Age-Specific Frequency of Clinical Features of Meningococcal Disease Before Hospital Admission

	<1 year	1–4 years	5–14 years	15–16 years
Early Features %				
Leg pain	5.1	30.6	62.4	53.3
Thirst	3.4	6.4	11.4	12.6
Diarrhea	9.9	7.8	3.1	5.5
Abnormal skin color	20.6	16.8	18.5	19.0
Breathing difficulty	16.2	9.7	7.1	12.1
Cold hands and feet	44.0	46.7	34.9	44.4
Classic Features %				
Hemorrhagic rash	42.3	64.2	69.8	65.9
Neck pain or stiffness	15.5	28.1	45.9	52.9
Photophobia	24.5	24.1	26.4	35.5
Bulging fontanelle	11.5	n/a	n/a	n/a
Late Features %				
Confusion or delirium	n/a	42.8	49.4	47.6
Seizure	8.9	12.8	7.8	7.3
Unconsciousness	7.0	9.1	5.9	15.1

34. **(c)** Bulging fontanelle

(Nelson's Textbook of Pediatrics, 18th edition)

Refer above table for explantion.

35. **(d)** All of the above

(Nelson's Textbook of Pediatrics, 18th edition)

The most common clinical manifestation, meningococcal meningitis, is distinguishable from other causes of bacterial meningitis. Headache, photophobia, lethargy, vomiting, and nuchal rigidity and other signs of meningeal irritation typically are present. Seizures and focal neurologic signs occur less frequently than in patients with meningitis caused by pneumococcus or Haemophilus influenzae type B. A meningoencephalitis-like picture can occur that may be associated with rapidly progressive cerebral edema, which may be more common with serogroup A infection.

36. **(d)** All of the above

(Nelson's Textbook of Pediatrics, 18th edition)

Meningococcal disease can appear similar to sepsis or meningitis caused by many other gram-negative bacteria, Streptococcus pneumoniae, Staphylococcus aureus, or group A streptococcus; Rocky Mountain spotted fever, ehrlichiosis, or epidemic typhus; and bacterial endocarditis. Viral and other etiologies of encephalitis should be considered in some cases. Autoimmune vasculitides (especially Henoch-Schönlein purpura), serum sickness, hemolytic-uremic syndrome, Kawasaki disease, idiopathic thrombocytopenic purpura, drug eruptions, and ingestion of various poisons can have features that overlap those of meningococcal infection. Infections with echoviruses (particularly types 6, 9 and 16), coxsackieviruses (primarily types A2, A4, A9 and A16), and other viruses also may have severe presentations that initially raise concerns about meningococcal infection.

37. **(b)** Ig M

(Nelson's Textbook of Pediatrics, 18th edition)

The earliest Ig to appear in fetus is IgM.

38. **(b)** Polio

(Nelson's Textbook of Pediatrics, 18th edition)

The pulse polio immunisation is done on fixed dates every year for children below 5 years of age.

39. **(b)** Gonorrhoea

(Nelson's Textbook of Pediatrics, 18th edition)

N. gonorrhoeae infection occurs only in humans. The organism is shed in the exudate and secretions of infected mucosal surfaces and is transmitted through intimate contact, such as sexual contact or parturition and, rarely, by contact with fomites. Gonococcal infections in the newborn period generally are acquired during delivery. Gonorrhea is the most common sexually transmitted infection found in sexually abused children.

40. **(a)** 1 to 4 days

(Nelson's Textbook of Pediatrics, 18th edition)

Gonococcal ophthalmitis may be unilateral or bilateral. It may occur in any age group after inoculation of the eye with infected secretions. Ophthalmia neonatorum due to N. gonorrhoeae usually appears from 1 to 4 days after birth. Ocular infection in older patients results from inoculation or autoinoculation from a genital site. The infection begins with mild inflammation and a serosanguineous discharge. Within 24 hours, the discharge becomes thick and purulent, and tense edema of the eyelids with marked chemosis occurs. If the disease is not treated promptly, corneal ulceration, rupture, and blindness may follow.

41. **(a)** V. cholerae

(Nelson's Textbook of Pediatrics, 18th edition)

Following colonization of the upper small intestine, V. cholerae O1 and O139 produce an enterotoxin that promotes the secretion of fluid and electrolytes into the lumen of the small intestine. The enterotoxin consists of 5 binding (B) subunits and 1 active (A) subunit. The (B) subunits bind to the GM1 ganglioside receptors in the small intestinal mucosa, allowing the (A) subunit to enter into the cell where it activates adenylate cyclase, leading to an increase in cyclic adenosine monophosphate (AMP). Cyclic AMP blocks the absorption of sodium chloride by the microvilli and promotes the secretion of chloride and water by the crypt cells. The result is massive outpouring of electrolyte-rich isotonic fluid into the small intestine. The large volume of fluid produced in the upper intestine overwhelms the absorptive capacity of the lower bowel, resulting in severe diarrhea. The diarrheal fluid contains large amounts of sodium, chloride, bicarbonate and potassium. Since the enterotoxin acts locally and does not invade the intestinal wall, few red blood cells and neutrophils are found in the stool. The loss of electrolyte-rich isotonic fluid leads to blood volume depletion with resulting low blood pressure and shock. Loss of bicarbonate and potassium leads to metabolic acidosis and hypokalemia.

Cholera is characterized by an acute onset of copious watery diarrhea and vomiting without abdominal cramps or fever. The stools are colorless with small flecks of mucus ("rice-water") and are sometimes described as having a fishy odor. At first, children may be restless or extremely thirsty, but if fluid and electrolyte losses are not replaced, they may become lethargic or unconscious. Other signs of dehydration may rapidly manifest, including poor skin turgor, sunken eyes, dry mouth and tongue, no urine output, delayed capillary refill, rapid or weak pulse, and low blood pressure. Severe dehydration, metabolic acidosis and hypokalemia can occur in 4–12 hours. The fluid losses may be so rapid that the child quickly develops hypovolemic shock, hypoglycemia, coma, and seizures and is at risk of dying within a few hours of onset.

42. **(d)** Herpes genitalis

(Nelson's Textbook of Pediatrics, 18th edition)

TORCH group of infections are most vital cause of mortality in intrauterine infections. Herpes is the most common cause.

43. **(b)** Natural passive immunity

(Nelson's Textbook of Pediatrics, 18th edition)

- Natural active immunity results from clinical or inapparent infection from parasite.
- A person who recovered from attack of chicken pox develop natural active immunity.
- Artificial active immunity is by vaccines.
- Artificial passive immunity is immune horse serum administration.

44. **(a)** Hookworm

(Nelson's Textbook of Pediatrics, 18th edition)

Two major genera of hookworms, which are nematodes or roundworms, infect humans. Necator americanus, the only representative of its genus, is a major anthropophilic hookworm and is the most common cause of human hookworm infection. Hookworms of the genus Ancylostoma includes the major anthropophilic hookworm Ancylostoma duodenale that also causes classic hookworm infection and the less common zoonotic species A. ceylanicum, A. caninum and A. braziliense.

Chronically infected children with moderate and heavy hookworm infections suffer from intestinal blood loss resulting in iron deficiency, which can lead to anemia as well as protein malnutrition. Prolonged iron deficiency associated with hookworms in childhood can lead to physical growth retardation and cognitive and intellectual deficits.

45. **(d)** None of these

(Nelson's Textbook of Pediatrics, 18th edition)

The earliest indicator is skeletal X-ray.

46. **(a)** Rotavirus

(Nelson's Textbook of Pediatrics, 18th edition)

Diarrhea is a leading cause of childhood mortality in the world, accounting for 5–10 million deaths per year. In early childhood, the single most important cause of severe dehydrating diarrhea is rotavirus infection.

Rotavirus, astrovirus, caliciviruses such as the Norwalk agent, and enteric adenovirus are the medically important pathogens of human viral gastroenteritis.

47. **(b)** < 48 hours

(Nelson's Textbook of Pediatrics, 18th edition)

Rotavirus infection typically begins after an incubation period of < 48 hours (range 1–7 days) with mild to moderate fever as well as vomiting followed by the onset of frequent, watery stools. All 3 symptoms are present in about 50–60% of cases. Vomiting and fever typically abate during the 2nd day of illness, but diarrhea often continues for 5–7 days. The stool is without gross blood or white cells. Dehydration may develop and progress rapidly, particularly in infants. The most severe disease typically occurs among children 4–36 months of age. Malnourished children and children with underlying intestinal disease such as short-bowel syndrome are particularly likely to acquire severe rotavirus diarrhea. Rarely, immunodeficient children experience severe and prolonged illness. Although most newborns infected with rotavirus are asymptomatic, some outbreaks of necrotizing enterocolitis.

48. **(a)** Isotonic dehydration with acidosis

(Nelson's Textbook of Pediatrics, 18th edition)

Isotonic dehydration with acidosis is the most common finding in children with severe viral enteritis. The stools are free of blood and leukocytes. Although the white blood cell count may be moderately elevated secondary to stress, the marked left shift seen with invasive bacterial enteritis is absent.

49. **(a)** Measles

(Nelson's Textbook of Pediatrics, 18th edition)

Measles is a serious infection characterized by high fever, an enanthem, cough, coryza, conjunctivitis, and a prominent exanthem. After an incubation period of 8–12 days, the prodromal phase begins with a mild fever followed by the onset of conjunctivitis with photophobia, coryza, a prominent cough and increasing fever. The enanthem, Koplik spots, is the pathognomonic sign of measles and appears 1 to 4 days prior to the onset of the rash. They first appear as discrete red lesions with bluish white spots in the center on the inner aspects of the cheeks at the level of the premolars. They may spread to involve the lips, hard palate and gingiva. They also may occur in conjunctival folds and in the vaginal mucosa. Koplik spots have been reported in 50–70% of measles cases but probably occur in the great majority.

50. **(c)** Both (a) and (b)

(Nelson's Textbook of Pediatrics, 18th edition)

The hallmarks of common HSV infections are skin vesicles and shallow ulcers. Classical infections present with small, 2–4 mm vesicles that may be surrounded by an erythematous base. These may persist for a few days before evolving into shallow, minimally erythematous ulcers. The vesicular phase tends to persist longer when keratinized epithelia is involved and be brief, sometimes fleeting, when moist mucous membranes are the site of infection. Because HSV infections are common and their natural history influenced by many factors, including portal of entry, immune status of the host, and whether it is an initial or recurrent infection, the typical manifestations are seldom classical. Most infections are asymptomatic or unrecognized, and nonclassical presentations such as small skin fissures and small erythematous nonvesicular lesions are common.

51. **(c)** Group B streptococci

(Nelson's Textbook of Pediatrics, 18th edition)

Bacterial	
Common	
Streptococcus pneumoniae	
Group B streptococci	Neonates
Group A streptococci	
Mycoplasma pneumoniae[*]	Adolescents; Summer-fall epidemics
Chlamydia pneumoniae[*]	Adolescents
Chlamydia trachomatis	Infants
Mixed anaerobes	Aspiration pneumonia
Gram-negative enteric	Nosocomial pneumonia

52. **(a)** Streptococcus viridans

(Nelson's Textbook of Pediatrics, 18th edition)

Acute suppurative thyroiditis is uncommon; it is usually preceded by a respiratory infection. The left lower lobe is affected predominantly. Abscess formation may occur. Anaerobic organisms, with or without aerobes, are the typical infectious agent. The most common organism is Streptococcus viridans, followed by Staphylococcus aureus and pneumococcus.

Chapter 34

Pediatric Pharmacology

1. **In N. meningitides for hospitalized patients the drug of choice is:**
   (a) Amikacin (b) Penicillin G
   (c) Amoxicillin (d) Penicillin V
2. **In age group <1 month drug used in treatment and postexposure prophylaxis for pertussis is:**
   (a) Erythromycin (b) Azithromycin
   (c) Clarithromycin (d) None
3. **In infection with respiratory syncytial virus treatment is:**
   (a) Humidified oxygen
   (b) Fluids administration
   (c) Ribavirin
   (d) All of the above
4. **Perinatal transmission from mother-to-child has been achieved by:**
   (a) Abacavir (b) Nevirapine
   (c) Zidovudine (d) Enfuvirtide
5. **In pediatrics, ________________have been used in combination with proton pump inhibitors to treat H. pylori infection.**
   (a) Antibiotics and bismuth salts
   (b) NSAIDs
   (c) H_2 receptor antagonists
   (d) None
6. **For school-aged children treatment of choice for atypical pneumonia:**
   (a) Azithromycin (b) Amoxicillin
   (c) Levofloxacin (d) Cefuroxime axetil
7. **For mildly ill children who do not require hospitalization treatment of choice is:**
   (a) Azithromycin (b) Amoxicillin
   (c) Gatifloxacin (d) Cefuroxime axetil
8. **________________ contraindicated in children with dysentery and probably have no role in the management of acute watery diarrhea.**
   (a) Zinc supplementation
   (b) Antimotility agents
   (c) ORS
   (d) None
9. **A child presents with acute onset of breathlessness, cough and fever, which of the following can be given:**
   (a) O_2 inhalation (b) Antipyretic
   (c) Ribavirin (d) All of the above
10. **Dose of metronidazole in children:**
    (a) 20 mg/kg/day in 3 doses × 10 days
    (b) 35-50 mg/kg/day in 3 doses × 7-10 days
    (c) 1 mg/kg/day × 6 days
    (d) 11 mg/kg (max 1 g) × 3 days
11. **Meningitis caused by GBS usually responds antibiotics within 24-48 hours and should be treated for ______________.**
    (a) 10-12 days (b) 14-21 days
    (c) 5-10 days (d) 21-30 days
12. **In neurocysticercosis antiparasitic drug of choice:**
    (a) Mebendazole (b) Tinidazole
    (c) Albendazole (d) None
13. **Rapid infusion of large doses can produce chest wall rigidity in children because of:**
    (a) Midazolam (b) Pentobarbital
    (c) Fentanyl (d) Ketamine
14. **For midazolam reversal agent in children is:**
    (a) Ketamine (b) Fentanyl
    (c) Flumazenil (d) Chloral hydrate

15. In children co-administration of ____________ with ketamine can reduce the risk of dysphoria or bad dreams.

(a) Midazolam (b) Fentanyl
(c) Pentobarbital (d) None

16. The WHO recommends single-dose of _______ for the treatment of trachoma in children.

(a) Doxycycline (b) Azithromycin
(c) Penicillin (d) Cefixim

17. Prophylactic therapy of childhood migraine includes:

(a) Propranolol (b) Flunarizine
(c) Both (d) None

18. Dose of acetaminophen in migraine headaches in children is:

(a) 15 mg/kg (b) 7.5-10 mg/kg
(c) 25 mg/kg (d) 1.5-5 mg/kg

19. _______ is the most commonly used intravenous induction agent in pediatric anesthesiology and has a rapid onset.

(a) Propofol (b) Ketamine
(c) Barbiturate (d) None

20. Management of the child with enuresis includes:

(a) Behavioral treatment (b) Imipramine
(c) Desmopressin acetate (d) All of the above

Answers

1. **(b)** Penicillin G

   (Nelson Textbook of Pediatrics, 18th ed.)

   For hospitalized patients, penicillin G (250,000–400,000 U/kg/day divided every 4–6 hours IV) remains the drug of choice. Cefotaxime (200 mg/kg/day) or ceftriaxone (100 mg/kg/day) are acceptable alternatives and are usually part of initial empiric regimens. Therapy in children is generally continued for 5–7 days.

2. **(b)** Azithromycin

   (Nelson Textbook of Pediatrics, 18th ed.)

   (See the following table)

3. **(d)** All of the above

   (Nelson Textbook of Pediatrics, 18th ed.)

   The treatment of uncomplicated cases of bronchiolitis is symptomatic. Humidified oxygen is usually indicated for hospitalized infants because most are hypoxic. Many infants are slightly to moderately dehydrated, and therefore fluids should be carefully administered in amounts somewhat greater than maintenance. Often intravenous or tube feeding is helpful when sucking is difficult due to tachypnea. Infants may breathe more easily when propped up at an angle of 10–30 degrees.

   There is disagreement among experts regarding the usefulness of epinephrine or β_2 agonists in RSV bronchiolitis. Corticosteroids are not indicated except in older children with an established diagnosis of asthma.

   In most instances of bronchiolitis, antibiotics are not useful. Interstitial pneumonia in infants 1–4 months old may be caused by *C. trachomatis,* and erythromycin (40 mg/kg/day) or clarithromycin (7.5 mg/kg every 12 hours) may be indicated.

   Ribavirin is an antiviral delivered through an oxygen hood, face mask, or endotracheal tube using the small particle aerosol generator (SPAG-2) for 12–20 hours/day for 3–5 days. Early trials showed a modest beneficial effect on the course of RSV pneumonia with some reduction in the duration of mechanical ventilation and days of hospitalization. Subsequent studies failed to document a clear beneficial effect of ribavirin.

4. **(c)** Zidovudine

   (Nelson Textbook of Pediatrics, 18th ed.)

Ans. 2 **Recommended Antimicrobial Treatment and Postexposure Prophylaxis for Pertussis by Age Group**

Age group	Primary agents			Alternate agent[*]
	Azithromycin	**Erythromycin**	**Clarithromycin**	**TMP-SMZ**
<1 month	Recommended agent. 10 mg/kg/day in a single dose for 5 days (only limited safety data available)	Not preferred. Erythromycin is associated with infantile hypertrophic pyloric stenosis Use if azithromycin is unavailable; 40–50 mg/kg/day in 4 divided doses for 14 days	Not recommended (safety data unavailable)	Contraindicated for infants aged <2 months (risk for kernicterus)
1–5 months	10 mg/kg/day in a single dose for 5 days	40–50 mg/kg/day in 4 divided doses for 14 days	15 mg/kg/day in 2 divided doses for 7 days	Contraindicated at age <2 months For infants aged < 2 months TMP 8 mg/kg/day, SMZ 40 mg/kg/day in 2 divided doses for 14 days
Infants (aged = 6 months) and children	10 mg/kg in a single dose on day 1 then 5 mg/kg/day (maximum 500 mg) on days 2–5	40–50 mg/kg/day (maximum 2 g/day) in 4 divided doses for 14 days	15 mg/kg/day in 2 divided doses (maximum 1 g/day) for 7 days	TMP 8 mg/kg/day, SMZ 40 mg/kg/day in 2 divided doses for 14 days
Adults	500 mg in a single dose on day 1 then 250 mg/day on days 2–5	2 g/day in 4 divided doses for 14 days	1 g/day in 2 divided doses for 7 days	TMP 320 mg/day, SMZ 1,600 mg/day in 2 divided doses for 14 days

Interruption of perinatal transmission from mother-to-child has been achieved by administering ZDV chemoprophylaxis (200 mg every 8 hours) to the pregnant woman (started as early as 4 weeks of gestation) and continued during delivery (2 mg/kg loading dose IV followed by 1 mg/kg/hr IV) and in the newborn for the 1st 6 weeks of life (2 mg/kg every 6 hours PO). In the developed world, such therapy has been documented to decrease the rate of perinatal HIV-1 transmission to <8%. Toxicity from ZDV therapy in both mothers and infants is minimal. Although this treatment was first given to untreated, asymptomatic, and immunologically intact women, epidemiologic data have confirmed the efficacy of ZDV chemoprophylaxis for reduction of perinatal transmission to offspring of women with advanced disease, low CD4 counts, and prior ZDV therapy. Rates of perinatal transmission have been as low as 2% among women who received HAART and all 3 components of the ZDV regimen, even in women with advanced HIV-1 disease. Therefore, the CDC recommends that women be treated with a HAART regimen appropriate for their own health during pregnancy, with collaboration between the HIV-specialist and the obstetrician. Women whose viral load at the time of delivery is >1,000 copies/mL should be counseled about the potential benefit of cesarean section in reducing the risk for vertical transmission.

5. **(a)** Antibiotics and bismuth salts

(Nelson Textbook of Pediatrics, 18th ed)

Treatment of *h. pylori*–Related Peptic Ulcer Disease

In pediatrics, antibiotics and bismuth salts have been used in combination with proton pump inhibitors to treat *H. pylori* infection. Eradication rates in children range from 68% to 92% when the dual or triple therapy is used for 4–6 wk. The ulcer healing rate ranges from 91% to 100%. Triple therapy yields a higher cure rate than dual therapy. The optimal regimen for the eradication of *H. pylori* infection in children has yet to be established, but the use of a proton pump inhibitor in combination with clarithromycin and amoxicillin or metronidazole for 2 weeks is a well-tolerated and recommended triple therapy. Although children < 5 years of age may become reinfected, the most common reason for treatment failure is poor compliance or antibiotic resistance.

6. **(a)** Azithromycin

(Nelson Textbook of Pediatrics, 18th ed.)

For school-aged children and in those in whom infection with *M. pneumoniae* or *C. pneumoniae* (atypical pneumonias) is suggested, a macrolide antibiotic such as azithromycin is an appropriate choice. In adolescents, a respiratory fluoroquinolone (levofloxacin, gatifloxacin, moxifloxacin, gemifloxacin) may be considered for atypical pneumonias.

7. **(b)** Amoxicillin

(Nelson Textbook of Pediatrics, 18th ed.)

For mildly ill children who do not require hospitalization, amoxicillin is recommended. In communities with a high percentage of penicillin-resistant pneumococci, high doses of amoxicillin (80–90 mg/kg/24 hr) should be prescribed.

8. **(b)** Antimotility agents

(Nelson Textbook of Pediatrics, 18th ed.)

Antimotility agents (loperamide) are contraindicated in children with dysentery and probably have no role in the management of acute watery diarrhea in otherwise healthy children. Similarly, antiemetic agents such as the phenothiazines are of little value and are associated with potentially serious side effects (lethargy, dystonia, malignant hyperpyrexia). Nonetheless, ondansetron is an effective and less toxic antiemetic agent. Because persistent vomiting may limit oral rehydration therapy, a single sublingual dose of an oral dissolvable tablet of ondansetron (2 mg children 8–15 kg; 4 mg children <15–30 kg; 8 mg children >30 kg) may be given. However, most children do not require specific antiemetic therapy; careful oral rehydration therapy is usually sufficient.

9. **(d)** All of the above

(Nelson Textbook of Pediatrics, 18th ed.)

- Treatment of an infant with wheezing depends on the underlying etiology. Response to bronchodilators is unpredictable, regardless of cause, but suggests a component of bronchial hyperreactivity. It is appropriate to administer albuterol aerosol and objectively observe the response.
- Infants with acute bronchiolitis who are experiencing respiratory distress should be hospitalized; the mainstay of treatment is supportive. If hypoxemic, the child should receive cool humidified oxygen. Sedatives are to be avoided because they may depress respiratory drive.
- Corticosteroids are not recommended in previously healthy infants with RSV. Ribavirin, an antiviral agent administered by aerosol, has been used for infants with congenital heart disease or chronic lung disease.

10. **(b)** 35–50 mg/kg/day in 3 doses × 7–10 days
(Nelson Textbook of Pediatrics, 18th ed.)
(See Table on the next page)

Amebiasis (*Entamoeba histolytica*)			
Asymptomatic			
Drug of choice:	Lodoquinol	650 mg tid × 20 days	30–40 mg/kg/day (max 2 g) in 3 doses × 20 days
OR	Paromomycin	25–35 mg/kg/day in 3 doses × 7 days	25–35 mg/kg/day in 3 doses × 7 days
Alternative:	Diloxanide furoate[2][*]	500 mg tid × 10 days	20 mg/kg/day in 3 doses × 10 days
Mild to moderate intestinal disease[3]			
Drug of choice[4]:	Metronidazole	500–750 mg tid × 7–10 days	35–50 mg/kg/day in 3 doses × 7–10 days
OR	Tinidazole[5]	2 g once daily × 3 days	50 mg/kg/day (max 2 g) in 1 dose × 3 days
Severe intestinal and extraintestinal disease[3]			
Drug of choice:	Metronidazole	750 mg tid × 7–10 days	35–50 mg/kg/day in 3 doses × 7–10 days
OR	Tinidazole[5]	2 g once daily × 5 days	50 mg/kg/day (max 2 g) × 5 days

11. **(b)** 14-21 days

(Nelson Textbook of Pediatrics, 18th ed.)

Meningitis caused by GBS usually responds within 24–48 hours and should be treated for 14–21 days. Gram-negative bacilli may continue to grow from repeated CSF samples for 72–96 hours after therapy despite the use of appropriate antibiotics. Treatment of gram-negative meningitis should be continued for 21 days or for at least 14 days after sterilization of the CSF, whichever is longer. *P. aeruginosa* meningitis should be treated with ceftazidime. Metronidazole is the treatment of choice for infection caused by *B. fragilis.* Prolonged antibiotic administration, with or without drainage for treatment and diagnosis, is indicated for neonatal cerebral abscesses. CT scans are recommended for patients with suspected ventriculitis, hydrocephalus, or cerebral abscess (initial and follow-up assessments) and for those with an unexpectedly complicated course (prolonged coma, focal neurologic deficits, persistent or recurrent fever). Neonatal herpes meningoencephalitis should be treated with acyclovir, and empirical therapy should be considered in symptomatic infants with a CSF mononuclear pleocytosis. Pleconaril was the treatment of choice for severe enteroviral infections such as meningoencephalitis, carditis or hepatitis.

12. **(c)** Albendazole

(Nelson Textbook of Pediatrics, 18th ed.)

Albendazole is the antiparasitic drug of choice (15 mg/kg/day PO divided bid for 28 days; maximum 800 mg/day). It can be taken with a fatty meal to improve absorption. Praziquantel is an alternative (50–100 mg/kg/day PO divided tid for 28 days). A worsening of symptoms can follow the use of either drug as the host responds to the dying parasite with increased inflammation. Corticosteroids for 2–3 days before and during drug therapy can ameliorate these effects but may decrease praziquantel levels by as much as 50%. An increase of praziquantel (to 100 mg/kg/day divided tid PO) or administration of cimetidine, an inhibitor of the cytochrome P450 system, has been advocated when both praziquantel and corticosteroids are used. Albendazole levels, in contrast, increase in the presence of corticosteroids.

13. **(c)** Fentanyl

(Nelson Textbook of Pediatrics, 18th ed.)

(See Table on the next page)

Fentanyl	0.5-μg/kg increments q 5 min up to 3–5 doses	Rapid infusion of large doses can produce chest wall rigidity
		Respiratory depression is amplified by co-administration of sedatives
Pentobarbital	1-mg/kg increments IV q 10 min up to 3 doses	Good sedative
	2–4 mg/kg IM	No analgesia
	4–6 mg/kg PO	Used often for radiologic procedures
		Can produce prolonged sedation

14. **(c)** Flumazenil

(Nelson Textbook of Pediatrics, 18th ed.)

(See the following Table)

Drugs used for conscious sedation in children

Drug	**Suggested starting dose(s)**	**Comments**
Midazolam	0.05-mg/kg incremental doses IV q 5–10 min up to 3–5 doses (to a maximum incremental dose of 1 mg)	Good anxiolytic Flumazenil is a reversal
	0.1–0.2 mg/kg IM (maximum dose, 10 mg)	Dose more cautiously when combined with opioids
	0.3–0.6 mg/kg PO (maximum dose, 20 mg)	

15. **(a)** Midazolam

(Nelson Textbook of Pediatrics, 18th ed.)

Ketamine	0.2–0.5-mg/kg increments q 10 min × 3	Co-administration of midazolam or other benzodiazepines can reduce the risk of dysphoria or bad dreams
	1–2 mg/kg IM	Use should be restricted to cases managed by physicians with deep sedation qualifications

16. **(b)** Azithromycin

(Nelson Textbook of Pediatrics, 18th ed.)

Poverty and lack of sanitation are important factors in the spread of trachoma. As socioeconomic conditions improve, the incidence of the disease decreases substantially. Endemic trachoma has been controlled in most instances by administering topical tetracyclines (or, rarely, erythromycin ointment) daily for periods of 6–10 weeks or intermittently over a 6 months period. Oral doxycycline is effective but is contraindicated in children < 9 years of age. Oral erythromycin requires frequent dosing, which is impractical in the control of endemic trachoma. One study reported that 1–6 doses of oral azithromycin were equivalent to 30 days of treatment with topical oxytetracycline/polymyxin ointment. The WHO recommends single-dose azithromycin (20 mg/kg, maximum 1 g) for the treatment of trachoma in children. A recent study from Tanzania demonstrated that mass treatment with a single dose of azithromycin to all the residents of a village dramatically reduced the prevalence and intensity of infection. This effect continued for 2 years after treatment, probably by interrupting the transmission of ocular *C. trachomatis* infection.

17. **(c)** Both

(Nelson Textbook of Pediatrics, 18th ed.)

The decision to use *continuous daily medication* (prophylactic therapy) is based on the severity and frequency of the headaches and on the impact of the migraine on the child's daily activities, including school attendance and performance as well as participation in recreation. The use of prophylactic drugs should be considered if a child experiences more than two to four severe episodes monthly or is unable to attend school regularly. Only two drugs have been subjected to rigorous controlled studies to test the efficacy and tolerability of these agents in reducing the severity and frequency of childhood migraine; propranolol, a β blocker, and flunarizine, a calcium channel blocking agent. The dose of propranolol is 10–20 mg tid (beginning with 10 mg/24 hours and gradually increasing the drug to the maximum dose or until the desired therapeutic effect is achieved) in children 7–8 years and older. A common mistake is to discontinue the drug prematurely, because it often takes several weeks to a month until the drug is effective. Flunarizine (not available in the United States) also has been shown to be an effective drug for the prophylaxis of pediatric migraine. The initial dose is 5 mg at bedtime and increased if necessary to 10 mg. The most frequent side effect is drowsiness. Additional drugs that show promise for the prophylaxis of pediatric migraine include sodium valproate, toprimate, levetiracetam, gabapentin, cyproheptadine, and amitriptyline.

18. **(a)** 15 mg/kg

(Nelson Textbook of Pediatrics, 18th ed.)

Management of an acute attack of migraine should include the use of analgesics and antiemetics. Most migraine headaches in children can be treated by the judicious use of *acetaminophen (15 mg/kg)* or *ibuprofen (7.5–10 mg/kg)* dispensed in the gel capsule formulation, particularly if the headaches are mild, infrequent, and of short duration.

19. **(a)** Propofol

(Nelson Textbook of Pediatrics, 18th ed.)

Propofol

Propofol is the most commonly used intravenous induction agent in pediatric anesthesiology and has a rapid onset. In doses of 2–3 mg/kg, propofol induces less respiratory depression than thiopental, but does produce hypotension. Propofol can sometimes burn and itch on injection; this frequently leads the child to withdraw or otherwise respond after a propofol bolus. After induction of anesthesia, propofol is also a useful agent for maintaining hypnosis and amnesia and can be used as a sole anesthetic agent for nonpainful procedures, such as radiation therapy, MRI and CT. Combined with opioids, it provides excellent, brief anesthesia for painful procedures, such as lumbar puncture and bone marrow aspiration. Propofol is a general anesthetic agent and obtunds airway reflexes, respiration, and hemodynamic function and should not be considered a "sedation agent". Although hemodynamic stability, and even spontaneous respirations, can be maintained with propofol sedation, its use for prolonged sedation over several hours to days in children younger than age 12 years is associated with hemodynamic collapse, metabolic acidosis, cardiac failure, profound shock and death. Its use for prolonged sedation (>12 hours) in the critical care setting in children is contraindicated.

20. **(d)** All of the above

(Nelson Textbook of Pediatrics, 18th ed.)

Management of the child with enuresis should begin with behavioral treatment.

Pharmacotherapy for enuresis is 2nd line treatment and should be reserved for cases in which behavioral treatment is unsuccessful. Comparison of the bell-and-pad system vs imipramine and desmopressin acetate (DDAVP) shows lower relapse rates for the bell-and-pad system, although the initial response rates are similar. Imipramine (Tofranil) at starting doses of 10–25 mg in children >5 years and maximum doses of 75 mg in adolescents before bedtime has a success rate of approximately 50%, with a relapse rate of 30% or more even after 6 months of treatment. Imipramine is associated with cardiac conduction disturbances and may be lethal in overdose. DDAVP can be administered orally or intranasally at bedtime. The fast action of DDAVP suggests a role for special occasions (such as overnight visits) when rapid control of enuresis is desired. Unfortunately, the relapse rate on discontinuation of DDAVP is very high, and 1 month of treatment typically costs as much as a bell-and-pad system (which can be used for several months, as necessary). DDAVP is also associated with rare side effects of hyponatremia and water intoxication, with resulting seizures.

Chapter 35

Physiology in Relation to Pediatrics

GENERAL

1. **Total Body Water (TBW) as a percentage of body weight for a term infant is:**
   (a) 55% of birth weight (b) 65% of birth weight
   (c) 75% of birth weight (d) 85% of birth weight

2. **The dominant cation and anion respectively in ECF are:**
   (a) Sodium and chloride
   (b) Sodium and phosphate
   (c) Potassium and chloride
   (d) Potassium and phosphate

3. **The plasma osmolality is maintained at:**
   (a) 265-275 mOsm/kg (b) 275-285 mOsm /kg
   (c) 285-295 mOsm/kg (d) 295-305 mOsm/kg

4. **Osmoreceptors are present in:**
   (a) Pituitary (b) Thalamus
   (c) Hypothalamus (d) Pons

5. **The minimum urine osmolality is approximately:**
   (a) 10-20 mOsm/kg (b) 30-50 mOsm/kg
   (c) 50-70 mOsm/kg (d) 70-90 mOsm/kg

6. **More than 40% of total body sodium is in:**
   (a) Muscles (b) Interstitial spaces
   (c) Intravascular spaces (d) Bones

7. **Principal site of sodium excretion is:**
   (a) Skin (b) Lung
   (c) Bowel (d) Kidney

8. **The majority of body potassium is contained in:**
   (a) Muscles (b) Bones
   (c) Tendons (d) Teeth

9. **Hormone which increases potassium movement into the cells:**
   (a) ADH (b) Insulin
   (c) ACTH (d) TSH

10. **The normal plasma magnesium concentration is:**
   (a) 1.5-2.3 mg/dL (b) 2.5-3.3 mg/dL
   (c) 3.5-4.3 mg/dL (d) 4.5-5.3 mg/dL

DIGESTIVE SYSTEM

1. **Nutritive sucking in a neonate first develops at:**
   (a) 32 weeks of gestation
   (b) 33weeks of gestation
   (c) 34 weeks of gestation
   (d) 35 weeks of gestation

2. **Regurgitation occurs in ___ year of life.**
   (a) 1st (b) 2nd
   (c) 3rd (d) 4th

3. **The tonic LES tone at rest is**
   (a) ~10 mm Hg (b) ~20 mmHg
   (c) ~30 mm Hg (d) ~40 mmHg

4. **The normal oesophageal peristaltic speed is:**
   (a) ~1 cm/sec (b) ~2 cm/sec
   (c) ~3 cm/sec (d) ~4 cm/sec

5. **Bile salts and vitamin B_{12} are absorbed in**
   (a) Distal ileum (b) Distal jejunum
   (c) Proximal ileum (d) Proximal jejunum

6. **Acetylcholine mediates the:**
   (a) Intestinal phase (b) Cephalic space
   (c) Both (d) None

7. **The stimulus for bicarbonate production is:**
   (a) CCK (b) Gastrin
   (c) Acetylcholine (d) Secretin

8. **Before excretion, cholic acid and chenodeoxycholic acid are conjugated with:**
   (a) Glycine and taurine (b) Glycine and tyrosine
   (c) Leucine and taurine (d) Leucine and tyrosine

9. Lipases liberate fatty acids from __and__ position of a triglyceride leaving a monoglyceride.
(a) 1 and 3 (b) 1 and 5
(c) 1 and 7 (d) 1 and 9

10. Swallowing is initiated by:
(a) Depression of the tongue
(b) Elevation of the tongue
(c) Both
(d) None

RESPIRATORY SYSTEM

1. The volume of gas remaining in the lung after maximum expiration is:
(a) Tidal lung capacity
(b) Expiratory reserve volume
(c) Vital capacity
(d) Residual volume

2. At rest, chest wall and lung recoil in:
(a) Same direction (b) Opposite direction
(c) None (d) Both

3. Elastance is calculated as:
(a) 8 lη ÷ πr4 (b) 2rvd ÷ η
(c) ΔP ÷ ΔV (d) ΔV ÷ ΔP

4. Autonomic control of respiration lies in:
(a) Brainstem
(b) Cerebellum
(c) Limbic forebrain structures
(d) Cerebral motor cortex

5. Inspiratory stridor is the hallmark of:
(a) Extrathoracic airway obstruction
(b) Intrathoracic–extrapulmonary airway obstruction
(c) Intrapulmonary airway obstruction
(d) Parenchymal pathology

6. Air movement in areas that are poorly perfused is called:
(a) Closing capacity
(b) Dead space ventilation
(c) Venous admixture
(d) Intrapulmonary right-left shunting

7. All are true *except:*
(a) Alveolar air is 100% humidified
(b) Oxygen delivery to the tissues is a product of oxygen content and cardiac output
(c) Venous blood brought to the lungs is "arterialized" after diffusion is complete
(d) When hemoglobin is near 100% saturated, the blood contains ≈10 mL oxygen per 100 mL or 100 mL/L

8. During intrauterine fetal development, the tunica media of pulmonary arteries become more muscular in:
(a) 1st trimester (b) 2nd trimester
(c) Last trimester (d) At the time of birth

9. The PVR is ≈50% of the systemic arterial resistance ___ days after birth.
(a) 3 (b) 4
(c) 5 (d) 6

10. In the lung, ________ are the chief architects of the early cytokine response.
(a) Alveolar macrophages
(b) Lymphocytes
(c) Eosinophils
(d) Neutrophils

CARDIOVASCULAR SYSTEM AND HAEMATOLOGY

1. The most effective means of increasing ventricular function in a fetus is:
(a) Increasing preload (b) Increasing heart rate
(c) Increasing afterload (d) None of the above

2. The total fetal cardiac output is;
(a) ~150 ml/kg/min (b) ~250 ml/kg/min
(c) ~350 ml/kg/min (d) ~450 ml/kg/min

3. The average central aortic pressure in a term neonate is:
(a) 75/50 mm of Hg (b) 85/50 mm of Hg
(c) 75/60 mm of Hg (d) 85/60 mm of Hg

4. Significant differences between the neonatal circulation and that of older infants include all *except:*
(a) Right-to-left or left-to-right shunting may persist across the patent foramen ovale
(b) In the presence of cardiopulmonary disease, continued patency of the ductus arteriosus may allow left-to-right, right-to-left, or bidirectional shunting
(c) The neonatal pulmonary vasculature constricts more vigorously in response to hypoxemia, hypercapnia and acidosis
(d) Newborn infants at rest have relatively low oxygen consumption

5. **In a full-term neonate, _____ is the most important factor controlling ductal closure.**
(a) Oxygen
(b) Endogenously produced prostaglandins
(c) Carbon dioxide
(d) None of the above

6. **By 6-8 weeks of gestation the _____replaces the yolk sac as the primary site of blood cell production.**
(a) Bone marrow (b) Liver
(c) Both (d) None

7. **All of the following are true *except:***
(a) In children and adults, neutrophils and macrophages originate from a common progenitor cell
(b) Neutrophils are first observed in the human fetus about 5 weeks postconception as small clusters of cells around the aorta
(c) From 14 weeks through term, the most common granulocytic cell type found in the fetal bone marrow space is the monocyte
(d) The fetal bone marrow space begins to develop around the 8th week postconception

8. **The gene that encodes TPO is located on the long arm of human chromosome:**
(a) 2 (b) 3
(c) 4 (d) 5

9. **Factor/s stimulating erythropoiesis is/are:**
(a) Hypoxia (b) Anaemia
(c) Both (d) None

10. **Factor VIII and platelets are stored in the:**
(a) Bone marrow (b) Liver
(c) Spleen (d) None of the above

ENDOCRINE SYSTEM

1. **All of the following stimulate release of GH *except:***
(a) Sleep (b) Exercise
(c) Hypoglycemia (d) Hypothyroidism

2. **PRL is consistently secreted unless it is actively inhibited by:**
(a) Dopamine (b) Oxytocin
(c) Thyroxine (d) Glucocorticoids

3. **_______ is the principal pigmentary hormone in humans.**
(a) ACTH (b) TSH
(c) TRH (d) CRH

4. **Before trapped iodide can react with tyrosine, it must be oxidized; this reaction is catalyzed by:**
(a) Thyroidal peroxidase (b) Thyroidal peptidase
(c) Thyroidal protease (d) None of the above

5. **Which of the following are true?**
(a) The metabolic potency of T3 is 3 to 4 times that of T4
(b) The metabolic potency of T4 is 3 to 4 times that of T3
(c) T3 and T4 are equipotent
(d) All are false

6. **The actions of PTH are:**
(a) Stimulates activity of 1α-hydroxylase in the kidney
(b) Increases intestinal absorption of calcium
(c) Mobilizes calcium by directly enhancing bone resorption
(d) All of the above

7. **Pulses of ACTH and cortisol occur every:**
(a) 30-120 mins (b) 30-220 mins
(c) 30-320 mins (d) 30-420 mins

8. **The rate of aldosterone synthesis, is regulated mainly by:**
(a) Renin-angiotensin system and by potassium levels
(b) Renin-angiotensin system and by sodium levels
(c) ACTH and by sodium levels
(d) ACTH and by potassium levels

9. **The most important estrogens produced by the ovary are:**
(a) Estradiol-17 and estrone
(b) Estradiol-17 and estriol
(c) Estradiol-16 and estrone
(d) Estradiol-16 and estriol

10. **The development of nocturnal pulsatile secretion of ____marks the advent of puberty.**
(a) LH (b) FSH
(c) Testosterone (d) Estrogen

Answers

GENERAL

1. **(c)** 75% of birth weight

(Nelson, 18th edition)

Total body water (TBW) as a percentage of body weight varies with age . The fetus has very high TBW, which gradually decreases to approximately 75% of birthweight for a term infant. Premature infants have higher TBW than term infants. During the 1st year. of life, TBW decreases to approximately 60% of body weight and basically remains at this level until puberty. At puberty, the fat content of females increases more than that of males, who acquire more muscle mass than females. Because fat has very low water content and muscle has high water content, by the end of puberty, TBW in males remains at 60%, but TBW in females decreases to approximately 50% of body weight.

2. **(a)** Sodium and chloride

(Nelson, 18th edition)

Sodium and chloride are the dominant cation and anion, respectively, in the ECF. Potassium is the most abundant cation in the ICF, and its concentration within the cells is approximately 30 times higher than in the ECF. Proteins, organic anions, and phosphate are the most plentiful anions in the ICF.

3. **(c)** 285-295 mOsm/kg

(Nelson, 18th edition)

The plasma osmolality is tightly regulated and maintained at 285–295 mOsm/kg. Modification of water intake and excretion maintains normal plasma osmolality. In the steady state, the combination of water intake and water produced by the body from oxidation balances water losses from the skin, lungs, urine and gastrointestinal tract.

4. **(c)** Hypothalamus

(Nelson, 18th edition)

Osmoreceptors in the hypothalamus sense the plasma osmolality. An elevated effective osmolality leads to secretion of antidiuretic hormone (ADH) by neurons in the supraoptic and paraventricular nuclei in the hypothalamus. The axons of these neurons terminate in the posterior pituitary.

5. **(b)** 30-50 mOsm/kg

(Nelson, 18th edition)

The minimum urine osmolality is approximately 30–50 mOsm/kg.The maximum urine osmolality is about 1,200 mOsm/kg.

6. **(d)** Bones

(Nelson, 18th edition)

More than 40% of total body sodium is in bone; the remainder is in the interstitial and intravascular spaces. The low intracellular sodium concentration, approximately 10 mEq/L, is maintained by Na+, K+-ATPase, which exchanges intracellular sodium for extracellular potassium.

7. **(d)** Kidney

(Nelson, 18th edition)

Sodium excretion occurs in stool and sweat, but the kidney regulates sodium balance and is the principal site of sodium excretion. There is some sodium loss in stool, but this is minimal unless diarrhea is present. Normally, sweat has 5–40 mEq/L of sodium. There is increased sweat sodium concentration in children with cystic fibrosis, aldosterone deficiency, or pseudohypoaldosteronism.

8. **(a)** Muscles

(Nelson, 18th edition)

The intracellular concentration of potassium, approximately 150 mEq/L, is much higher than the plasma concentration . The majority of body potassium is contained in muscle. As muscle mass increases, there is an increase in body potassium. There is thus an increase in body potassium during puberty, and it is more significant in males. The majority of extracellular potassium is in bone; <1% of total body potassium is in plasma.

9. **(b)** Insulin

(Nelson, 18th edition)

Insulin increases potassium movement into cells by activating the Na+, K+-ATPase. Because hyperkalemia stimulates insulin secretion, this may have a protective effect during hyperkalemia.

10. **(a)** 1.5-2.3 mg/dL

(Nelson, 18th edition)

Magnesium is the 4th most common cation in the body and the 3rd most common intracellular cation. Between 50% and 60% of body magnesium is in bone, where it serves as a reservoir because 30% is exchangeable, allowing movement to the extracellular space. Most intracellular magnesium is bound to proteins; only approximately 25% is exchangeable. Because cells with higher metabolic rates have higher magnesium concentrations, most intracellular magnesium is present in muscle and liver.The normal plasma magnesium concentration is 1.5–2.3 mg/dL (1.2–1.9 mEq/L; 0.62–0.94 mmol/L), with some variation between clinical laboratories.

DIGESTIVE SYSTEM

1. **(c)** 34 weeks of gestation

(Nelson, 18th edition)

A fetus can swallow amniotic fluid as early as 12 weeks gestation, but nutritive sucking in neonates 1st develops at about 34 weeks gestation. The coordinated oral and pharyngeal movements necessary for swallowing solids develop within the 1st few months of life.

2. **(a)** 1st

(Nelson, 18th edition)

Regurgitation, the result of gastroesophageal reflux, occurs commonly in the 1st year of life. In an otherwise healthy infant with regurgitation, volumes of emesis are commonly ≈15–30 mL but may occasionally be larger. Regurgitation gradually resolves in 80% of infants by 6 months of age and in 90% by 12 months.

3. **(b)** ~20 mm Hg

(Nelson, 18th edition)

At rest, the tonic LES pressure is normally ≈20 mm Hg; values <10 mm Hg are usually considered abnormal, although it seems that competence against retrograde flow of gastric material is maintained if the LES pressure is >5 mm Hg. The LES pressure rises during intragastric pressure amplifications, whether caused by gastric contractions, abdominal wall muscle contractions ("straining"), or external pressure applied to the abdominal wall. It also rises in response to cholinergic stimuli, gastrin, gastric alkalization, and certain drugs (bethanechol, metoclopramide, cisapride). The UES pressure is more variable and often higher than that of the LES; it decreases almost to zero during deep sleep but increases markedly during stress and straining.

4. **(c)** ~3cm/sec

(Nelson, 18th edition)

The normal esophageal peristaltic speed is ≈3 cm/sec; the wave takes at least 4 sec to traverse the 12 cm esophagus of a young infant and considerably longer in a larger child. Facial stimulation by a puff of air can induce swallowing and esophageal peristalsis in healthy young infants, comprising a reflex termed the Santmyer swallow.

5. **(a)** Distal ileum

(Nelson, 18th edition)

Carbohydrates, protein, and fat are normally absorbed by the upper half of the small intestine; the distal segments represent a vast reserve of absorptive capacity. Most of the sodium, potassium, chloride, and water are absorbed in the small bowel. Bile salts and vitamin B_{12} are selectively absorbed in the distal ileum, and iron is absorbed in the duodenum and proximal jejunum. Intraluminal digestion depends on the exocrine pancreas. Secretin and cholecystokinin stimulate synthesis and secretion of bicarbonate and digestive enzymes, which are released by the upper intestinal mucosa in response to various intraluminal stimuli, among them components of the diet.

6. **(b)** Cephalic space

(Nelson, 18th edition)

Acetylcholine mediates the cephalic phase; cholecystokinin (CCK) mediates the intestinal phase.

7. **(d)** Secretin

(Nelson, 18th edition)

The stimulus for bicarbonate production is secretin in concert with CCK. Secretin cells are abundant in the duodenum.

8. **(a)** Glycine and taurine

(Nelson, 18th edition)

In humans, the two primary bile acids, cholic acid and chenodeoxycholic acid, are synthesized in the liver. Before excretion, they are conjugated with glycine and taurine.

9. **(a)** 1 and 3

(Nelson, 18th edition)

Pancreatic lipase requires colipase, a coenzyme also found in pancreatic fluid, for activity. Lipase liberates fatty acids from the one and three positions of triglycerides, leaving a monoglyceride.

10. **(b)** Elevation of the tongue

(Nelson, 18th edition)

Swallowing is initiated by elevation of the tongue, propelling the bolus into the pharynx. The larynx elevates and moves anteriorly, pulling open the relaxing UES, while the opposed aryepiglottic folds close. The epiglottis drops back to cover the larynx and direct the bolus over the larynx and into the UES. The soft palate occludes the nasopharynx. The primary peristalsis thus initiated is a contraction originating in the oropharynx that clears the esophagus aborally.

RESPIRATORY SYSTEM

1. **(d)** Residual volume

(Nelson, 18th edition)

Lung volumes are traditionally measured with a spirogram . Tidal volume (VT) is the amount of air moved in and out of the lungs during each breath. At rest, it is usually 6–7 mL/kg body weight. Inspiratory capacity (IC) is the amount of air inspired by maximum inspiratory effort after tidal expiration. Expiratory reserve volume (ERV) is the amount of air exhaled by maximum expiratory effort after tidal expiration. The volume of gas remaining in the lungs after maximum expiration is residual volume (RV). Vital capacity (VC) is defined as the amount of air moved in and out of the lungs with maximum inspiration and expiration. VC, IC, and ERV are decreased in lung pathology but are also effort dependent. Total lung capacity (TLC) is the volume of gas occupying the lungs after maximum inhalation.

2. **(b)** Opposite direction

(Nelson, 18th edition)

Since the chest wall and the lungs recoil in opposite directions at rest, FRC is reached at the point where the outward elastic recoil of the thoracic cage counterbalances the inward lung recoil.

3. **(c)** $\Delta P \div \Delta V$

(Nelson, 18th edition)

Elastance refers to the property of a substance to oppose deformation or stretching. It is calculated as a change in pressure (ΔP) ÷ change in volume (ΔV). Compliance ($\Delta V \div \Delta P$) is the reciprocal of elastance.

Resistance to laminar flow is governed by Poiseuille's law stated as: $R = 8\ l\eta \div \pi r4$ where R is resistance, l length, η viscosity, and r radius. Turbulence depends to a great extent on the Reynolds number (Re), a dimensionless entity, which is calculated as $Re = 2rvd \div \eta$ where r is radius, v velocity, d density, and η viscosity. Turbulence in gas flow is most likely to occur when Re exceeds 2000.

4. **(a)** Brainstem

(Nelson, 18th edition)

Voluntary control of respiration resides in the cerebral motor cortex and limbic forebrain structure. Automatic control of respiration resides in the brainstem.

5. **(a)** Extrathoracic airway obstruction

(Nelson, 18th edition)

Rapid and shallow respirations (tachypnea) are characteristic of parenchymal pathology, in which the elastic work of breathing is increased disproportionately to the resistive work of breathing. Chest wall, intercostal, and suprasternal retractions are most striking, with increased negative intrathoracic pressure during inspiration. This occurs in extrathoracic airway obstruction as well as diseases of decreased compliance. Inspiratory stridor is a hallmark of extrathoracic airway obstruction. Expiratory wheezing is characteristic of intrathoracic airway obstruction, either extrapulmonary or intrapulmonary. Grunting is produced by expiration against a partially closed glottis and is an attempt to maintain positive airway pressure during expiration for as long as possible.

6. **(b)** Dead space ventilation

(Nelson, 18th edition)

The lung volume at which the dependent airways start to close is referred to as the closing capacity. Air movement in areas that are poorly perfused is referred to as dead space ventilation. Examples of dead space ventilation include pulmonary thromboembolism and hypovolemia. Perfusion of poorly ventilated alveoli is referred to as intrapulmonary right-to-left shunting or venous admixture. Examples include pneumonia, asthma, and hyaline membrane disease. In intrapulmonary airway obstruction, the closing capacity is abnormally increased and may exceed the FRC. In such situations, perfusion of poorly ventilated alveoli during tidal respiration results in venous admixture.

7. **(d)** When hemoglobin is near 100% saturated, the blood contains ≈ 10 mL oxygen per 100 mL or 100 mL/L

(Nelson, 18th edition)

Alveolar air is 100% humidified and, therefore, for alveolar gas calculations, the inspired gas is also presumed to be 100% humidified.Oxygen delivery to the tissues is a product of oxygen content and cardiac output. Venous blood brought to the lungs is "arterialized" after diffusion is complete.When hemoglobin is near 100% saturated, the blood contains ≈ 20 mL oxygen per 100 mL or 200 mL/L.

8. **(c)** Last trimester

(Nelson, 18th edition)

During intrauterine fetal development, the tunica media of pulmonary arteries become more muscular in the last trimester of pregnancy.

9. **(a)** 3

(Nelson, 18th edition)

The PVR is ≈ 50% of the systemic arterial resistance 3 days after birth. In the next several weeks after birth, there is a further decline in PVR and, therefore, the pulmonary artery pressure, as pulmonary arterial musculature in the tunica media involutes. Two to 3 months after birth, the PVR and the pulmonary artery pressure are ≈ 15% of the systemic values, a relationship that exists through childhood and adolescence. Pulmonary vasculature constricts in response to hypoxemia, acidosis, and hypercarbia, and dilates with increased alveolar and arterial PO_2, alkalosis, and hypocarbia. Younger infants, with their relatively muscular pulmonary arteries, are especially susceptible to pulmonary vasoconstrictive stimuli.

10. **(a)** Alveolar macrophages

(Nelson, 18th edition)

In the lung, alveolar macrophages are the chief architects of the early cytokine response, producing tumor necrosis factor-α (TNF-α) and interleukin 1β (IL-1β).

CARDIOVASCULAR SYSTEM AND HAEMATOLOGY

1. **(b)** Increasing heart rate

(Nelson, 18th edition)

Fetal cardiac function is poorly responsive to changes in both preload (filling volume) and afterload (systemic resistance). The most effective means of increasing ventricular function in a fetus is through increasing the heart rate. After birth and with further maturation, preload and afterload play an increasing role in regulating cardiac function.

2. **(d)** ~450 ml/kg/min

(Nelson, 18th edition)

The total fetal cardiac output—the combined output of both the left and right ventricles—is ≈ 450 mL/kg/min. Approximately 65% of descending aortic blood flow returns to the placenta; the remaining 35% perfuses the fetal organs and tissues.

3. **(a)** 75/50 mm of Hg

(Nelson, 18th edition)

The average central aortic pressure in a term neonate is 75/50 mm Hg.

4. **(d)** Newborn infants at rest have relatively low oxygen consumption

(Nelson, 18th edition)

Significant differences between the neonatal circulation and that of older infants include: (1) right-to-left or left-to-right shunting may persist across the patent foramen ovale; (2) in the presence of cardiopulmonary disease, continued patency of the ductus arteriosus may allow left-to-right, right-to-left, or bidirectional shunting; (3) the neonatal pulmonary vasculature constricts more vigorously in response to hypoxemia, hypercapnia and acidosis; (4) the wall thickness and muscle mass of the neonatal left and right ventricles are almost equal; and (5) newborn infants at rest have relatively high oxygen consumption, which is associated with relatively high cardiac output.

5. **(a)** Oxygen

(Nelson, 18th edition)

During fetal life, patency of the ductus arteriosus appears to be maintained by the combined relaxant effects of low oxygen tension and endogenously produced prostaglandins, specifically prostaglandin E2. In a full-term neonate, oxygen is the most important factor controlling ductal closure. When the PO_2 of the blood passing through the ductus reaches about 50 mmHg, the ductal wall constricts. The effects of oxygen on ductal smooth muscle may be direct or mediated by its effects on prostaglandin synthesis. Gestational age also appears to play an important role; the ductus of a premature infant is less responsive to oxygen, even though its musculature is developed.

6. **(b)** Liver

(Nelson, 18th edition)

Developmental hematopoiesis occurs in three anatomic stages: mesoblastic, hepatic and myeloid. Mesoblastic hematopoiesis occurs in extraembryonic structures, principally in the yolk sac, and begins between the 10th and 14th days of gestation. By 6–8 weeks of gestation the liver replaces the yolk sac as the primary site of blood cell production, and by 10–12 weeks extraembryonic hematopoiesis has essentially ceased. Hepatic hematopoiesis occurs in the liver throughout the remainder of gestation, although production begins to diminish during the second trimester as bone marrow (myeloid) hematopoiesis increases. The liver remains the predominant hematopoietic organ through 20–24 weeks of gestation.

7. **(c)** From 14 weeks through term, the most common granulocytic cell type found in the fetal bone marrow space is the monocyte

(Nelson, 18th edition)

Neutrophils are first observed in the human fetus about 5 weeks postconception as small clusters of cells around the aorta. From 14 weeks through term, the most common granulocytic cell type found in the fetal bone marrow space is the neutrophil. The fetal bone marrow space begins to develop around the 8th week postconception.

8. **(b)** 3

(Nelson, 18th edition)

Thrombopoietin (TPO) is the physiologic regulator of platelet production and acts as a potent stimulator of all stages of megakaryocyte growth and development. The gene that encodes TPO is located on the long arm of human chromosome 3.

9. **(c)** Both

(Nelson, 18th edition)

The regulation of EPO gene expression involves an oxygen-sensing mechanism, and both hypoxia and anemia stimulate erythropoiesis by stimulating mRNA transcription and EPO production.

10. **(c)** spleen

(Nelson, 18th edition)

Factor VIII and platelets are stored in the spleen and can be released by stress or epinephrine injection. Thrombocytosis and leukocytosis occur with loss of the splenic reservoir function.

ENDOCRINE SYSTEM

1. **(d)** Hypothyroidism

(Nelson, 18th edition)

Sleep, exercise, physical stress, trauma, acute illness, puberty, fasting and hypoglycemia stimulate the release of GH, whereas hyperglycemia, hypothyroidism, and glucocorticoids inhibit GH release.

2. **(a)** Dopamine

(Nelson, 18th edition)

The regulation of PRL is unique because PRL is consistently secreted unless it is actively inhibited by dopamine, which is produced by neurons in the hypothalamus. Disruption of the hypothalamus or pituitary stalk can result in elevated PRL levels. Dopamine antagonists, states of primary hypothyroidism, administration of thyrotropin-releasing hormone (TRH), physiologic stress (shock) and pituitary tumors result in increased serum levels of PRL. Dopamine agonists and processes causing destruction of the pituitary cause reduced levels of PRL.

3. **(a)** ACTH

(Nelson, 18th edition)

ACTH also appears to be the principal pigmentary hormone in humans.

4. **(a)** Thyroidal peroxidase

(Nelson, 18th edition)

Before trapped iodide can react with tyrosine, it must be oxidized; this reaction is catalyzed by thyroidal peroxidase. T4 and T3 are liberated from thyroglobulin by activation of proteases and peptidases.

5. **(a)** The metabolic potency of T3 is 3 to 4 times that of T4

(Nelson, 18th edition)

The metabolic potency of T3 is 3 to 4 times that of T4.

6. **(d)** All of the above

(Nelson, 18th edition)

When serum levels of calcium fall, the signal is transduced through the calcium-sensing receptor and secretion of PTH increases. PTH stimulates activity of 1α-hydroxylase in the kidney, enhancing production of 1,25-dihydroxycholecalciferol (1,25[OH]2D3). The increased level of 1,25[OH]2D3 induces synthesis of a calcium-binding protein (calbindin-D) in the intestinal mucosa with resultant absorption of calcium.

PTH also mobilizes calcium by directly enhancing bone resorption, an effect that requires 1,25[OH]2D3. The effects of PTH on bone and kidney are mediated through binding to specific receptors on the membranes of target cells and through activation of a transduction pathway involving a G-protein coupled to the adenylate cyclase system.

7. **(a)** 30-120 mins

(Nelson, 18th edition)

ACTH is released in secretory bursts of varying amplitude throughout the day and night. The normal diurnal rhythm of cortisol secretion is caused by the varying amplitudes of ACTH pulses. Pulses of ACTH and cortisol occur every 30–120 min, are highest at about the time of waking, are low in late afternoon and evening, and reach their lowest point 1 or 2 hours after sleep begins.

8. **(a)** Renin-angiotensin system and by potassium levels

(Nelson, 18th edition)

The rate of aldosterone synthesis, which is normally 100- to 1000- fold less than that of cortisol synthesis, is regulated mainly by the renin-angiotensin system and by potassium levels, with ACTH having only a short-term effect.

9. **(a)** Estradiol-17 and estrone

(Nelson, 18th edition)

The most important estrogens produced by the ovary are estradiol-17 (E2) and estrone (E1); estriol is a metabolic product of these two, and all three estrogens may be found in the urine of mature females.

10. **(a)** LH

(Nelson, 18th edition)

The development of nocturnal pulsatile secretion of LH marks the advent of puberty.

Chapter 36

Pediatric Pathology

1. **Juvenile rheumatoid arthritis is characterized pathologically by:**
   (a) Villous hypertrophy and hyperplasia
   (b) Vascular endothelial hyperplasia
   (c) Pannus formation
   (d) All of the above

2. **Lupus in newborns results from transfer of:**
   (a) IgA autoantibodies (b) IgG autoantibodies
   (c) IgM autoantibodies (d) None of the above

3. **Juvenile dermatomyositis is associated with:**
   (a) HLA Class 1 (b) HLA Class 2
   (c) HLA Class 3 (d) None

4. **In epidemic outbreak pneumocystis carinii, seen as:**
   (a) Infantile interstitial plasma cell pneumonitis
   (b) Infantile interstitial polymorphonuclear cell pneumonitis
   (c) Diffuse desquamative alveolar pneumonitis
   (d) Diffuse squamative alveolar pneumonitis

5. **The Warthin-Finkeldey giant cells that are pathognomonic for:**
   (a) Mumps (b) Measles
   (c) Rubella (d) Varicella-zoster virus

6. **Intussusceptions most common site is:**
   (a) Colic (b) Ileocolic
   (c) Ilum (d) Colon

7. **Cases of acute appendicitis demonstrate luminal obstruction on histologic examination:**
   (a) 50 (b) <50
   (c) 60 (d) 80

8. **In juvenile polyposis seen:**
   (a) Adenoma (b) Hamartoma
   (c) Both (d) None

9. **α_1-Antitrypsin deficiency in children cause:**
   (a) Emphysema (b) Liver disease
   (c) Lung Ca (d) Kidney disease

10. **α1-antitrypsin PiM protein is secreted by**
    (a) Lung (b) Liver
    (c) Kidney (d) Pancreas

11. **Bronchiolitis obliterans organizing pneumonia (BOOP) is:**
    (a) Interstitial lung disease
    (b) Fibrosing lung disease
    (c) Necroting lung disease
    (d) Parenchymal lung disease

12. **Hypersensitivity pneumonitis (HP) or extrinsic allergic alveolitis subacute presentation characterized by:**
    (a) Classical caseating granuloma
    (b) Classical non caseating granuloma
    (c) Classical necrotising granuloma
    (d) Classical non necrotising granuloma

13. **Williams-Campbell syndrome there is absence of:**
    (a) Annular bronchial cartilage
    (b) Annular alveolar cartilage
    (c) Lung parenchyma
    (d) Alveolar septa

14. **Most severe form of bronchiectasis is:**
    (a) Cylindrical (b) Saccular
    (c) Varicose (d) All of the above

15. **Primary pulmonary abscesses found commonly on:**
    (a) Right side (b) Left side
    (c) Both (d) None

16. **In cystic fibrosis early pathological lesion is:**
    (a) Bronchiolitis (b) Bronchitis
    (c) Bronchiolectasis (d) Bronchiolectasis

17. Interstitial lung disease most common form in children is:
(a) Usual interstitial pneumonitis
(b) Lymphocytic interstitial pneumonitis
(c) Desquamative pneumonitis
(d) Pulmonary interstitial glycogenosis

18. Pulmonary hemosiderosis seen:
(a) Hemosiderin-laden macrophages
(b) Thickening of alveolar septae
(c) Hypertrophy of type II pneumocytes
(d) All of the above

19. In Goodpasture syndrome, anti-basement membrane antibody (ABMA) binds to the basement membrane:
(a) Alveolus (b) Glomerulus
(c) Both (d) None

20. Thrombus formation include:
(a) Injury to the vessel endothelium
(b) Hemostasis
(c) Hypercoagulability
(d) All of the above

21. Loculation of the fluid, with thickening of the parietal pleura occur in which stage of empyema?
(a) Exudative stage (b) Fibrinopurulent stage
(c) Organizational stage (d) Squamative stage

22. Pathological change of Eisenmenger syndrome occur in:
(a) Arterioles (b) Vein
(c) Capillary (d) Lymphatic system

23. Heath-Edwards classification of Eisenmenger syndrome, medial hypertrophy and intimal hyperplasia occur in:
(a) Grade 1 (b) Grade 2
(c) Grade 3 (d) Grade 4

24. Congenital hypoplastic anemia also called as
(a) Diamond-Blackfan anemia
(b) Pearson Marrow-Pancreas syndrome
(c) Transient erythroblastopenia of childhood
(d) Red cell aplasia

25. Children with Beckwith-Wiedemann syndrome (BWS) are predisposed to which neoplasm?
(a) Wilm's tumour (b) ALL
(c) GIST (d) Malignant melanoma

26. In transient erythroblastopenia of childhood all occur, *except:*
(a) Decreased in RBC production
(b) Reticulocytes count decreased
(c) Bone marrow erythroid precursors are decreased
(d) Platelet count decreased

27. Most common variant of CDA (congenital dyserythropoietic anemias) is:
(a) CDA Class 1 (b) CDA Class 2
(c) CDA Class 3 (d) CDA Class 4

28. HEMPAS (hereditary erythroblastic multinuclearity with a positive acidified serum test is other name of which CDA class?
(a) Class 1 (b) Class 2
(c) Class 3 (d) Class 4

29. 'CUP' shaped RBC are seen in:
(a) Hereditary spherocytosis
(b) Hereditary elliptocytosis
(c) Hereditary stomatocytosis
(d) None

30. Sickle cell disease, the primary pathology is:
(a) Quantity change in globulin
(b) Quality change in globulin
(c) Both
(d) None

31. Beta-thalassemia, the primary pathology is:
(a) Quantity change in globulin
(b) Quality change in globulin
(c) Both
(d) None

32. Primary polycythemia (Polycythemia Rubra Vera) the major criteria is:
(a) Increased red cell mass
(b) Platelet count of $>400 \times 10^9/L$
(c) Leukocytosis of $>12 \times 10^9/L$
(d) Increased leukocyte alkaline phosphatase

33. Constitutional (Inherited) pancytopenia syndromes are:
(a) Fanconi anemia
(b) Schwachman-Diamond syndrome
(c) Amegakaryocytic thrombocytopenia
(d) All of the above

34. In hemophilia A deficiency of factor:
(a) V (b) VIII
(c) IX (d) X

35. In hemophilia B deficiency of factor:
(a) V (b) VIII
(c) IX (d) X

36. Prolongation of both PT and PTT occur in deficiency of factor:
(a) II (b) V
(c) X (d) All of the above

37. Most common form of VWD (von Willebrand disease) is:
(a) Type 1 (b) Type 2
(c) Type 3 (d) Type 4

38. Reduction of the platelet-binding function of VWF seen in which type?
(a) 2A (b) 2B
(c) 2M (d) 2N

39. Acute lymphoblastic leukemia all are correct *except:*
(a) Childhood ALL was the first disseminated cancer shown to be curable
(b) Acute leukemia occurs about 14 times more frequently in children with Down syndrome
(c) ALL caused by Philadelphia chromosome
(d) None

40. Most common pathological subtypes of childhood and adolescent NHL (non-Hodgkin's lymphoma) is:
(a) Lymphoblastic lymphoma (LL)
(b) Burkitt lymphoma (BL)
(c) Diffuse large B-cell lymphoma (DLBCL)
(d) Anaplastic large cell lymphoma (ALCL)

41. Childhood brain tumors based on histology most common type is:
(a) Medulloblastoma
(b) Juvenile pilocytic astrocytoma
(c) Craniopharyngioma
(d) Both (a) and (b)

42. Most common astrocytoma in children is:
(a) Juvenile pilocytic astrocytoma
(b) Low-grade astrocytoma
(c) High-grade astrocytoma
(d) Fibrillary infiltrating astrocytoma

43. Most common bone tumor occur in children is:
(a) Osteosarcoma (b) Ewing sarcoma
(c) Chondroblastoma (d) Bone cyst

44. Most common gynaecological tumor occur in childhood is:
(a) Breast tumor (b) Ovarian tumor
(c) Uterine tumor (d) Cervical tumor

45. Most common malignant ovarian tumor in adolescent:
(a) Germ cell tumor (b) Sex cord stromal tumor
(c) Epithelial tumor (d) Squamous cell tumor

46. α - fetoprotein tumor marker seen in:
(a) Endodermal sinus tumors
(b) Choriocarcinoma
(c) Dysgerminoma
(d) Sertoli cell tumors

47. Vaginal carcinoma that occurs primarily in pediatric age is:
(a) Sarcoma botryoides
(b) Adenocarcinoma of the corpus
(c) Squamous carcinoma
(d) All of the above

48. True about subacute thyroiditis (Hashimoto's thyroiditis) is:
(a) Lymphocytic infiltration
(b) Giant cells, granulomas
(c) Abscess formation
(d) Abscess formation

49. Most common thyroid carcinoma is:
(a) Papillary (b) Follicular
(c) Medullary (d) Anaplastic

50. RET proto-oncogene is seen in which type of thyroid ca?
(a) Papillary ca (b) Medullary ca
(c) Anaplastic ca (d) Follicular ca

51. Adrenal medullary hyperplasia or pheochromocytoma and parathyroid hyperplasia is seen in:
(a) MEN 1 (b) MEN 2 A
(c) MEN 2 B (d) MEN 2 C

52. Most common intramedullary tumor of spinal cord is:
(a) Low grade astrocytoma
(b) High grade astrocytoma
(c) Ganglioglioma
(d) Ependyoma

Answers

1. **(a)** All of the above

(Nelson Textbook of Pediatrics, 18th ed.)

The synovitis of JRA is characterized pathologically by villous hypertrophy and hyperplasia with hyperemia and edema of the subsynovial tissues. Vascular endothelial hyperplasia is prominent and characterized by infiltration of mononuclear and plasma cells. Pannus formation, which is an inflammatory exudate over the synovial lining, occurs in advanced uncontrolled disease and results in progressive erosion of articular cartilage and contiguous bone.

2. **(b)** IgG autoantibodies

(Nelson Textbook of Pediatrics, 18th ed.)

Lupus in newborns results from maternal transfer of IgG autoantibodies, usually anti-Ro/SSA or anti-La/SSB, between the 12th and 16th week of gestation. Only a small percentage of offspring of mothers with autoantibodies to Ro and/or La develop disease. Maternal or fetal factors must have an added role. Symptoms usually derive from a single organ, although multiple organ involvement may occur and include congenital heart block, cutaneous lesions, hepatitis, thrombocytopenia, neutropenia, and pulmonary and neurologic disease. Cutaneous lesions occur after ultraviolet exposure at about 6 weeks of life and last 3–4 months. The rash most frequently occurs on the face and scalp, and 25% of rashes scar. Treatment is supportive. Most manifestations resolve, although congenital heart block is permanent and often requires cardiac pacing, either after birth or, when detected and severe, antenatally. Corticosteroid treatment of the pregnant mother after heart block is detected early in utero and postnatal steroids may be effective. Even infants of asymptomatic mothers with lupus may have slightly prolonged PR intervals. Cardiomyopathy is a rare serious sequela, sometimes requiring heart transplantation.

Neonatal lupus must be distinguished from neonatal onset multisystem inflammatory disease, a rare syndrome characterized by fever, rash, arthropathy, chronic meningitis, seizures, uveitis, and lymphadenopathy. This autoinflammatory syndrome, resulting from defective IL-1 regulation in the innate immune system, is difficult to treat and requires long-term immunomodulation Anakinra, an IL-1 antagonist, has been very successful in the treatment of a small cohort of these patients.

3. **(b)** HLA Class 2

(Nelson Textbook of Pediatrics, 18th ed.)

Susceptibility to JDM appears to be associated with the class II HLA antigen, DQA1*0501, which is found in >80% of children with JDM in the United States, and may interact with DRB*0301 to define the antigen binding site. Chronicity of JDM is associated with the tumor necrosis factor (TNF)–α-308A allele, which is a substitution of an A for a G in position -308 of the promoter region for the TNF-α gene. Children with JDM who have the TNF-α-308A allele, compared with children with JDM without this allele, frequently have increased cellular production of TNF-α, a chronic disease course requiring immunosuppressive therapy for >36 months, and increased frequency of pathologic calcifications.

4. **(a)** Infantile interstitial plasma cell pneumonitis

(Nelson Textbook of Pediatrics, 18th ed.)

The histopathologic features of P. carinii pneumonia are of 2 types. The 1st type is infantile interstitial plasma cell pneumonitis, which is seen in epidemic outbreaks in debilitated infants 3–6 months of age. Extensive infiltration with thickening of the alveolar septum occurs, and plasma cells are prominent. The 2nd type is a diffuse desquamative alveolar pneumonitis found in immunocompromised children and adults. The alveoli contain large numbers of P. carinii in a foamy exudate with alveolar macrophages active in the phagocytosis of organisms. The alveolar septum is not infiltrated to the extent it is in the infantile type, and plasma cells are usually absent.

5. **(b)** Measles

(Nelson Textbook of Pediatrics, 18th ed.)

TheWarthin-Finkeldey giant cells that are pathognomonic for measles, with up to 100 nuclei and intracytoplasmic and intranuclear inclusions.

6. **(b)** Ileocolic

(Nelson Textbook of Pediatrics, 18th ed.)

Intussusceptions are most often ileocolic, less commonly cecocolic, and rarely exclusively ileal. Very rarely, the appendix forms the apex of an intussusception.

7. **(b)** <50

(Nelson Textbook of Pediatrics, 18th ed.)

The finding that <50% of specimens from cases of acute appendicitis demonstrate luminal obstruction on histologic examination has lead to investigations of alternative etiologies. Enteric infection likely plays a role in many cases in association with mucosal ulceration and invasion of the appendiceal wall by bacteria.

8. **(b)** Hamartoma

(Nelson Textbook of Pediatrics, 18th ed.)

See the following Table

9. **(b)** Liver disease

(Nelson Textbook of Pediatrics, 18th ed.)

Homozygous deficiency of α_1-antitrypsin (α-AT) is an important cause of the early onset of severe panacinar pulmonary emphysema in adults in the 3rd and 4th decades of life and an important cause of liver disease in children; it rarely causes lung disease in children.

10. **(b)** Liver

(Nelson Textbook of Pediatrics, 18th ed.)

The normal α_1-antitrypsin PiM protein is secreted by the liver into the circulation at a rate of ≈ 34 mg/kg/day. Mutant protein is not produced (null), or is misfolded (PiZ and others); it may polymerize in the endoplasmic reticulum or be degraded, with subsequent low serum levels. Early adult-onset emphysema associated with α_1-antitrypsin deficiency occurs most frequently with PiZZ (mutation in SERPINA1 gene), although Pi (null) (null) and, to a lesser extent, other mutant Pi types such as SZ have been associated with emphysema.

11. **(b)** Fibrosing lung disease

(Nelson Textbook of Pediatrics, 18th ed.)

Bronchiolitis obliterans organizing pneumonia (BOOP) is a fibrosing lung disease that includes the histologic features of BO with extension of the inflammatory process from distal alveolar ducts into alveoli and proliferation of fibroblasts. Bronchiolitis obliterans syndrome (BOS) is a clinical entity that relates to graft deterioration after transplantation due to progressive airway disease that appears histologically similar to BO.

12. **(b)** Classical non caseating granuloma

(Nelson Textbook of Pediatrics, 18th ed.)

HP can present as an acute, subacute, or chronic illness. These forms can be distinguished based on the morphologic features of the pulmonary involvement. In the acute stage, alveolar walls are infiltrated by neutrophils, lymphocytes, plasma cells, and macrophages. The alveolar lumen may contain a proteinaceous exudate mixed with inflammatory cells.

Ans. 8

General Features of the Inherited Colorectal Cancer Syndromes

Syndrome	Polyp Histology	Polyp Distribution	Age of Onset	Risk of Colon Cancer	Genetic Lesion	Clinical Manifestations	Associated Lesions
Familial adenomatous polyposis	Adenoma	Large intestine	16 yr (range 8–34 yr)	100%	5q (APC gene)	Rectal bleeding, abdominal pain, bowel obstruction	Desmoids, CHRPE
Gardner syndrome	Adenoma	Large and small intestine	16 yr (range 8–34 yr)	100%	5q (APC gene)	Rectal bleeding, abdominal pain, bowel obstruction	Desmoids, CHRPE
Peutz-Jeghers syndrome	Hamartoma	Large and small intestine	1st decade	Increased	19p (STK11)	Possible rectal bleeding, abdominal pain, intussusception	Orocutaneous melanin pigment spots
Juvenile polyposis	Hamartoma (rarely adenoma)	Large and small intestine	1st decade	~10–50%	PTEN, SMAD4, BMPR1	Possible rectal bleeding, abdominal pain, intussusception	Congenital abnormalities in 20% of the nonfamilial type
Heriditary nonpolyposis colon cancer	Adenoma	Large intestine	40 yr (range 18–65 yr)	30%	Mismatch repair genes[*]	Rectal bleeding, abdominal pain, bowel obstruction	Other tumors (e.g., ovary, ureter, pancreas, stomach)

Repeated or continuous exposure may result in a subacute presentation characterized by the classic non-caseating granuloma associated with HP.

13. **(a)** Annular bronchial cartilage

(Nelson Textbook of Pediatrics, 18th ed.)

Bronchiectasis can also be congenital, as in Williams-Campbell syndrome, in which there is an absence of annular bronchial cartilage, and Marnier-Kuhn syndrome (congenital tracheobronchomegaly), in which there is a connective tissue disorder. Other disease entities associated with bronchiectasis include right middle lobe syndrome (chronic extrinsic compression of right middle lobe bronchus by hilar lymph nodes) and yellow nail syndrome (pleural effusion, lymphedema, discolored nails).

14. **(a)** Cylindrical

(Nelson Textbook of Pediatrics, 18th ed.)

Bronchiectasis can present in any combination of three pathologic forms, best defined by high-resolution CT (HRCT) scan. In cylindrical bronchiectasis, the bronchial outlines are regular, but there is diffuse dilatation of the bronchial unit. The bronchial lumen ends abruptly because of mucous plugging. In varicose bronchiectasis, the degree of dilatation is greater and local constrictions cause an irregularity of outline resembling varicose veins. There may also be small sacculations. In saccular (cystic) bronchiectasis, bronchial dilatation progresses and results in ballooning of bronchi that end in fluid- or mucus-filled sacs. This is the most severe form of bronchiectasis.

15. **(a)** Right side

(Nelson Textbook of Pediatrics, 18th ed.)

Primary abscesses are found most often on the right side, whereas secondary lung abscesses, particularly in immunocompromised patients, have a predilection for the left side.

16. **(a)** Bronchiolitis

(Nelson Textbook of Pediatrics, 18th ed.)

The earliest pathologic lesion in the lung is that of bronchiolitis (mucous plugging and an inflammatory response in the walls of the small airways). With time, mucus accumulation and inflammation extend to the larger airways (bronchitis). Goblet cell hyperplasia and submucosal gland hypertrophy become prominent pathologic expressions of a hypersecretory state, which is most likely a response to chronic airway infection. Organisms appear to be confined to the endobronchial space; invasive bacterial infection is not characteristic. With long-standing disease, evidence of airway destruction such as bronchiolar obliteration, bronchiolectasis, and bronchiectasis becomes prominent.

17. **(b)** Lymphocytic interstitial pneumonitis

(Nelson Textbook of Pediatrics, 18th ed.)

Lymphocytic interstitial pneumonitis (LIP), the most common form of ILD in children, is a form of pulmonary lymphoproliferative disease. LIP usually develops in association with conditions of impaired immunity, such as an autoimmune disease or immunodeficiency (HIV infection). The pulmonary interstitium is invaded by a diffuse infiltrate of mature lymphocytes. Fibrosis is rare.

18. **(c)** All of the above

With repeated episodes of pulmonary hemorrhage, lung tissue appears brown secondary to the presence of hemosiderin. The finding of blood in the airways or alveoli is representative of a recent hemorrhage. Hemosiderin-laden macrophages are seen with recovering, recurrent, or chronic pulmonary hemorrhage. It takes 48–72 hours for the alveolar macrophages to convert iron from erythrocytes into hemosiderin. Hemosiderin-laden macrophages may be detectable for weeks after a hemorrhagic event. Other nonspecific pathologic findings can include thickening of alveolar septae and hypertrophy of type II pneumocytes. Fibrosis may be seen with chronic disease.

19. **(c)** Both

(Nelson Textbook of Pediatrics, 18th ed.)

In Goodpasture syndrome, anti-basement membrane antibody (ABMA) binds to the basement membrane of both the alveolus and the glomerulus. At the alveolar level, immunoglobulin G (IgG), IgM, and complement are deposited at alveolar septae. Electron microscopy shows disruption of basement membranes and vascular integrity, thereby allowing blood to escape into alveolar spaces.

20. **(d)** All of the above

(Nelson Textbook of Pediatrics, 18th ed.)

Favorable conditions for thrombus formation include injury to the vessel endothelium, hemostasis, and hypercoagulability.

21. **(b)** Fibrinopurulent stage

(Nelson Textbook of Pediatrics, 18th ed.)

Empyema has 3 stages: exudative, fibrinopurulent, and organizational. During the exudative stage, fibrinous exudate forms on the pleural surfaces. In the fibrinopurulent stage, fibrinous septae form, causing loculation of the fluid, with thickening of the parietal pleura. If the pus is not drained, it may dissect through the pleura into lung parenchyma, producing bronchopleural fistulas and pyopneumothorax, or into the abdominal cavity. Rarely, the pus dissects through the chest wall (i.e., empyema necessitatis). During the organizational stage, there is fibroblast proliferation, and pockets of loculated pus may develop into thick-walled abscess cavities or the lung may collapse and become surrounded by a thick, inelastic envelope (peel).

22. **(a)** Arterioles

(Nelson Textbook of Pediatrics, 18th ed.)

The pathologic changes of Eisenmenger syndrome occur in the small pulmonary arterioles and muscular arteries (<300 mm) and are graded on the basis of histologic characteristics (Heath-Edwards classification): Grade I changes involve medial hypertrophy alone, grade II consists of medial hypertrophy and intimal hyperplasia, grade III involves near obliteration of the vessel lumen, grade IV includes arterial dilatation, and grades V and VI include plexiform lesions, angiomatoid formation, and fibrinoid necrosis. Grades IV–VI indicate irreversible pulmonary vascular obstructive disease.

23. **(b)** Grade 2

(Nelson Textbook of Pediatrics, 18th ed.)

The pathologic changes of Eisenmenger syndrome occur in the small pulmonary arterioles and muscular arteries (<300 mm) and are graded on the basis of histologic characteristics (Heath-Edwards classification): Grade I changes involve medial hypertrophy alone, grade II consists of medial hypertrophy and intimal hyperplasia, grade III involves near obliteration of the vessel lumen, grade IV includes arterial dilatation, and grades V and VI include plexiform lesions, angiomatoid formation, and fibrinoid necrosis. Grades IV–VI indicate irreversible pulmonary vascular obstructive disease.

24. **(a)** Diamond-Blackfan anemia

25. **(a)** Wilm's tumour

(Nelson Textbook of Pediatrics, 18th ed.)

The children of Beckwith-Wiedemann syndrome are predisposed to a specific subset of childhood neoplasms, including Wilm's tumor and adrenocortical carcinoma.

26. **(d)** Platelet count decreased

(Nelson Textbook of Pediatrics, 18th ed.)

The most common acquired red cell aplasia occurring in children, transient erythroblastopenia of childhood (TEC) is more common than congenital hypoplastic anemia. This syndrome of severe, transient hypoplastic anemia occurs mainly in previously healthy children between 6 months and 3 years of age, with most of the children older than 12 months at onset. Only 10% are >3 years of age. The cause of this decrease in red blood cell (RBC) production is a transient immunologic suppression of erythropoiesis. It often follows a viral illness, although no specific virus has been identified. Parvovirus B_{19} infections, which may cause hypoplasia in children with chronic hemolytic anemia, are not responsible for TEC. Reticulocytes and bone marrow erythroid precursors are markedly decreased, although examination of the bone marrow rarely is needed to make the diagnosis. Some degree of neutropenia may occur in up to 20% of cases while platelet numbers are normal or elevated.

27. **(b)** CDA Class 2

(Nelson Textbook of Pediatrics, 18th ed.)

Type II CDA, an autosomal recessive disorder, is the most common variant of CDA. The gene for type II CDA has been mapped to chromosome 20q11.2. The clinical and laboratory features are similar to those of type I CDA, but the anemia usually is more severe.

28. **(b)** Class 2

(Nelson Textbook of Pediatrics, 18th ed.)

Pathognomonic findings in type II CDA are that the patient's RBCs are lysed by acidified serum. Type II CDA is known by the acronym HEMPAS (hereditary erythroblastic multinuclearity with a positive acidified serum test) because it features both erythroblast multinuclearity and circulating RBCs that are sensitive to lysis by acidified normal serum.

29. **(c)** Hereditary stomatocytosis

(Nelson Textbook of Pediatrics, 18th ed.)

Hereditary stomatocytosis is a rare condition in which the red blood cells (RBCs) are cup-shaped. On stained blood film, they present a mouthlike slit in place of the usual circular area of central pallor. Acquired stomatocytosis may be seen in several conditions, especially liver disease. Hereditary stomatocytosis is associated with increased RBC membrane permeability to $Na^+$and $K^+$and alterations in RBC hydration status.

30. **(b)** Quality change in globulin

(Nelson Textbook of Pediatrics, 18th ed.)

The primary pathology in thalassemia stems from the quantity of globin gene production, whereas in sickle cell disease, the primary pathology is the quality of globin production.

31. **(a)** Quantity change in globulin

(Nelson Textbook of Pediatrics, 18th ed.)

The primary pathology in thalassemia stems from the quantity of globin gene production, whereas in sickle cell disease, the primary pathology is the quality of globin production.

32. **(d)** Increased leukocyte alkaline phosphatase

(Nelson Textbook of Pediatrics, 18th ed.)

Major criteria
1. Increased red cell mass (see text)
2. Arterial O_2 saturation of ≥ 92%[*]
3. Palpable splenomegaly
Minor criteria
1. Platelet count of >400 × 10^9/L
2. Leukocytosis of >12 × 10^9/L
3. Increased leukocyte alkaline phosphatase
4. Increased vitamin B_{12} (>900 pg/mL) or unbound B_{12} binding capacity (>2,200 pg/mL)

33. **(d)** All of the above

(Nelson Textbook of Pediatrics, 18th ed.)

Constitutional (Inherited) Pancytopenia Syndromes
• Fanconi anemia
• Shwachman-Diamond syndrome
• Dyskeratosis congenita
• Amegakaryocytic thrombocytopenia
• Other genetic syndromes
• Down syndrome
• Dubowitz syndrome
• Seckel syndrome
• Reticular dysgenesis
• Schimke immuno-osseous dysplasia
• Familial aplastic anemia (non-Fanconi)
• Pearson syndrome
• Reticular dysgenesis
• Noonan's syndrome

34. **(b)** VIII

35. **(c)** IX

(Nelson Textbook of Pediatrics, 18th ed.)

Hemophilia A (factor VIII deficiency) and hemophilia B (factor IX deficiency) are the most common and serious congenital coagulation factor deficiencies. The clinical findings in hemophilia A and hemophilia B are virtually identical. Hemophilia C is the bleeding disorder associated with reduced levels of factor XI.

36. **(a)** All of the above

(Nelson Textbook of Pediatrics, 18th ed.)

Deficiencies in the factors of the common pathway (factors I, II, V, and X) causing prolongation of both PT and PTT.

37. **(a)** Type 1

(Nelson Textbook of Pediatrics, 18th ed.)

Type 1 VWD is the most common form and accounts for 85% of cases.

38. **(c)** 2M

(Nelson Textbook of Pediatrics, 18th ed.)

Type 2M VWD is caused by mutations that result in reduction of the platelet-binding function of VWF. Thus, levels of VWF activity are significantly lower than the levels of VWF antigen. Binding of this protein to factor VIII is normal; thus, factor VIII levels are similar to those of VWF antigen. DDAVP will increase VWF and factor VIII levels, but the released type 2M VWF may not have sufficient activity to cause cessation of bleeding. Thus, VWF replacement therapy may need to be used.

39. **(c)** ALL caused by Philadelphia chromosome

(Nelson Textbook of Pediatrics, 18th ed.)

CML is a clonal disorder of the hematopoietic tissue that accounts for 2–3% of all cases of childhood leukemia. About 99% of the cases are characterized by a specific translocation, t(9;22)(q34;q11), known as the Philadelphia chromosome.

40. **(b)** Burkitt lymphoma (BL)

(Nelson Textbook of Pediatrics, 18th ed.)

The four major pathological subtypes of childhood and adolescent NHL are Burkitt lymphoma (BL), constituting 40% of NHL; lymphoblastic lymphoma (LL), accounting for 30%; diffuse large B-cell lymphoma (DLBCL), constituting 20%; and anaplastic large cell lymphoma (ALCL), accounting for 10%.

41. **(a)** Medulloblastoma

(Nelson Textbook of Pediatrics, 18th ed.)

Distribution of Childhood Brain Tumors Based on Histology

Histology	Distribution (% of total)
Medulloblastoma/primitive neuroectodermal tumor	20
Juvenile pilocytic astrocytoma	20
Low-grade astrocytoma	15
High-grade astrocytoma	7
Ependymoma	7
Craniopharyngioma	7
Unclassified primary tumors	7
Choroid plexus tumors, germ cell tumors, oligodendroglioma, meningioma, mixed tumors, pineal parenchymal tumors	1–2 (each histologic group)

42. **(a)** Juvenile pilocytic astrocytoma

(Nelson Textbook of Pediatrics, 18th ed.)

Juvenile pilocytic astrocytoma (JPA) is the most common astrocytoma in children, accounting for 20% of all brain tumors. Based on clinicopathologic features using the WHO Classification System.

43. **(b)** Ewing sarcoma

(Nelson Textbook of Pediatrics, 18th ed.)

Ewing sarcoma is more common than osteosarcoma. Both tumor types are most likely to occur in the second decade of life. Osteosarcoma is the most common primary malignant bone tumor in children and adolescents

44. **(b)** Ovarian tumor

(Nelson Textbook of Pediatrics, 18th ed.)

The most common gynecologic neoplasm found in children is of ovarian origin and usually presents as an abdominal mass. Ovarian neoplasms constitute 1% of all childhood malignancies, and 8% of all malignant and abdominal tumors in children are of ovarian origin.

45. **(a)** Germ cell tumor

(Nelson Textbook of Pediatrics, 18th ed.)

Malignant Ovarian Tumors in Adolescents

Germ Cell (Most common)
• Dysgerminoma • Immature teratoma • Endodermal sinus tumor • Choriocarcinoma • Embryonal carcinoma
Sex Cord Stromal Tumors
• Granulosa stroma cell tumor • Sertoli-Leydig cell tumor • Lipoid cell tumor • Gynandroblastoma
Epithelial Tumors

46. **(a)** Endodermal sinus tumors

(Nelson Textbook of Pediatrics, 18th ed)

Serum Tumor Markers

Marker	Associated Tumor
CA 125	Epithelial tumors (especially serous) Immature teratoma (rare)
α-Fetoprotein	Endodermal sinus tumors Embryonal carcinomas Mixed germ cell tumors Immature teratoma (rare) Polyembryoma (rare)
Human chorionic gonadotropins	Choriocarcinoma Embryonal carcinomas Mixed germ cell tumors Polyembryoma Dysgerminoma (rare)
Lactate dehydrogenase	Dysgerminoma Mixed germ cell tumors
Estradiol	Thecomas Adult granulosa cell tumors
Testosterone	Sertoli cell tumors Leydig (hilus) cell tumors
F9 embryoglycan	Embryonal carcinoma Yolk sac tumor Choriocarcinoma Immature teratoma
Inhibin	Granulosa—theca cell tumor
Müllerian-inhibiting substance	Granulosa—theca cell tumor

47. **(a)** Sarcoma botryoides

(Nelson Textbook of Pediatrics, 18th ed.)

Sarcoma botryoides, a vaginal carcinoma that occurs primarily in pediatric patients.

48. **(b)** Giant cells, granulomas

(Nelson Textbook of Pediatrics, 18th ed.)

See Table on the next page.

49. **(a)** Papillary

(Nelson Textbook of Pediatrics, 18th ed.)

Histologically, the carcinomas are papillary (80%), follicular (17%), medullary (2%), or mixed differentiated tumors. These are usually slow-growing tumors and may remain dormant for years.

Ans. 48

Characteristics of thyroiditis syndromes

Characteristic	Hashimoto's Thyroiditis	Painless Postpartum Thyroiditis	Painless Sporadic Thyroiditis	Painful Subacute Thyroiditis	Suppurative Thyroiditis	Riedel's Thyroiditis
Sex ratio (F : M)	8–9 : 1	—	2 : 1	5 : 1	1 : 1	3–4 : 1
Cause	Autoimmune	Autoimmune	Autoimmune	Unknown	Infectious	Unknown
Pathologic findings	Lymphocytic infiltration, germinal centers, fibrosis	Lymphocytic infiltration	Lymphocytic infiltration	Giant cells, granulomas	Abscess formation	Dense fibrosis

50. **(b)** Medullary ca

(Nelson Textbook of Pediatrics, 18th ed.)

The susceptibility for all these disorders has been associated with germ line mutations of the RET proto-oncogene on chromosome 10q11.2. When the tumor occurs sporadically, it is usually unicentric, but in the familial form, it is usually multicentric, and it begins as hyperplasia of parafollicular cells.

51. **(b)** MEN 2 A

(Nelson Textbook of Pediatrics, 18th ed.)

When hyperplasia or carcinoma of C cells is associated with adrenal medullary hyperplasia or pheochromocytoma and parathyroid hyperplasia, it is known as multiple endocrine neoplasia (MEN) IIA.

52. **(a)** Low grade astrocytoma

(Nelson Textbook of Pediatrics, 18th ed.)

In children, spinal cord tumors account for ≈ 20% of neuraxial tumors and are classified according to anatomic position. Intramedullary tumors arise within the substance of the cord and grow slowly by infiltration, usually in the cervical region. The most common intramedullary tumor is a low-grade astrocytoma, followed by ganglioglioma and ependymoma. Extramedullary intradural tumors tend to be benign and arise from neural crest tissue. Tumors in this area include neurofibroma, ganglioneuroma and meningioma. Extramedullary extradural tumors characteristically are metastatic lesions, particularly neuroblastoma, sarcoma.

Chapter 37

Preventive Pediatrics

1. **National Youth Day is celebrated on:**
(a) January 12 (b) February 6
(c) March 13 (d) July 22

2. **World Leprosy Eradication Day is celebrated on:**
(a) January 30 (b) April 13
(c) July 22 (d) May 26

3. **Street Children's Day is celebrated on:**
(a) June 8 (b) December 28
(c) February 5 (d) January 31

4. **International Day of Zero Tolerance to Female Genital Mutilation is celebrated on:**
(a) May 26 (b) July 18
(c) February 6 (d) December 13

5. **Measles Immunization Day is celebrated on:**
(a) March 7 (b) February 7
(c) September 14 (d) October 2

6. **International Women's Day is celebrated on:**
(a) March 8 (b) 1 May
(c) March 11 (d) June 23

7. **International Nurses Day is celebrated on:**
(a) May 12 (b February 25
(c) April 12 (d) August 15

8. **National Vaccination Day is celebrated on:**
(a) March 16 (b) May 25
(c) September 2 (d) July 18

9. **World Down Syndrome Day is celebrated on:**
(a) February 22 (b) March 21
(c) May 3 (d) June 13

10. **World TB Day is celebrated on:**
(a) January 12 (b) April 29
(c) May 18 (d) March 24

11. **World Autism Awareness Day is celebrated on:**
(a) February 2 (b) June 8
(c) August 17 (d) April 2

12. **World Health Day is celebrated on:**
(a) April 7 (b) June 18
(c) August 15 (d) January 26

13. **World Hemophilia Day is celebrated on:**
(a) March 3 (b) June 29
(c) April 17 (d) December 13

14. **World Malaria Day is celebrated on:**
(a) April 25 (b) January 18
(c) May 4 (d) November 2

15. **Child Labour Day is celebrated on:**
(a) November 23 (b) September 25
(c) April 30 (d) December 12

16. **World Thalassemia Day is celebrated on:**
(a) May 8 (b) March 23
(c) July 22 (d) August 25

17 **International Family Day is celebrated on:**
(a) May 15 (b) April 01
(c) August 5 (d) November 5

18. **World Family Doctors' Day is celebrated on:**
(a) January 23 (b) May 19
(c) November 9 (d) August 24

19. **International Missing Children's Day is celebrated on:**
(a) July 22 (b) April 25
(c) November 4 (d) May 25

20. **International Children's Day is celebrated on:**
(a) February 7 (b) March 16
(c) June 1 (d) August 28

21. **National Cancer Survivors Day is celebrated on:**
(a) June 13 (b) June 1
(c) August 18 (d) December 3

22. **World Blood Donor Day is celebrated on:**
(a) January 23 (b) March 4
(c) June 14 (d) November 15

23. Autistic Pride Day is celebrated on:
(a) June 18 (b) August 4
(c) November 2 (d) December 25

24. International Day Against Drug Abuse and Illicit Trafficking is celebrated on:
(a) January 5 (b) February 23
(c) June 26 (d) November 14

25. Doctor's Day is celebrated on:
(a) March 25 (b) April 12
(c) July 1 (d) December 25

26. World Hepatitis Day is celebrated on:
(a) January 5 (b) February 2
(c) March 28 (d) July 28

27. World ORS Day is celebrated on:
(a) July 29 (b) October 22
(c) December 2 (d) May 24

28. Breast Feeding Week is celebrated on:
(a) 1 August to 7 August (b) March 1st week
(c) April 1st week (d) Nov 1st week

29. World Mosquito Day is celebrated on:
(a) January 15 (b) August 20
(c) May 23 (d) December 18

30. International Youth Day is celebrated on:
(a) August 12 (b) February 12
(c) April 23 (d) May 16

31. World Polio Day is celebrated on:
(a) October 24 (b) March 24
(c) June 12 (d) November 18

32. World Cancer Awareness Day is celebrated on:
(a) January 7 (b) March 9
(c) November 7 (d) July 22

33. World Immunization Day is celebrated on:
(a) January 15 (b) November 10
(c) December 2 (d) April 23

34. Pregnancy and Infant Loss Remembrance Day is celebrated on:
(a) January 14 (b) March 26
(c) May 20 (d) October 15

35. World Pneumonia Day is celebrated on:
(a) November 12 (b) February 12
(c) July 22 (d) May 30

36. Children's Day/ World Diabetics Day is celebrated on:
(a) February 2 (b) April 23
(c) November 14 (d) December 20

37. World prematurity day is celebrated on:
(a) April 13 (b) November 17
(c) July 5 (d) August 18

38. UNICEF Day is celebrated on:
(a) December 11 (b) February 24
(c) June 23 (d) November 4

39. World AIDS Day is celebrated on:
(a) December 1 (b) October 7
(c) May 6 (d) April 4

40. Who were Registrar General and Commissioner of 2011 Indian Census?
(a) Shri Shrikant Yadav
(b) W. W. M. Yeatts
(c) R. A. Gopalaswami
(d) Shri C. Chandramouli

41. What is 0-6 years sex ratio in 2011?
(a) 904 females per 1000 males
(b) 914 females per 1000 males
(c) 925 females per 1000 males
(d) 940 females per 1000 males

Child Sex ratio (0-6 age group) per 1000 males–914 females.

42. What is literacy rate of India as per 2011 census?
(a) 74.04% (b) 68.23%
(c) 55.63% (d) 83.45%

43. What is infant mortality rate in India?
(a) 74 per 1000 births (b) 49 per 1000 births
(c) 58 per 1000 births (d) 52 per 1000 births

44. What was population in the age group of 0-6 of India as per 2011 census?
(a) 1,58,789,287 (b) 82,952,135
(c) 12,848,375 (d) 75,837,152

45. What is population of India above the age of 7 years as per 2011 census?
(a) 1,051,404,135 (b) 540,772,113
(c) 510,632,022 (d) 99,524,597

46. What was annual birth rate of India during 2005-2010?
(a) 510,632,022 (b) 99,524,597
(c) 27,271,000 (d) 1,58,789,287

47. What was crude birth rate of India during 2005-2010?
(a) 21.2 per 1000 (b) 23.1 per 1000
(c) 30.9 per 1000 (d) 45 per 1000

48. What was crude death rate of India during 2005-2010?
(a) 4.5 per 1000 (b) 6 per 1000
(c) 8.3 per 1000 (d) 9.2 per 1000

49. What was total fertility rate (number of children per woman) of India during 2005-2010?
(a) 1.25 (b) 2.24
(c) 2.73 (d) 3.12

50. What was infant mortality rate of India during 2005-2010?
(a) 41.1 per 1000 (b) 46.9 per 1000
(c) 51.2 per 1000 (d) 52.9 per 1000

51. What was 2011 census regarding India's live births?
(a) 18,268,000 (b) 20,0658,000
(c) 23,0941,000 (d) 27,092,000

52. What was crude birth rate of India during 2011?
(a) 15.6 per 1000 (b) 21.8 per 1000
(c) 24.3 per 1000 (d) 26.1 per 1000

53. What was crude death rate of India during 2011?
(a) 4.1 per 1000 (b) 6.3 per 1000
(c) 7.1 per 1000 (d) 9.7 per 1000

54. What was total fertility rate (number of children per woman) of India during 2005-2010?
(a) 1.25 (b) 1.75
(c) 2.44 (d) 2.85

55. What is birth rate of Maharashtra as per 2011 census?
(a) 17.1 (b) 18.6
(c) 19.7 (d) 21.4

56. What is infant mortality rate as per 2011 census?
(a) 28 (b) 21
(c) 32 (d) 41

57. As per 2001 census what is percent wise population of 0-14 year's age group in India?
(a) 30.8% (b) 32.5%
(c) 36.1% (d) 38.7%

58. As per 2001 census what is percent wise sex ratio at birth in India?
(a) 1.01 males/female (b) 1.12 males/female
(c) 2.15 males/female (d) 2.30 males/female

59. What is life expectancy at birth in India as per 2011 census?
(a) 58.2 years (b) 61.3 years
(c) 65.8 years (d) 72.8 years

60. What is total fertility rate in 2009 of India?
(a) 2.34 children born/woman
(b) 2.72 children born/woman
(c) 3.12 children born/woman
(d) 3.26 children born/woman

61. What is world's average child population involved in prostitution?
(a) 6 million (b) Around 10 million
(c) 7.2 million (d) 8 million

62. What is India's average child population involved in prostitution?
(a) 3.25 million (b) 2.80 million
(c) 2.13 million (d) 1.2 million

63. Which is apex governmental body regarding to women and child development in India?
(a) Ministry of Social Welfare
(b) Ministry of Health Science
(c) Ministry of Women and Child Development
(d) None

64. Under terminology of maternal death what is the duration after termination of pregnancy?
(a) 42 days (b) 40 days
(c) 35 days (d) 28 days

Answers

1. (a) January 12
2. (a) January 30
3. (d) January 31
4. (c) February 6
5. (a) March 7
6. (a) March 8
7. (a) May 12
8. (a) March 16
9. (b) March 21
10. (d) March 24
11. (d) April 2
12. (a) April 7
13. (c) April 17
14. (a) April 25
15. (c) April 30
16. (a) May 8
17. (a) May 15
18. (b) May 19
19. (d) May 25
20. (c) June 1
21. (b) June 1
22. (c) June 14
23. (a) June 18
24. (c) June 26
25. (c) July 1
26. (d) July 28
27. (a) July 29
28. (a) 1 August to 7 August
29. (b) August 20
30. (a) August 12
31. (a) October 24
32. (c) November 7
33. (b) November 10
34. (d) October 15
35. (a) November 12
36. (c) November 14
37. (b) November 17
38. (a) December 11
39. (a) December 1
40. (d) Shri C. Chandramouli
41. (b) 914 females per 1000 males
42. (a) 74.04%

Census year	Total (%)	Male (%)	Female (%)
2011	74.04	82.14	65.46

43. (b) 49 per 1000 births

Year	Infant (0-1 year) Male	Infant (0-1 year) Female
1998	70	74
2005	56	58
2009	49	52

44. (c) 12,848,375

	Person	Males	Females
Maharashtra	12,848,375	6,822,262	6,026,113
India	158,789,287	82,952,135	75,837,152

What is population of India above the age of 7 years as per 2011 census?

45. (a) 1,051,404,135

India/State/UT	Persons	Males	Females
Maharashtra	99,524,597	51,539,135	47,985,462
India	1,051,404,135	540,772,113	510,632,022

46. (c) 27,271,000
47. (b) 23.1 per 1000
48. (c) 8.3 per 1000

49. **(c)** 2.73

50. **(d)** 52.9 per 1000

Period	Births per year	Deaths per year	Natural change per year	CBR[1]	CDR[1]	NC[1]	TFR[1]	IMR[1]
2005–2010	27,271,000	9,757,000	17,514,000	23.1	8.3	14.8	2.73	52.9[1]

CBR = crude birth rate (per 1000); CDR = crude death rate (per 1000); NC = natural change (per 1000); TFR = total fertility rate (number of children per woman); IMR = infant mortality rate per 1000 births.

51. **(d)** 27,092,000

52. **(b)** 21.8 per 1000

53. **(c)** 7.1 per 1000

54. **(c)** 2.44

2011 Average population (x 1000)	Live births[1]	Deaths[1]	Natural change	Crude birth rate (per 1000)	Crude death rate (per 1000)	Natural change (per 1000)	Total fertility rate
1,242,738	27,092,000	8,823,000	18,268,000	21.8	7.1	14.7	2.44

55. **(a)** 17.1

56. **(a)** 28

State	Birth Rate	BR Rural	BR Urban	Death Rate	DR Rural	DR Urban	NGR	NGR Rural	NGR Urban	IMR
Maharashtra	17.1	17.6	16.4	6.5	7.5	5.3	1.06%	1.02%	1.11%	28

57. **(a)** 30.8%

2001 Census–Age structure
0–14 years: 30.8%
Male: 188,208,196; Female: 171,356,024

58. **(b)** 1.12 males/female

2001 Census–Sex ratio
At birth: 1.12 male(s)/female
Under 10 years: 1.14 male(s)/female
15–24 years: 1.09 male(s)/female

59. **(c)** 65.8 years

60. **(b)** 2.72 children born/woman

Total fertility rate–2.72 children born/woman (2009 est.) although more up to date statistics indicate that India's TFR was 2.6 in 2008. The TFR (Total number of children born per woman) according to Religion in 2001 was: Hindus — 2.0, Muslims — 3.4, Sikhs — 2.1, Christians — 2.1, Buddhists — 2.1, Jains — 1.4, Animists and Others — 2.99, Tribals — 3.16, Scheduled Castes — 2.89

61. **(b)** Around 10 million

Country	Number of children involved in prostitution
Worldwide	10,000,000
India	1,200,000

Children account for 40% of prostitutes in India.

62. **(d)** 1.2 million

63. **(c)** Ministry of Women and Child Development

The Ministry of Women and Child Development, a branch of the Government of India, is the apex body for formulation and administration of the rules and regulations and laws relating to women and child development in India.

64. **(a)** 42 days

According to the World Health Organization (WHO), maternal death is defined as the death of a woman while pregnant or within 42 days of termination of pregnancy, irrespective of the duration and site of the pregnancy, from any cause related to or aggravated by the pregnancy or its management but not from accidental or incidental causes.

Chapter 38

Nursing in Pediatrics

1. **Eriksons theory of development is based on:**
(a) Psychosocial development
(b) Social development
(c) Spiritual development
(d) Cognitive development

2. **WHO day is celebrated at:**
(a) 10th April (b) 7th April
(c) 6th May (d) 2nd May

3. **The major stressor of hospitalization for infant and young children is:**
(a) Pain (b) Separation anxiety
(c) Loss of control (d) Body injury

4. **A 2 years old child grabs handful of cake from the plate and puts in his mouth according to Freud the child is satisfying his:**
(a) Id (b) Ego
(c) Superego (d) Unconscious mind

5. **Neonates are less likely to get infections if their nutrition is provided by:**
(a) Breast milk (b) Water
(c) Formula feed (d) Soft food

6. **At what point during the first year of life you would expect bonding to occur:**
(a) Soon after birth (b) At 6 months
(c) At 3 weeks (d) Not until 12 months

7. **Piagots theory relates to:**
(a) Moral development
(b) Cognitive development
(c) Spiritual development
(d) Interpersonal development

8. **Children generally double their weight by:**
(a) Heredity (b) State of health
(c) Development (d) Physical growth

9. **Based on Freuds theory the preschooler is:**
(a) Phallic stage (b) Anal stage
(c) Oral stage (d) Latency stage

10. **Cardinal feature of kwashiorkor is:**
(a) Hepatomegaly (b) Anasarca
(c) Tricrome sign (d) Healthy skin

11. **Bitots spot occur in deficiency of:**
(a) A (b) B
(c) C (d) D

12. **The most common form of PEM is:**
(a) Kwashiorkor
(b) Nutritional marasmus
(c) Marasmic kwashiorkor
(d) None

13. **Pigeon chest is due to deficiency of vitamin:**
(a) A (b) D
(c) E (d) K

14. **Deficiency of vitamin B_2 causes:**
(a) Scurvy
(b) Angular stomatitis
(c) Pellagra
(d) Megaloblastic anemia

15. **Beriberi is caused by:**
(a) Vit B_6 (b) C
(c) B_{12} (d) B_1

16. **The following are sign of kwashiorkor *except:***
(a) Diarrhea (b) Irritability
(c) Loose wrinkled skin (d) Sparse thin hair

17. **When comparing breast milk with cow which of the following statement is true?**
(a) Carbohydrate content is greater in breast milk
(b) Carbohydrate content is less in breast milk

(c) Each type has equal amount of carbohydrate
(d) Each has different kind of carbohydrate

18. Food allergies most common in:
(a) Old age infant
(b) Women
(c) Infant and younger children
(d) Same in all age group

19. Mid Day Meal programme started in:
(a) 1950 (b) 1961
(c) 1975 (d) 1980

20. Neural tube defect can be due to:
(a) Folate deficiency in pregnancy
(b) Vit A deficiency in pregnancy
(c) Vit C deficiency in pregnancy
(d) Iron deficiency in pregnancy

21. Pellagra is a deficiency of:
(a) Vitamin C (b) Riboflavin
(c) Niacin (d) Thiamine

22. Which of the following not a feature of marasmus:
(a) Muscle wasting
(b) Edema
(c) Apathy
(d) Severe subcutaneous tissue loss

23. Human milk is deficient in:
(a) Vitamin C (b) Iron
(c) Proteins (d) Lactose

24. The beneficiaries of ICDS proramme are:
(a) Children below 6 years, adolescent girl and lactating mother
(b) Children upto 1-3 years, adolescent boys and lactating women
(c) Children upto 1-3 years and 3-10 years
(d) Pregnant and lactating female from slum areas

25. While feeding animal milk adjustment of fat content is done by:
(a) Cow's milk (b) Goat milk
(c) Dried powder milk (d) Buffalo milk

26. The lunch for school children suggested by regional nutritional committee South East Asia provides how much calories?
(a) 300 kcal (b) 400
(c) 500 (d) 250

27. Children suffering from moderate malnutrition treated in:
(a) Anganwadi
(b) Secondary level hospital
(c) Nutrition supplementary hospital
(d) Nutrition rehabilitation centre

28. Lactose content of human milk is:
(a) 1% (b) 4%
(c) 7% (d) 10%

29. Vitamin D deficiency in children leads to:
(a) Scurvy (b) Rickets
(c) Obesity (d) Night blindness

30. Dose of vitamin A prophylaxis for infant is:
(a) 50,000 IU (b) 1 lakh IU
(c) 2 lakh IU (d) 3 lakh IU

31. ICDS started in the year:
(a) 1956 (b) 1975
(c) 1978 (d) 1954

32. In Mid Day Meal Programme meal should supply at least:
(a) 1/3rd of total energy (b) 2/3rd of total energy
(c) 2/5th of total energy (d) ½ of total energy

33. Infancy as a Sensor Motor stage suggested by:
(a) Freud (b) Jung
(c) Pavlov (d) Jean Piaget

34. In mental retardation the IQ falls:
(a) Below 50 (b) Below 70
(c) Between 90-110 (d) None

35. The formula for calculating IQ is:
(a) MA/CA×100 (b) CA/MA×100
(c) CA/100×MA (d) MA/100×CA

36. With arrival of new baby in the family the 5 years old child may refuse to go to school and cling to his mother the defense mechanism is:
(a) Regression (b) Repression
(c) Withdrawl (d) Reaction formation

37. A physically weak child who turns into a bully and hurts other children may be using the defence mechanism of:
(a) Projection (b) Rationalization
(c) Sublimation (d) Compensatiom

38. A young child's pleasure in collecting stamps might rise from the movie for:
(a) Acquisition (b) Mastery
(c) Activity (d) Gregariousness

39. Erbs palsy is due to injury of:
(a) 3 and 4 cervical nerve
(b) 4 and 5 cervical nerve
(c) 5 and 6 cervical nerve
(d) 1 and 6 cervical nerve

40. The test to assess foetal distress is:
(a) NST (b) MSAFP
(c) CVS (d) Amniocentesis

41. Number of blood vessel in umbilical cord is:
(a) 2 artery one vein (b) 2 artery 2 vein
(c) 1 artery 1 vein (d) 1 artery 2 vein

42. Vitamin K given to newborn to:
(a) Reduce bilirubin level
(b) Increase RBC production
(c) Increase blood clotting
(d) Stimulate surfactant formation

43. IUGR is present in babies whose weight is below:
(a) 10th percentile (b) 15th percentile
(c) 20th percentile (d) 25th percentile

44. After birth baby should pass meconium in:
(a) 24 hours (b) 48 hours
(c) 36 hours (d) 72 hours

45. Anterior fontanelle closes by:
(a) 6 weeks (b) 6 months
(c) 9 months (d) 18 months

46. Caput succedanum subsides by:
(a) 24 hours after birth (b) Within 2 or 3 days
(c) 5 days after birth (d) 7 days after birth

47. All major structure of foetus formed by:
(a) 4-[illegible]eeks (b) 6-8 weeks
(c) 8-[illegible]weeks (d) 10-12 weeks

48. [illegible]itamin K is given to newborn to:
(a) [illegible]duced bilirubin level
(b) [illegible]creased produced level of red blood cells
(c) [illegible]nhance ability of blood to clot
(d) Stimulate the formation of surfactant

49.. The 'fencing posture' a newborn assumes when is supine and turns his head to left side:
(a) Moro reflex (b) Cremastric reflex
(c) Tonic reflex (d) Babinski reflex

50. Which of the following action of breast feeding mother indicates the need for further instruction?
(a) Holds breath with four fingers along bottom and thumb at top
(b) Leans forward to bring breast towards baby
(c) Stimulates rooting reflex then inserts nipple and areola in newborn's mouth
(d) Puts her finger in newborn's mouth before removing breast

51. Common problem associated with monochorionic twins is:
(a) Anemia (b) Heart disease
(c) Polyhydramnios (d) Pre-eclampsia

52. Flaring of the toe when the sole of newborn is stroked:
(a) Cremastric reflex (b) Tonic reflex
(c) Babinski reflex (d) Moro reflex

53. Normal foetal heart sound per minute (FHS):
(a) 120-140 per minute (b) 150-170 per minute
(c) 110-140 per minute (d) 80-90 per minute

54. Shape of anterior fontanels:
(a) Round (b) Diamond
(c) Triangular (d) Rectangular

55. When weighing a newborn the nurse should:
(a) Leave its diaper on comfort
(b) Place sterile sheet on the scale
(c) Keep hand on newborn's abdomen
(d) Weigh newborn at the same time everyday

56. During the extra uterine life umbilical vein becomes:
(a) Ligamentum venosum
(b) Ligamentum arteriosum
(c) Fossa ovalis
(d) Ligamentum teres

57. One of the common problem associated with monochorionic twins:
(a) Anemia
(b) Heart disease
(c) Polyhydramnios
(d) Pressure symptoms

58. IUGR is present in babies whose birth weight is below 10th percentile of average for gestational age:
(a) 10th (b) 15th
(c) 20th (d) 25th

Answers

1. (a) Psychosocial development
2. (b) 7th April
3. (b) Separation anxiety
4. (a) Id
5. (a) Breast milk
6. (a) Soon after birth
7. (b) Cognitive development
8. (a) Heredity
9. (a) Phallic stage
10. (b) Anasarca
11. (a) A
12. (c) Marasmic kwashiorkor
13. (b) D
14. (b) Angular stomatitis
15. (d) B_1
16. (c) Loose wrinkled skin
17. (a) Carbohydrate content is greater in breast milk
18. (c) Infant and younger children
19. (a) 1950
20. (a) Folate deficiency in pregnancy
21. (d) Thiamine
22. (d) Severe subcutaneous tissue loss
23. (a) Vit C
24. (a) Children below 6 years, adolescent girl and lactating mother
25. (a)
26. (a) 300 kcal
27. (a) Anganwadi
28. (c) 7%
29. (b) Rickets
30. (b) 1 lakh IU
31. (b) 1975
32. (a) 1/3rd of total energy
33. (d) Jean Piaget
34. (b) Below 70
35. (a) MA/CA×100
36. (d) Reaction formation
37. (a) Projection
38. (d) Gregariousness
39. (a) 3 and 4 cervical nerve
40. (a) NST
41. (a) 2 artery one vein
42. (c) Increase blood clotting
43. (a) 10th percentile
44. (b) 48hours
45. (d) 18 months
46. (a) 24 hours after birth
47. (a) 4-6 weeks
48. (c) Enhance ability of blood to clot
49. (c) Tonic reflex
50. (d) Puts her finger in newborn's mouth before removing breast
51. (a) Anemia
52. (c) Babinski reflex
53. (a) 120-140 per minute
54. (b) Diamond
55. (d) Weigh newborn at the same time everyday
56. (a) Ligamentum venosum
57. (a) Anemia
58. (a) 10th

Chapter 39

Miscellaneous Pediatrics

1. **Intramuscular injections are given with________ degree angle between skin and needle.**
   (a) 90° (b) 45°
   (c) <25° (d) <15°

2. **Subcutaneous injections are given with_______ degree angle between skin and needle.**
   (a) 45° (b) 90°
   (c) <25° (d) <15°

3. **Intravenous injections are given with_______ degree angle between skin and needle.**
   (a) 25° (b) <10
   (c) 90° (d) <15°

4. **Intradermal injections are given with________ degree angle between skin and needle.**
   (a) 10-15° (b) 25°
   (c) 90° (d) 120°

5. **Site for bone marrow aspiration:**
   (a) Iliac crest (b) Sternum
   (c) Tibial tuberosity (d) All of the above

6. **Ideal site for lumbar puncture in children is:**
   (a) L3-4 interspaces (b) L1-2 interspaces
   (c) L5-6 interspaces (d) S3-4 interspaces

7. **Normal CSF pressure is (mm H20):**
   (a) 80-120 (b) <80
   (c) 70-180 (d) >180

8. **Contraindication for renal biopsy:**
   (a) Uncontrolled blood pressure
   (b) Solitary kidney
   (c) Anatomical abnormalities of the kidney
   (d) All of the above

9. **The first liver aspirate was performed by:**
   (a) Ralph Benjamin (b) Paul Ehrlich
   (c) Robert W. Cahn (d) Richard

10. **First exchange transfusion via umbilical vein was done by:**
    (a) Thomas Adams
    (b) Walter
    (c) Louis K. Diamond
    (d) George Frederick Barker

11. **What are indications for exchange transfusion?**
    (a) Removal of antibody-coated red blood cells in hemolytic disease
    (b) Removal of excessive unconjugated bilirubin
    (c) For correction of severe anemia
    (d) All of the above

12. **Laryngoscope blade size for preterm babies:**
    (a) 0.5 (b) Zero
    (c) 1 (d) 5

13. **Which is contraindication for bag and mask ventilation?**
    (a) Diaphragmatic hernia (b) TGA
    (c) CHPS (d) Cyanosis

14. **Which is contraindication for bag and mask ventilation?**
    (a) Meconium aspiration
    (b) TAPVC
    (c) CHPS
    (d) Bradycardia

15. **What is endotracheal tube size for three kilogram baby?**
    (a) 2.5 mm (b) 3.0 mm
    (c) 4.0 mm (d) 3.5 mm

16. **Contraindication of umbilical vessel cannulation:**
    (a) Omphalitis
    (b) Omphalocele
    (c) Necrotizing enterocolitis
    (d) All of the above

17. Complications of umbilical vessel cannulation:
(a) Thromboembolism
(b) Infection
(c) Disseminated intravascular coagulation
(d) All of the above

18. What is dose of cefixime? (mg/kg/day od/bd)
(a) 5 (b) 8
(c) 10 (d) 100

19. What is dose of ceftazidine?
(a) 25 mg/kg/day (b) 100-150 mg /kg/day
(c) 50 mg/kg/day (d) None

20. Contraindication for ceftriaxone is:
(a) Meningitis
(b) Neonatal hyperbilirubinemia
(c) Septisemia
(d) Pneumonia

21. Gray baby syndrome is caused by:
(a) Ceftriaxone (b) Ceftazidine
(c) Chloramphenicol (d) Penicillin

22. What is dose of Gentamicin?
(a) 2.5 mg/kg/day (b) 5 to 7.5 mg /kg/day
(c) 10-25 mg/kg/day (d) 100 mg/kg/day

23. What is dose of Amikacin?
(a) 7.7-10 mg/kg/day (b) 15 to 25 mg/kg/day
(c) 50 mg/kg/day (d) 75-100 mg/kg/day

24. Indication for use Metronidazole;
(a) Abdominal surgery (b) Osteomyelitis
(c) Amoebiasis (d) All of the above

25. What is dose of Isoniazid ?
(a) 0.1 mg/kg/day (b) 10 mg/kg/day
(c) 25-25 mg/kg/day (d) 50 mg/kg/day

26. What is dose of Rifampicin ?
(a) 1 mg/kg/day (b) 10 mg/kg/day
(c) 15 to 25 mg/kg/dose (d) 10 mg/kg/dose

27. Which is first line ATT having good CSF penetration?
(a) Pyrazinamide (b) Isoniazide
(c) Ethambutol (d) Streptomycin

28. Side effect of Ethambutol:
(a) Retrobulbarneuritis
(b) Constriction of visual field
(c) Color blindness
(d) All of the above

29. Contraindication for streptomycin:
(a) Myasthenia gravis (b) T.B.
(c) SLE (d) S.M.A.

30. After what age mebendazole is advised?
(a) Two years (b) 6 months
(c) 3 years (d) 5 years

31. Which is deworming drug given below two years of age?
(a) Mebendazole (b) Ivermectin
(c) Albendazole (d) Meconazole

32. Adverse reaction of chloroquine is:
(a) Hypotension (b) Retinal damage
(c) Psychosis (d) All of the above

33. What is adverse effect of iron therapy?
(a) Bleeding
(b) Malabsorption syndrome
(c) Staining of teeth
(d) Cyanosed nails

34. What is dose of paracetamol?
(a) 15 mg/kg/dose (b) 25 mg/kg/dose
(c) 15 mg/kg/day (d) 50 mg/kg/day

35. One TSF (15 ml) MCT oil (Medium Chain Tryglyceride) has how much calories?
(a) 14 kcal (b) 50 kcal
(c) 1000 kcal (d) 115 kcal

36. Contraindication for Atropine:
(a) Paralytic ileus (b) Pyloric stenosis
(c) Thyrotoxicosis (d) All of the above

37. Soda bicarbonate is diluted with equal amount of:
(a) Distal water (b) NS
(c) RL (d) Given undiluted

38. Indication for use of digoxin:
(a) Congestive cardiac failure
(b) Supraventricular tachycardia
(c) Cardiac arrhythmia
(d) All of the above

39. Side effect of salbutamol:
(a) Fine tremors (b) Palpitation
(c) Tachycardia (d) All of the above

40. Drug of choice in apnea of prematurity in neonate:
(a) Theophylline (b) Atropine
(c) Adrenaline (d) Aminophylline

41. **Side effect of furosemide:**
(a) Muscle cramp (b) Hypokalaemia
(c) Deafness (d) All of the above

42. **Contraindication for Carbamazepine:**
(a) AV block
(b) Bone marrow depression
(c) Porphyria
(d) All of the above

43. **Drug of choice for neonatal seizure:**
(a) Valparine (b) Phenytoin sodium
(c) Phenobarbitone sodium (d) Lorazepam

44. **What is dose of phenytoin sodium?**
(a) 0.1 mg/kg/day (b) 0.5 mg/kg/day
(c) 0.5 to 0.8 mg/kg/day (d) 5-8 mg/kg/day

45. **What is dose of sodium valproate?**
(a) 0.10 to 0.15 mg/kg/day (b) 1 to 1.5 mg/kg/day
(c) 100 mg/kg/dose (d) 10-15 mg/kg/day

46. **Commonly orally used drug for restless child is:**
(a) Triclofos (b) Phenobarbitone
(c) Diazepam (d) Distilled water

47. **Extra pyramidal reaction occurs commonly due to:**
(a) Dopamine (b) Metoclopramide
(c) Dobutamine (d) Domperidone

48. **Commonly used antiemetic after chemotherapy is:**
(a) Metoclopramide (b) Domperidone
(c) Ondansatron (d) None

49. **Drug of choice in staphylococcus infection:**
(a) Cloxacillin (b) Penicillin
(c) Azithromycin (d) Cephalosporine

50. **What is oral dose of benzathine penicillin?**
(a) 12,500 units/kg/day (b) 25,000 units/kg/day
(c) 6 lakh IU (d) 12 lakh IU

51. **Drug of choice in anthrax infection:**
(a) Procaine penicillin (b) Cephalosporine
(c) Chloroquine (d) Fluconazole

52. **Penicillin sensitivity test is done by which route?**
(a) Intradermal (b) Intramuscular
(c) Subcutaneous (d) Per rectal

53. **What is PH of Isolyte P?**
(a) 6 (b) 7
(c) 8 (d) 3

54. **Which IV fluid solution is isotonic with blood?**
(a) Normal saline (b) Ringer lactate
(c) Isolyte-P (d) Distilled water

55. **What is PH of normal saline?**
(a) 5 (b) 7
(c) 9 (d) 1

56. **What is contraindication for normal saline fluid administration?**
(a) PDA (b) Large VSD
(c) Pulmonary edema (d) Anaemia

57. **Who is father of immunization?**
(a) Joseph Brant (b) Robert William Briggs
(c) Edward Anthony Jenner (d) Robert Koch

58. **When expanded programme on immunization was started?**
(a) 1882 (b) 1974
(c) 1996 (d) 2004

59. **When Universal Immunization Programme (UIP) was started in India?**
(a) 1985 (b) 1987
(c) 1997 (d) 2010

60. **Cold chain consists of:**
(a) Walk in freezer (b) Walk in cold rooms
(c) Ice lined refrigerators (d) All of the above

61. **Recommended storage of oral polio vaccine in the refrigerator:**
(a) Freezing compartment (b) Middle compartment
(c) Door (d) Outside

62. **Which vaccines are stored in top compartment of refrigerator?**
(a) BCG (b) Measles
(c) MMR (d) All of the above

63. **Which is live vaccine?**
(a) BCG (b) Sabin Polio
(c) Measels (d) All of the above

64. **BCG vaccine was invented by:**
(a) Albert Calmette
(b) John B. Calhoun
(c) David Callaway
(d) James Edward Campbell

65. **BCG vaccine protects against:**
(a) Filariasis (b) Brucellosis
(c) Ricketsial fever (d) TB meningitis

66. **Protective efficacy of BCG vaccine for pulmonary tuberculosis is:**
(a) >75% (b) 50%
(c) <20% (d) 97%

67. By which route BCG vaccine is administered?
(a) Intramuscular (b) Intravenous
(c) Oral (d) Intradermal

68. When the scar of BCG appears?
(a) <24 hours (b) 6-12 weeks
(c) >3 months (d) After 5 years

69. What is dose of BCG vaccine in neonate?
(a) .01 ml (b) 0.1 ml
(c) 0.05 ml (d) 0.5 ml

70. What is universal site for BCG vaccine administration?
(a) Left deltoid (b) Any deltoid
(c) Thigh (d) Gluteus medius

71. Oral Polio Vaccine was invented by:
(a) Harold Cummins
(b) Joseph Augustine Cushman
(c) Richard H
(d) Albert Bruce Sabin

72. What is shelf life of Oral Polio Vaccine at a temperature of -20°C?
(a) 7 days (b) 2 years
(c) 6 months (d) Unlimited

73. What is dose of Oral Polio Vaccine?
(a) 0.1 ml (b) 0.5 ml
(c) Two drops (d) 8 drops

74. Oral Polio Vaccine is contraindicated in:
(a) Immunodeficiency (b) HIV
(c) Active viral infections (d) All of the above

75. Inactivated Polio Vaccine was invented by:
(a) Joseph Brant
(b) Robert William Briggs
(c) Edward Anthony Jenner
(d) Jonas Edward Salk

76. What is dose of Inactivated Polio Vaccine?
(a) 0.5 ml (b) 0.1 ml
(c) 1.0 ml (d) 2 drops

77. What is adjuvant in DPT vaccine?
(a) Aluminum hydroxide/phosphate

78. What is lowest age limit at which DPT vaccine is given?
(a) 6 weeks
(b) 10 weeks
(c) 14 weeks
(d) 6 months

79. What is dose of DPT vaccine?
(a) 2 drops (b) 0.5 ml
(c) 0.1 ml (d) 1.0 ml

80. What is contraindication for DPT vaccine?
(a) Cerebral palsy
(b) Meningitis
(c) Spinal canal stenosis
(d) Progressive neurological disease

81. Maurice Ralph Hilleman invented which vaccine?
(a) Measles (b) Mumps
(c) Hepatitis A (d) All of the above

82. By which route measles vaccine is given?
(a) Subcutaneously (b) Intravenous
(c) Intradermal (d) Oral

83. What is the most common side effect of measles vaccine?
(a) Orchitis
(b) Staphylococcal toxic shock syndrome
(c) Otitis media
(d) None

84. MMR vaccine is contraindicated in patients with:
(a) Severe immunodeficiency
(b) Pregnancy
(c) History of serious allergy to vaccine
(d) All of the above

85. What is dose of hepatitis B vaccine in children? (/ 10 μg)
(a) 0.1 ml (b) 1.0 ml
(c) 0.5 ml (d) 5 ml

86. What is oral typhoid vaccine strain name?
(a) Ty 21b (b) Ty 21a
(c) Edmonston (d) Dannish 1331

87. At what age Hib vaccine is given?
(a) Day 1 of life (b) 6 weeks
(c) 12 weeks (d) 6 months

88. What is strain in varicella vaccine?
(a) Ty 21a
(b) Dannish 1331
(c) Oka strain
(d) None

89. What is strain in Hepatitis A vaccine?
(a) HM175 (b) Ty 21a
(c) Oka strain (d) All of the above

90. Indication for pneumococcal vaccine:
(a) HIV (b) Asplenia
(c) Sickle cell anemia (d) All of the above

91. By which route rotavaccine is administered?
(a) Oral (b) Intravenous
(c) Intradermal (d) Per rectal

92. What is dose of human papilloma virus vaccine?
(a) 0.1 ml (b) 0.5 ml
(c) 1.0 ml (d) 1.5 ml

93. What is measurement in one cup?
(a) 240 ml (b) 100 ml
(c) 150 ml (d) 1 litre

94. What is measurement in one glass?
(a) 200 ml (b) 500 ml
(c) 1 litre (d) Any of the above

95. One teaspoon means:
(a) 1 ml (b) 10 ml
(c) 2.5 ml (d) 5 ml

96. One tablespoon means:
(a) 5 ml (b) 10 ml
(c) 15 ml (d) 25 ml

97. What is biological value of an egg?
(a) 60 (b) 96
(c) 70 (d) 100

98. What is net protein utilization of an egg?
(a) 60 (b) 70
(c) 96 (d) 77

99. What is biological value of wheat?
(a) 74 (b) 66
(c) 85 (d) 96

100. Caloric content of cashew nuts (100 gm):
(a) 150 (b) 596
(c) 259 (d) 1000

101. Caloric content of kishmish (100 gm):
(a) 125 (b) 299
(c) 350 (d) 500

102. What is protein content per 100 gms of soyabean seeds?
(a) 25.2 grams (b) 28.9 grams
(c) 30 grams (d) 43.2 grams

103. What is protein content per 100 gms of rajma seeds?
(a) 25.2 grams (b) 28.9 grams
(c) 30 grams (d) 22.9 grams

104. What is protein content per 100 gms of bajra seeds?
(a) 28 grams (b) 100 grams
(c) 52 grams (d) 11.6 grams

105. What is protein content per 100 gms of rice?
(a) 1.25 grams (b) 5 grams
(c) 15 grams (d) 7.5 grams

106. Identify this instrument:

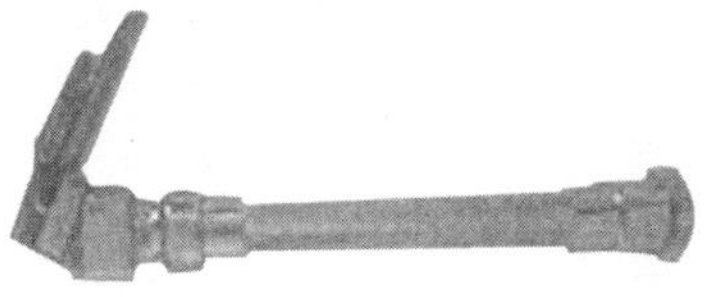

(a) Laryngoscope (b) Tracheostomy tube
(c) Ambu bag (d) None

107. Which structures is seen through?
(a) Base of tongue (b) Epiglottis
(c) Arypeiglottic folds (d) All of the above

108. Direct laryngoscopy is done in:
(a) Cord palsy (b) Anatomical lesion
(c) Foreign body (d) All of the above

109. How much increase in the FiO_2 of the oxygen occurs by ambu bag?
(a) 10% (b) 20%
(c) 30% (d) 40%

110. Identify the instrument:

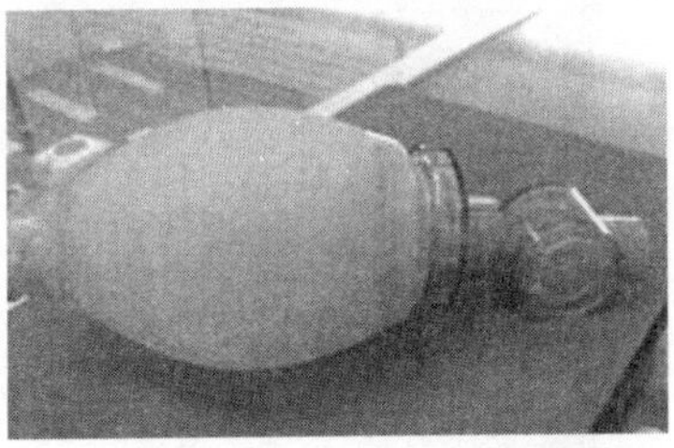

(a) Bag valve mask (b) Foot junction
(c) Laryngoscope (d) None

111. Use of infant feeding tube:
(a) Diagnosis of tracheo-oesophageal fistula
(b) Nasogastric feeds
(c) As a tourniquet
(d) All of the above

112. **Identify the instrument:**

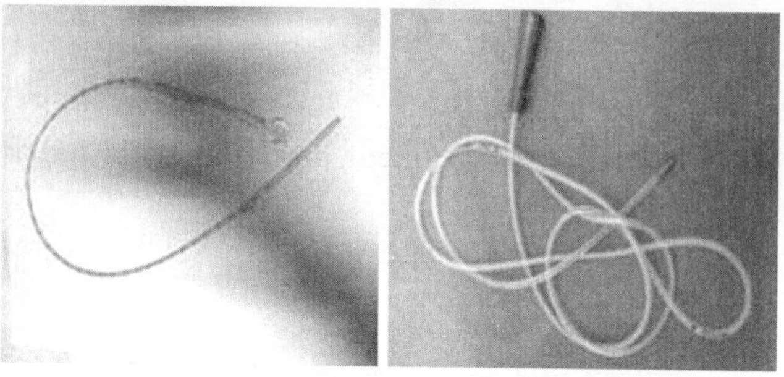

(a) Bag valve mask
(b) Foot junction
(c) Infant feeding tube
(d) Laryngoscope

113. **Identify this instrument:**

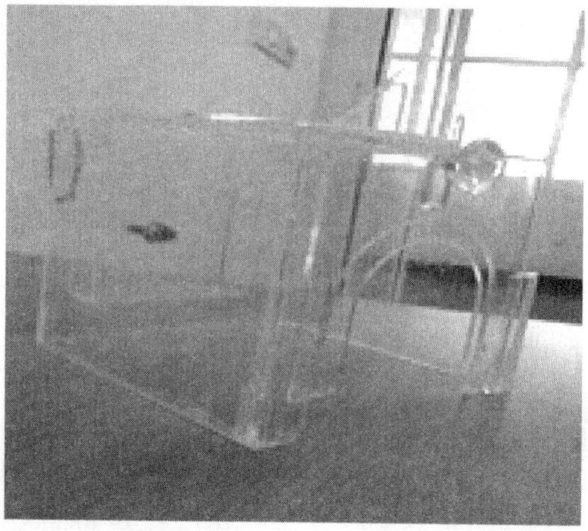

(a) Bag and mask
(b) Oxygen hood
(c) Warmer
(d) Massager

114. **Identify this instrument:**

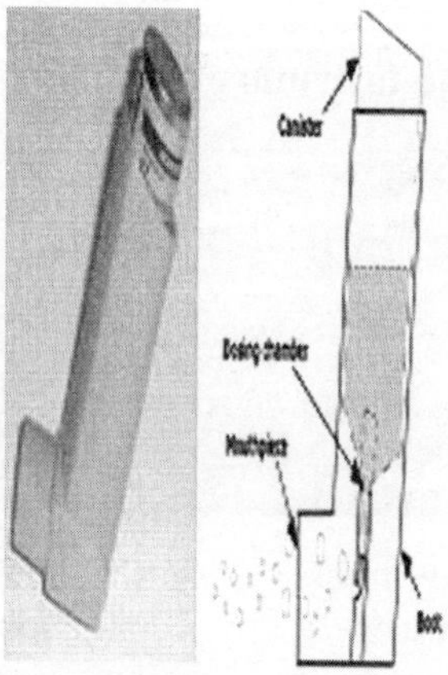

(a) Hand junction
(b) Hood box
(c) Syringe pump
(d) Metered dose inhaler

115. **Identify this instrument:**

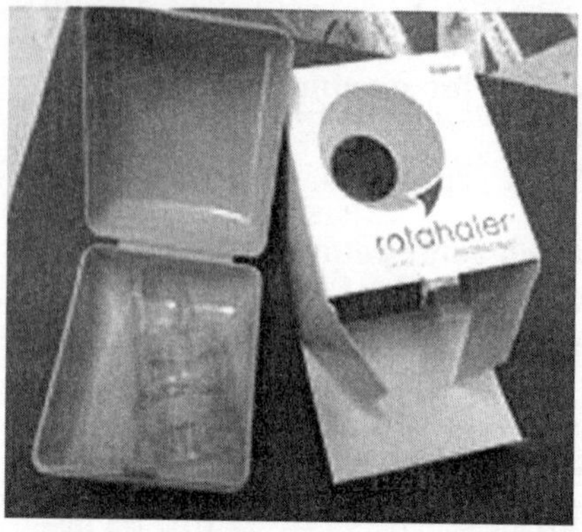

(a) Hand junction
(b) Syringe pump
(c) Metered dose inhaler
(d) Rotahaler

116. **Identify the instrument:**

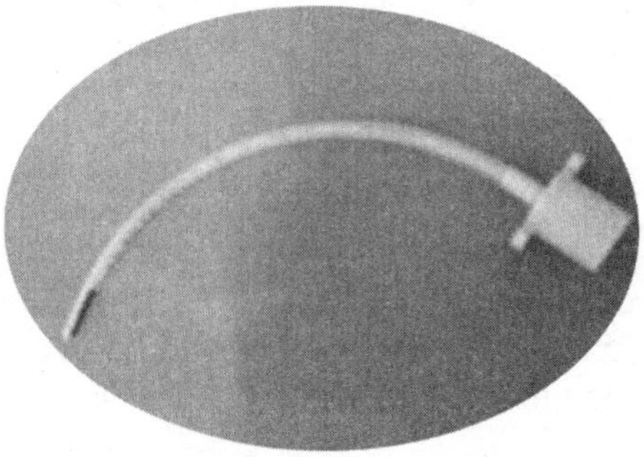

(a) Endotracheal tube
(b) Syringe pump
(c) Hand junction
(d) Nasogastric tube

117. **In routine IV set 1 ml has how many drops?**
(a) 16
(b) 10
(c) 20
(d) 60

118. **In microdrip set 1 ml has how many drops?**
(a) 60
(b) 20
(c) 16
(d) 100

119. **In blood set 1 ml has how many drops?**
(a) 10
(b) 20
(c) 5
(d) 40

120. **In intrauterine life systemic circulation depends on which side of heart?**
(a) Not on any side
(b) Both sides
(c) Left side
(d) Right side

121. In intrauterine life which chamber of human heart is dominant?

(a) Right ventricle (b) Left ventricle
(c) Right atrium (d) Left atrium

122. In newborn which chamber of heart is larger?

(a) Left ventricle (b) Right ventricle
(c) Right atrium (d) Left atrium

123. In the newborns the ECG will show which axis deviation?

(a) Left (b) Straight
(c) Right (d) Any of the above

124. After first 1-3 years of life, on ECG the findings shows:

(a) QRS axis shift from rightward to a more leftward axis
(b) R wave amplitude decreases in leads V1 and V2
(c) Right ventricle increases in leads V5 and V6
(d) All of the above

125. In neonates, the normal PR interval duration is:

(a) 40 (b) 80
(c) 120 (d) 20

126. In neonates, the normal QRS complex duration is:

(a) 5 ms (b) 10 ms
(c) 20 ms (d) 30 ms

127. Upright T waves at birth indicates:

(a) Right ventricular hypertrophy
(b) Left ventricular hypertrophy
(c) Right atrial hypertrophy
(d) Left atrial hypertrophy

128. The "juvenile pattern" of T wave inversion usually seen in the anterior leads (leads V1-V3) typically lasts up to what age?

(a) 1 year (b) 2 years
(c) 8 years (d) 18 years

129. Increased R wave amplitude in leads V1, V2 is suggestive of:

(a) Left atrial hypertrophy
(b) Left ventricular hypertrophy
(c) Right atrial hypertrophy
(d) Right ventricular hypertrophy

130. Right ventricular hypertrophy is seen in:

(a) Early neonatal period
(b) Pulmonary stenosis
(c) Tetralogy of Fallot
(d) All of the above

131. Left ventricular hypertrophy is seen in:

(a) Aortic stenosis (b) Co-arctation of aorta
(c) Patent ductus arteriosus (d) All of the above

132. Right atrial enlargement is seen in:

(a) Atrial septal defect
(b) Tricuspid atresia
(c) Ebstein's anomaly
(d) All of the above

133. Left atrial enlargement is seen in:

(a) Mitral stenosis or insufficiency
(b) Left heart obstruction
(c) Complete AV canal defects
(d) All of the above

134. Right axis deviation is seen in:

(a) Tetralogy of Fallot
(b) Co-arctation of aorta
(c) Transposition of great arteries
(d) All of the above

135. Left axis deviation is seen in:

(a) Large ventricular septal defect
(b) Tricuspid atresia
(c) Transposition of great arteries
(d) All of the above

136. Atrial septal defect (secondum) have ECG findings of:

(a) Right atrial enlargement
(b) Tall R waves V_{1-3} and corresponding deep S waves in V_{4-6}
(c) Right axis deviation with T waves are flat in V_1
(d) All of the above

137. Ventricular septal defect have ECG findings of :

(a) QRS axis: RAD with BVH
(b) QRS configuration: Normal or RSR′
(c) Right atrial enlargement
(d) All of the above

138. Patent ductus arteriosus have ECG findings of:
(a) PR interval increased
(b) Deep S V_1, tall R V_5 and V_6 in QRS complex
(c) Left atrial enlargement
(d) All of the above

139. Pulmonary stenosis have ECG findings of:
(a) Normal PR interval
(b) Right atrial enlargement
(c) Right ventricular hypertrophy
(d) All of the above

140. Coarctation of aorta have ECG findings of:
(a) Normal pr interval (b) Normal QRS axis
(c) Left atrial enlargement (d) All of the above

141. Tetralogy of Fallot has ECG findings of:
(a) Right ventricular hypertrophy
(b) Upright T waves in V_{1-2}
(c) Right axis deviation
(d) All of the above

142. Preterm baby has ECG finding of:
(a) Short QRS duration (b) Short PR
(c) Short QT interval (d) All of the above

143. Name the congenital anomalies in picture:

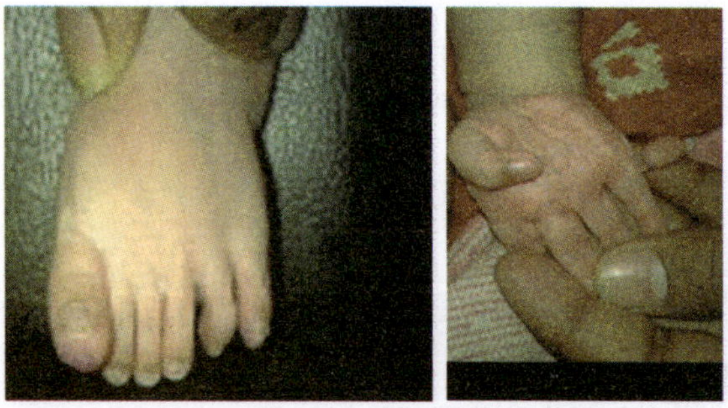

(a) Syndactyle (b) Simian crease
(c) Polydactyle (d) None

144. Name the congenital anomalies in picture:

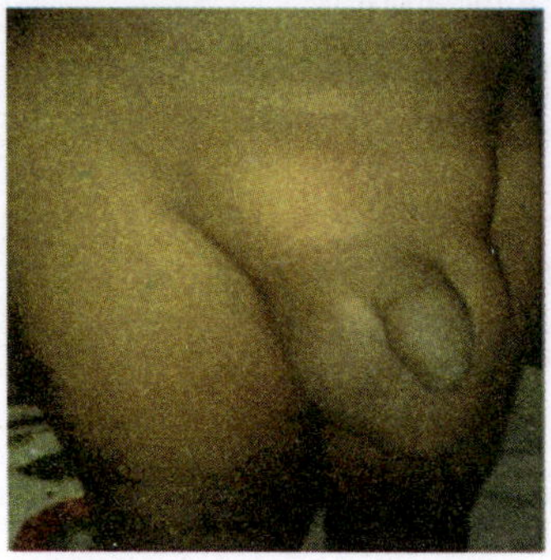

(a) Bilateral inguinal hernia
(b) Unilateral inguinal hernia
(c) Femoral hernia
(d) Undescended testis

145. Name the congenital anomalies in picture:

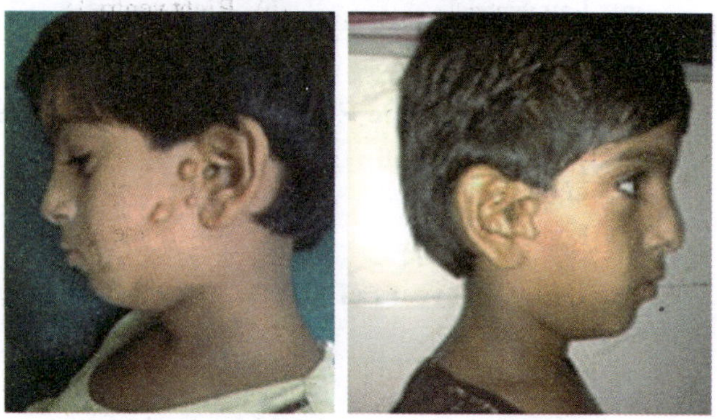

(a) Preauricular skin tag (b) Lipoma
(c) Sebacious cyst (d) None

146. Name the congenital anomalies in picture:

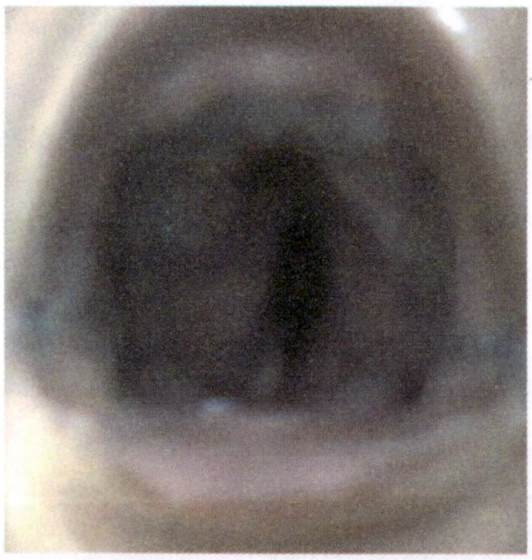

(a) Vocal cord agenesis (b) Unerupted teeth
(c) Cleft palate (d) Anal atresia

147. Name the congenital anomalies in picture:

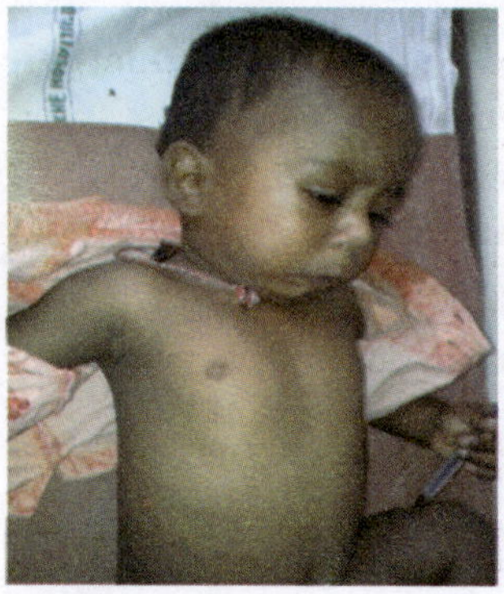

(a) Macrognathia (b) Micrognathia
(c) Agnathia (d) None

148. Name the congenital anomalies in picture:

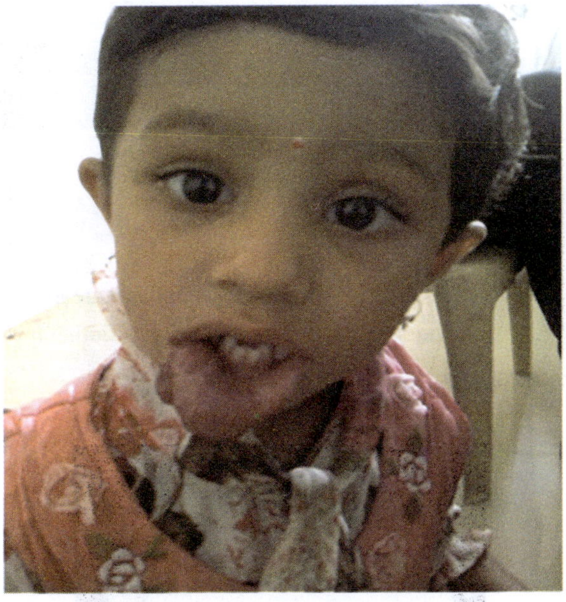

(a) Lipoma
(b) Cavernous hemangioma
(c) Strawberry hemangioma
(d) None

149. What is diagnosis from picture?

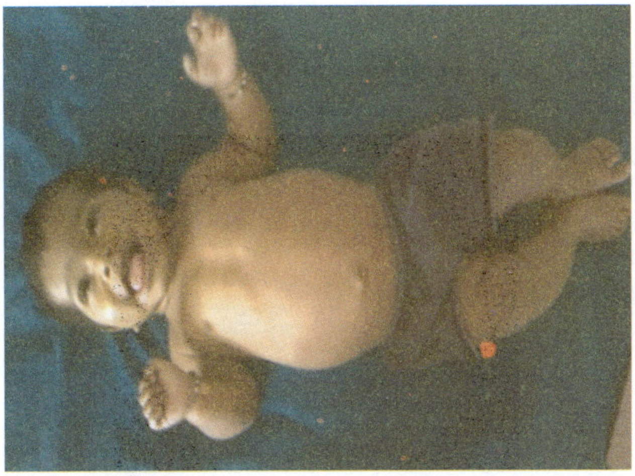

(a) Congenital hypothyroidism
(b) Down's syndrome
(c) Hyperthyroidism
(d) PEM

150. Which drug commonly causes this condition of congenital rudimentary forearms?

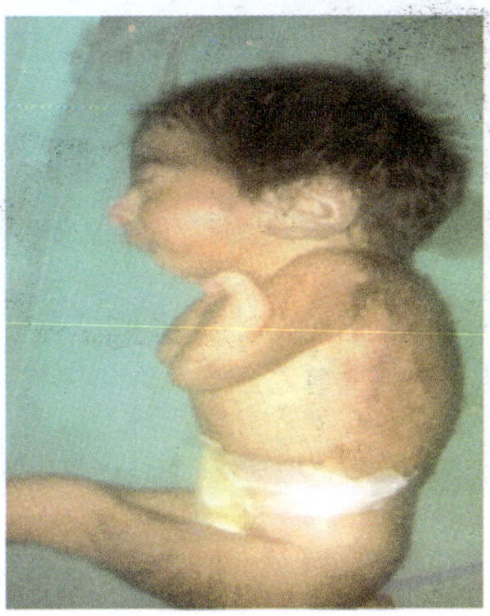

(a) Streptomycin (b) Levamisol
(c) Fluconazole (d) Thalidomide

151. Name the condition in picture:

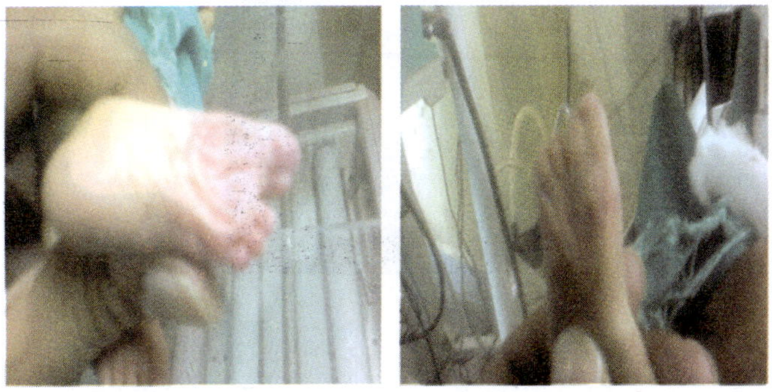

(a) Syndactyle (b) Polydactyle
(c) Flat foot (d) CTEV

152. What is this condition?

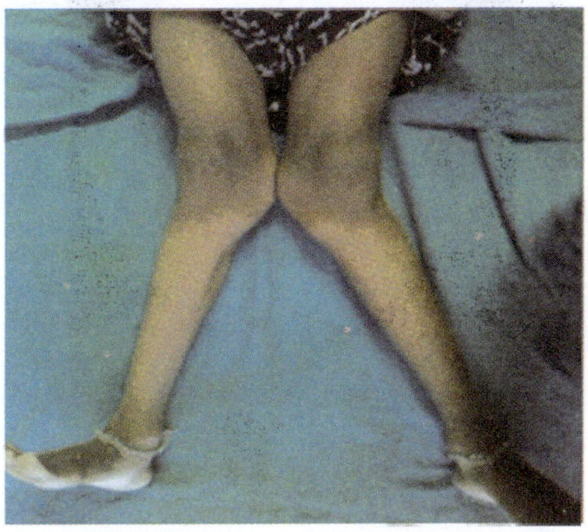

(a) Hallux valgus (b) Genu varus
(c) Genu valgum (d) CDH

153. Diagnose the condition:

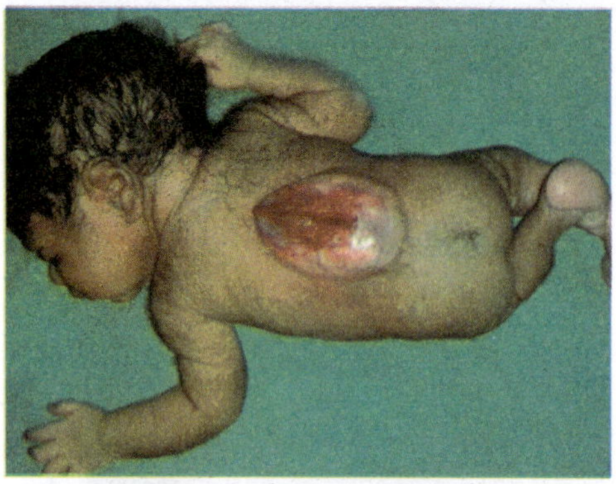

(a) Spina bifida (b) Neural tube defect

154. Lable the congenital anomoly:

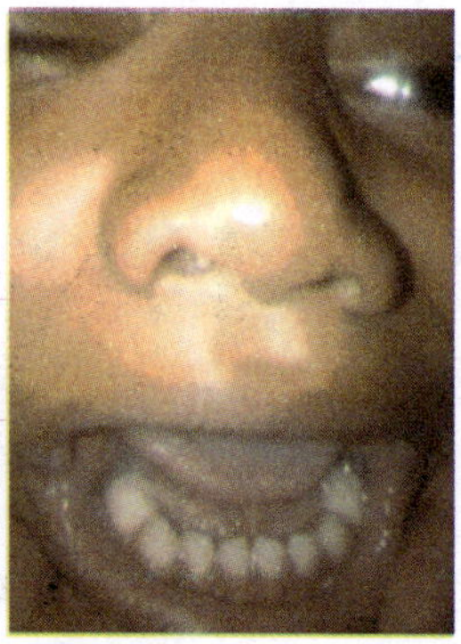

(a) DNS (b) Cleft lip
(c) Cleft palate (d) Tongue tie

155. Prof. Dr. H.C. Andrea Prader invented:

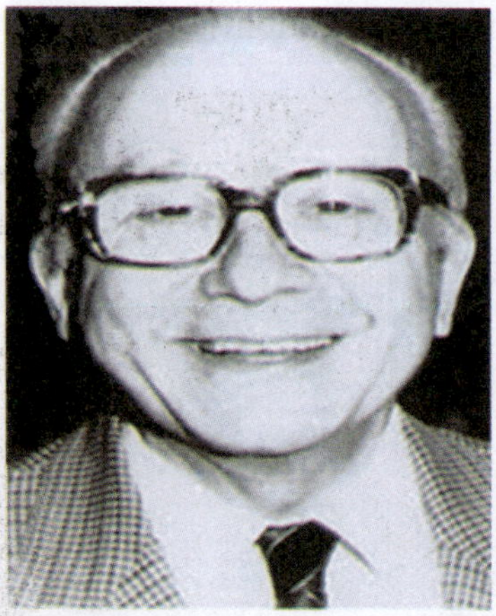

(a) Stethoscope (b) Tunning fork
(c) Orchidometer (d) Oxygen hood

156. Identify this instrument:

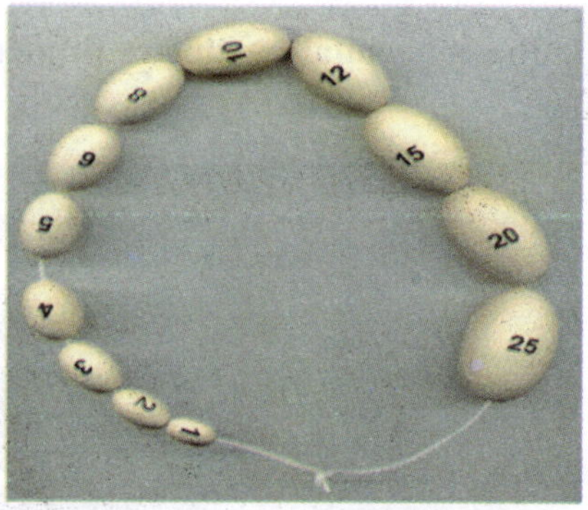

(a) Sahils tape (b) Umbilical thread
(c) Orchidometer (d) Chest physiotherapy unit

157. Identify the peripheral blood smear:

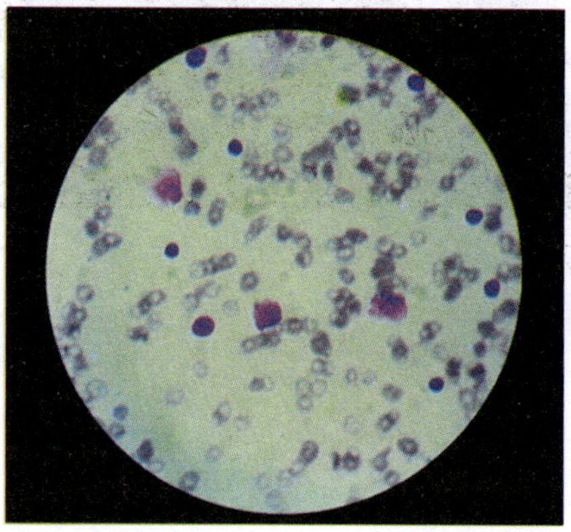

(a) CML smudge cell (b) PMN
(c) Hodgkin's cells (d) Reticulocytes

158. Identify the peripheral blood smear:

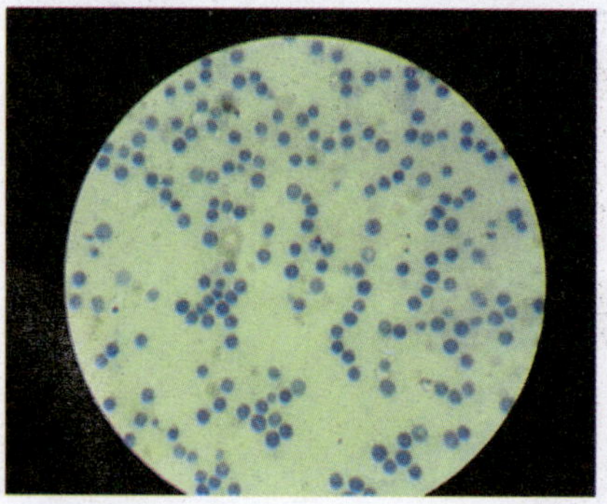

(a) CML smudge cell
(b) Reticulocytosis—hemolytic anemia
(c) Malarial parasite ring form
(d) Hodgkin's cells

159. Identify the peripheral blood smear:

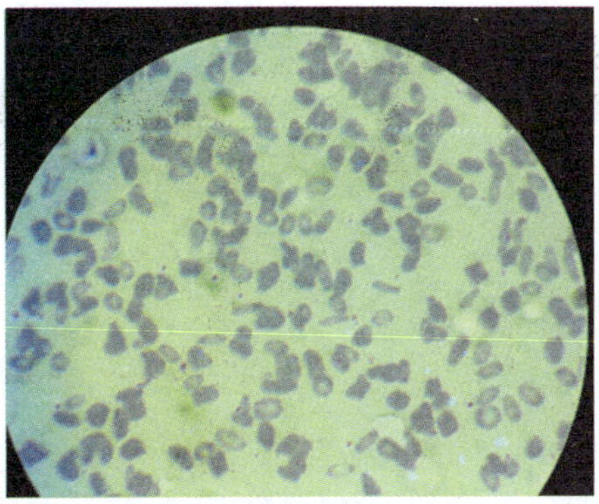

(a) Hodgkin's cells
(b) Eliptocytes
(c) Malarial parasite ring form
(d) Macrocytes

160. Identify the peripheral blood smear:

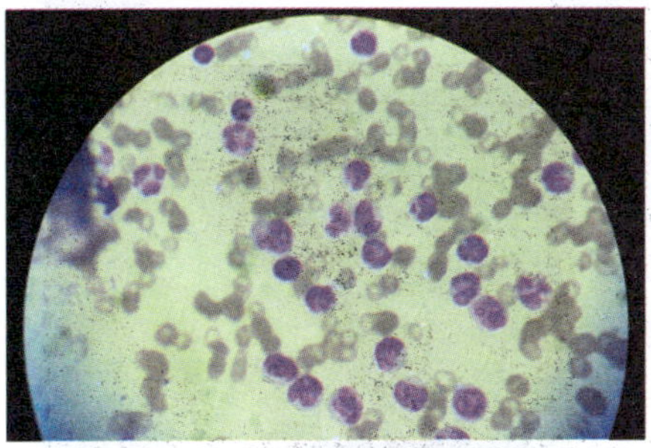

(a) Acute myeloid leukemia
(b) Macrocytes
(c) Hodgkin's cells
(d) Malarial parasite ring form

161. Identify the peripheral blood smear:

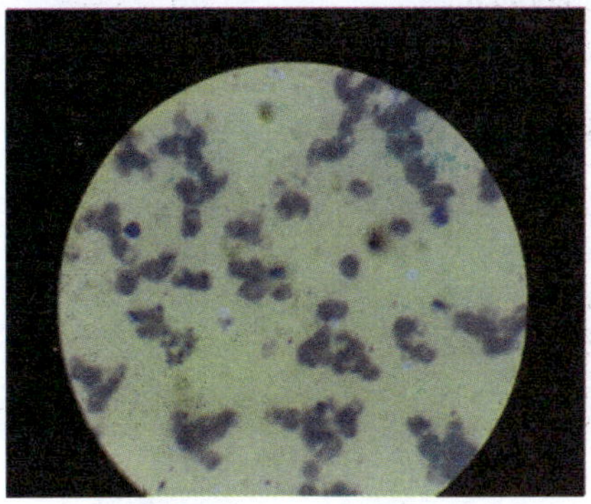

(a) Malarial parasite ring form
(b) Hodgkin's cells
(c) Macrocytes
(d) Malarial parasite ring form

162. Identify the peripheral blood smear:

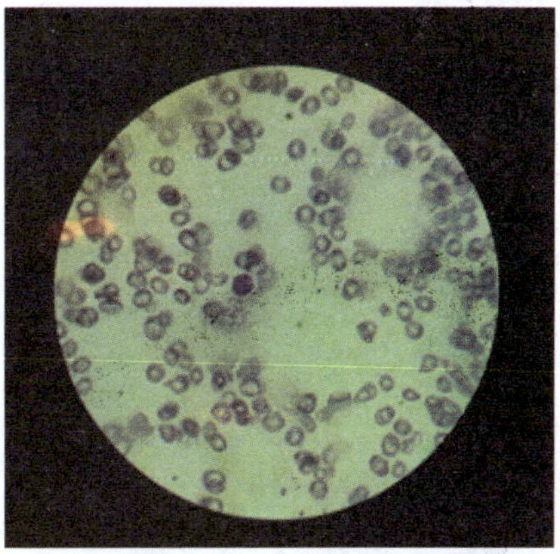

(a) Malarial parasite ring form
(b) Mast cells
(c) Sickled RBCs
(d) Hypersegmented neutrophil—megaloblastic anemia

163. Identify the peripheral blood smear:

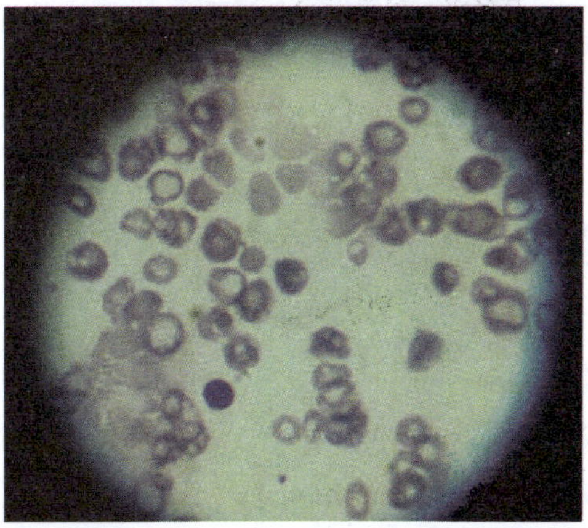

(a) RE cells
(b) Sickled RBCs
(c) Plasma cells
(d) Macrocytes–macrocytic anemia

164. Identify the peripheral blood smear:

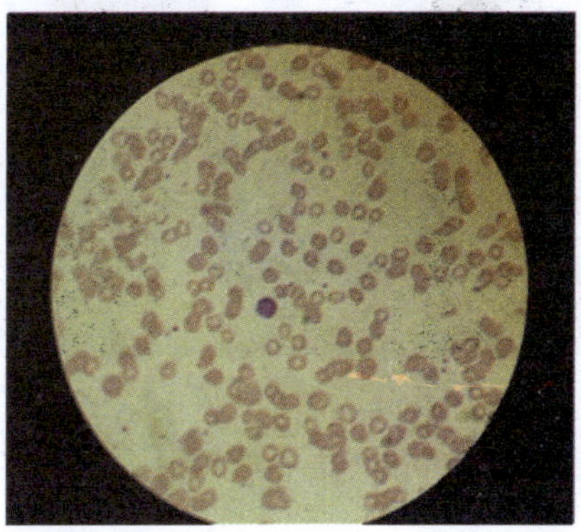

(a) Sickled RBCs
(b) Sickle cells
(c) Malarial parasite ring form
(d) Microcyte-microcytic hypochromic anemia

165. Identify this condition:

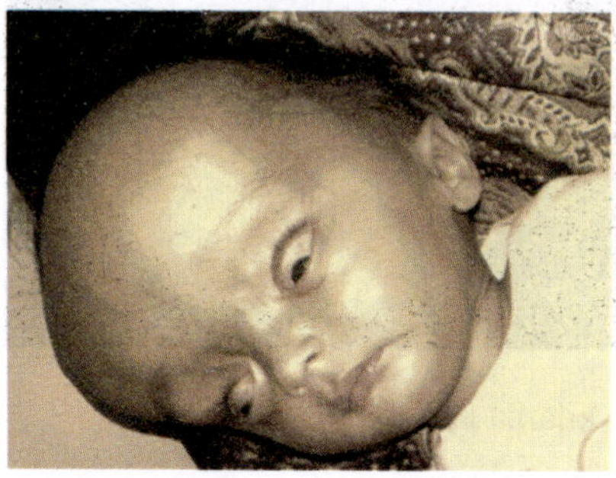

(a) Hydrocephalus (b) Meningitis
(c) Down's (d) Hypothyroidism

166. Which sign is present in the eye?

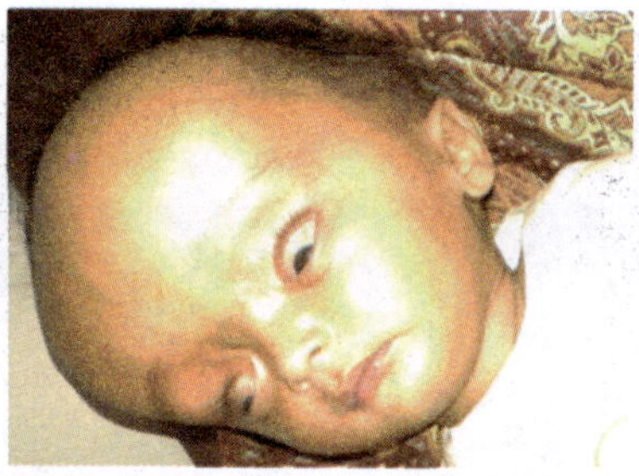

(a) Sunset sign (b) Sunrise sign
(c) Meckel's sign (d) Herald sign

167. Diagnose the condition:

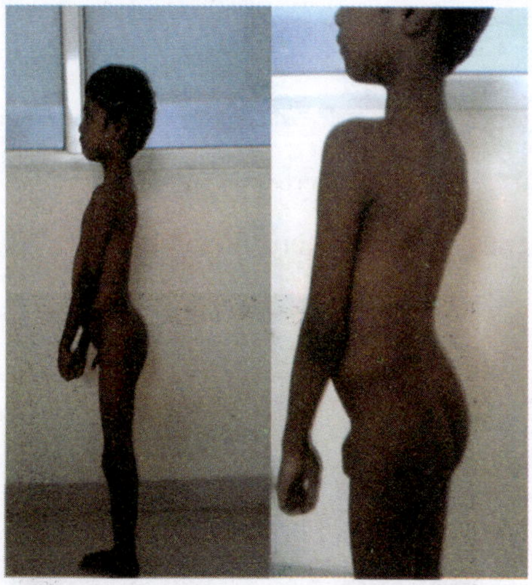

(a) Pegion chest (b) Lordosis
(c) Jenson's sign (d) Kyphoscoliosis

168. Diagnose the condition:

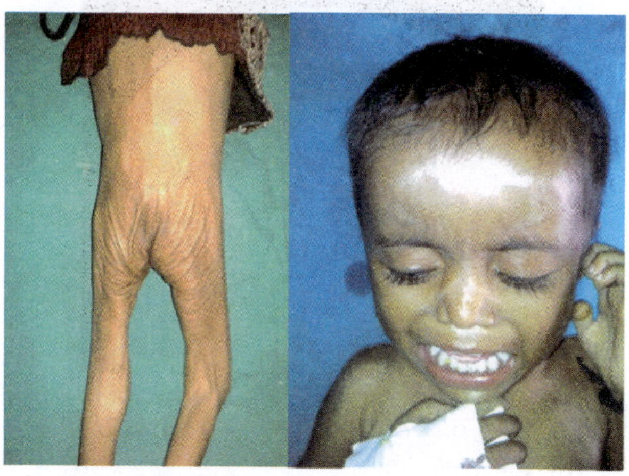

(a) Kwashiorkor (b) Marasmus
(c) Hypothyroidism (d) Dermatitis

169. Diagnose the condition:

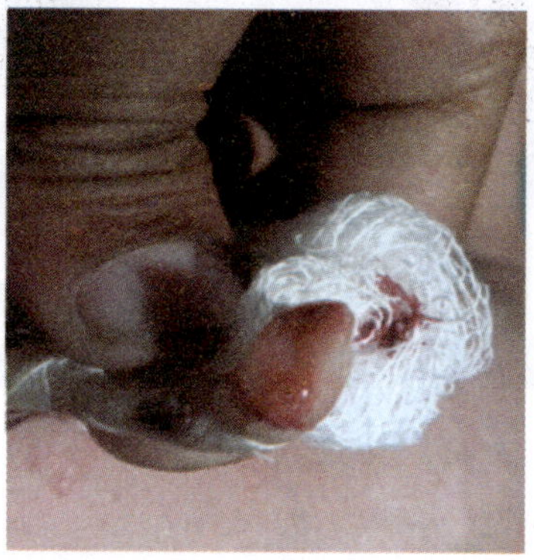

(a) Single umbilical artery
(b) Umbilical vein thrombosis
(c) Embolism
(d) None

170. Diagnose the condition:

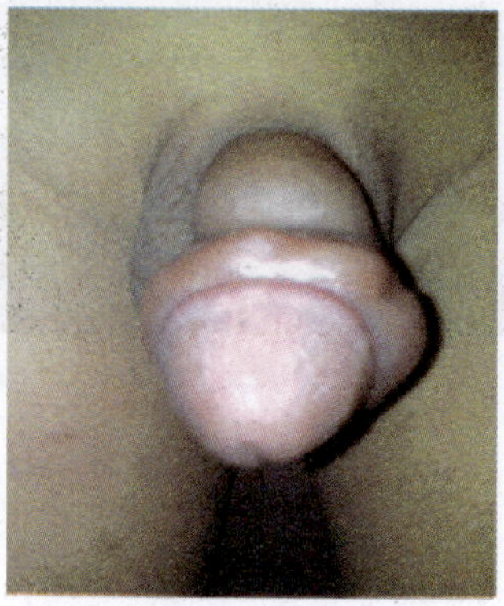

(a) Phimosis (b) Paraphimosis
(c) CA testis (d) Both (a) and (b)

171. Diagnose the condition:

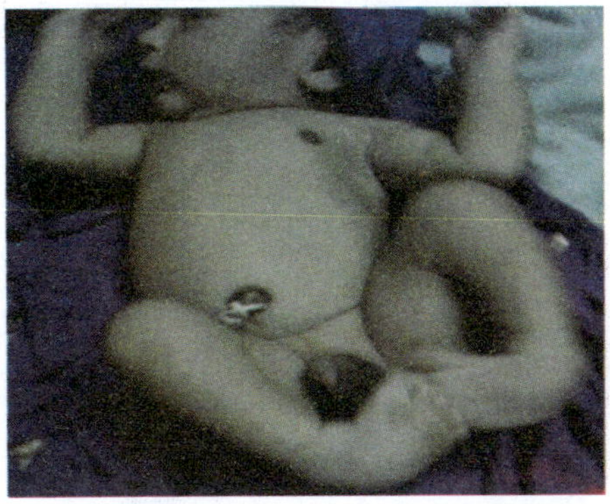

(a) Gynecomastia (b) CDH
(c) Muscular atrophy (d) Bilateral CTEV

172. Diagnose the condition:

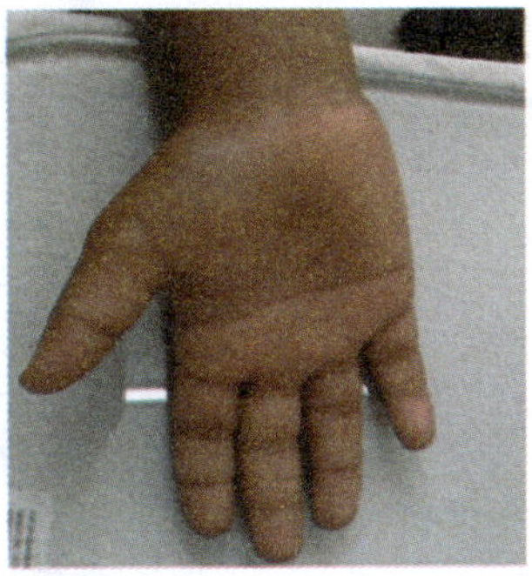

(a) Simian crease (b) Syndactyly
(c) Polydactyly (d) None

173. Facial appearance is suggestive of:

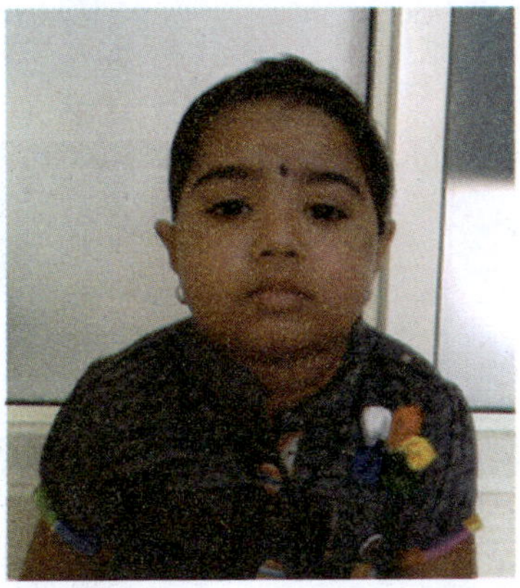

(a) Steroid therapy (b) Nephrotic syndrome
(c) Nephritic syndrome (d) Squint

174. Diagnose the condition:

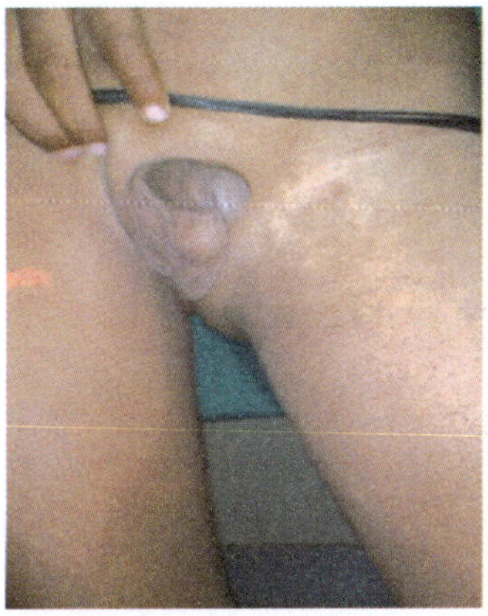

(a) Femoral hernia
(b) Phimosis
(c) Left sided undescended testis
(d) Right sided undescended testis

175. This CT scan brain is suggestive of:

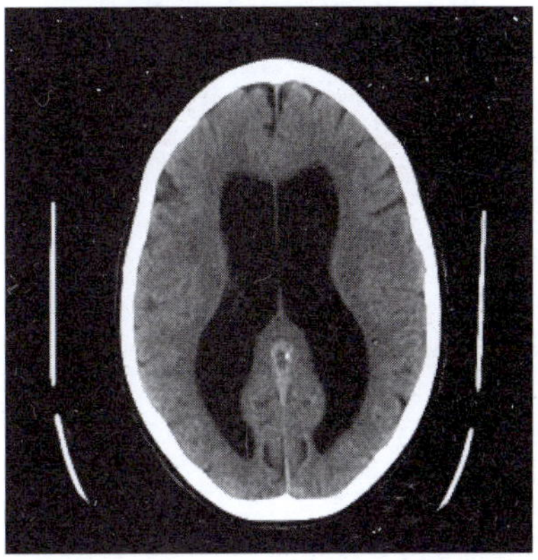

(a) Hydrocephalous (b) TBM
(c) Tuberous sclerosis (d) Normal

176. This CT scan brain is suggestive of:

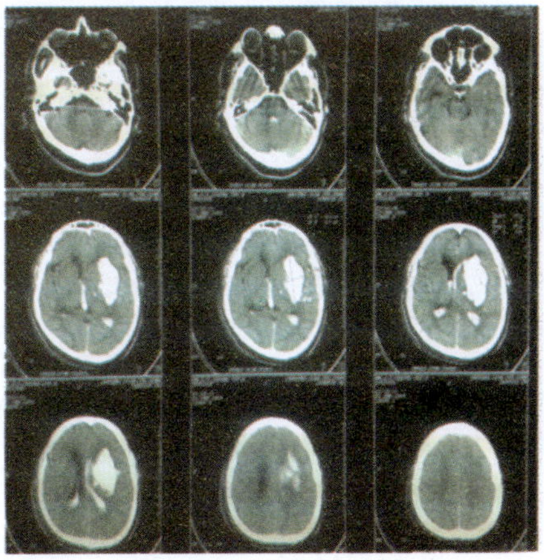

(a) Hydrocephalous (b) Maple syrup urine disease
(c) SMA (d) Normal appearance

177. This chest X-ray cardiac shadow suggestive of:

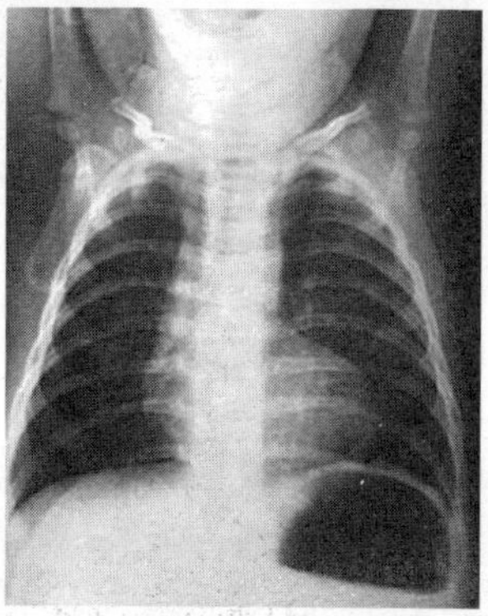

(a) TGA (b) TAPVC
(c) Fallot's tetralogy (d) MAS

178. What is X-ray diagnosis?

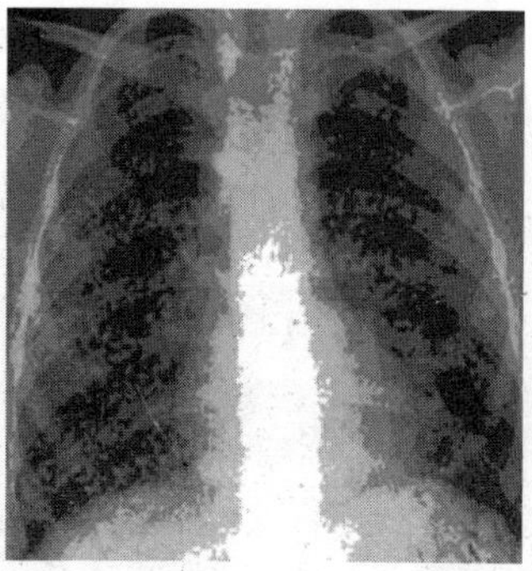

(a) Miliary tuberculosis
(b) Canon ball secondary
(c) Ground glass appearance
(d) Fallot's tetralogy

179. What is X-ray diagnosis?

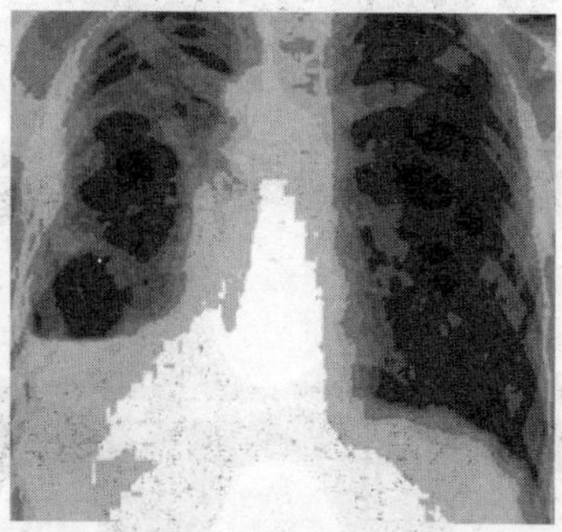

(a) Right side pyopneumothorax
(b) Left sided consolidation
(c) Right sided consolidation
(d) Bilateral ghona foci

180. What is X-ray diagnosis?

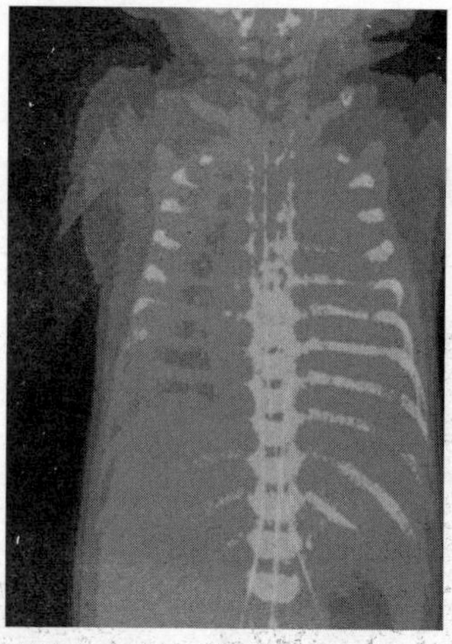

(a) Hyaline membrane disease
(b) Pleural effusion right
(c) Pleural effusion left
(d) Cavitary lesion

181. What is X-ray diagnosis?

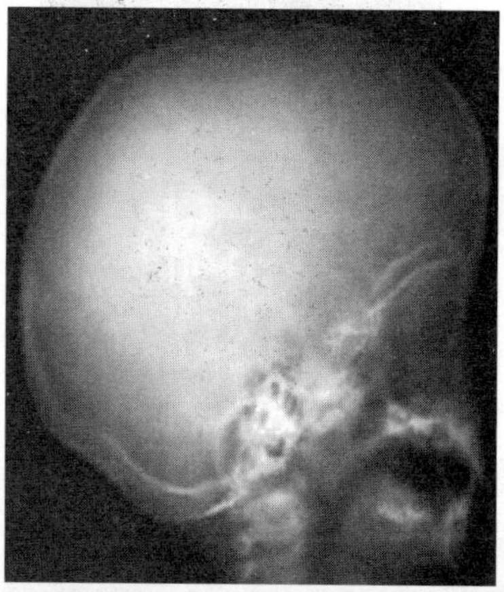

(a) Hypothyroidism (b) Thalassemia
(c) Sutural dehiscence (d) Hydrocephalous

182. What is X-ray diagnosis?

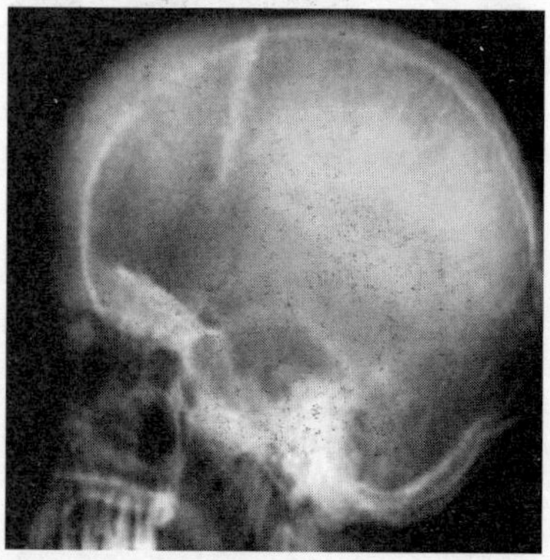

(a) Thalassemia (b) Hypothyroidism
(c) Temporal outer table # (d) Encephalitis

183. What is X-ray diagnosis?

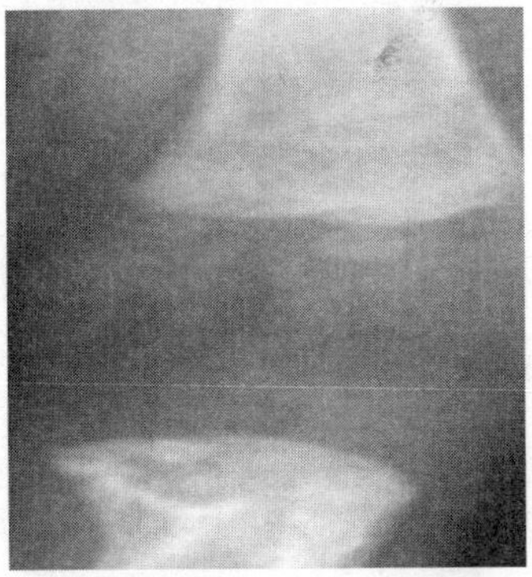

(a) Rickets (b) Thalassemia
(c) Rheumatoid arthritis (d) Congenital syphilis

184. What is X-ray diagnosis?

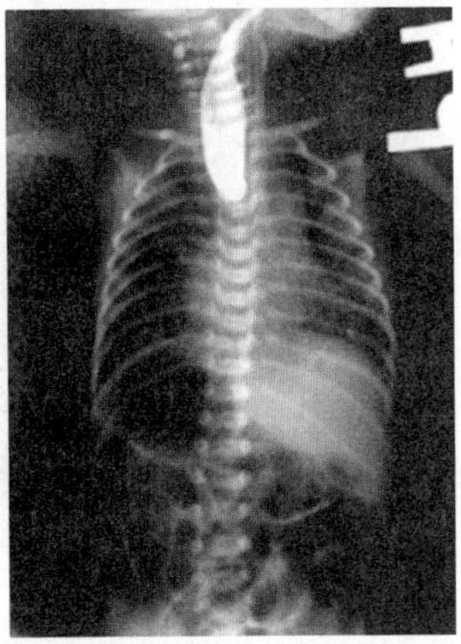

(a) TOF (b) Diaphragmatic hernia
(c) Esophageal atresia (d) CA esophagus

185. What is X-ray diagnosis?

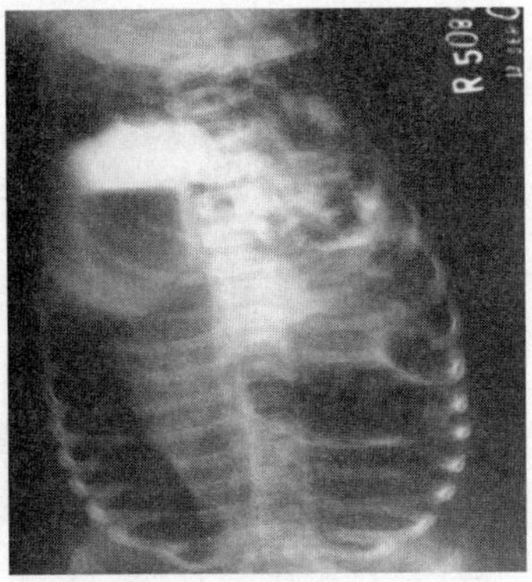

(a) Congenital diaphragmatic hernia
(b) Eventration
(c) Esophageal atresia
(d) Esophageal fistula

186. What is X-ray diagnosis?

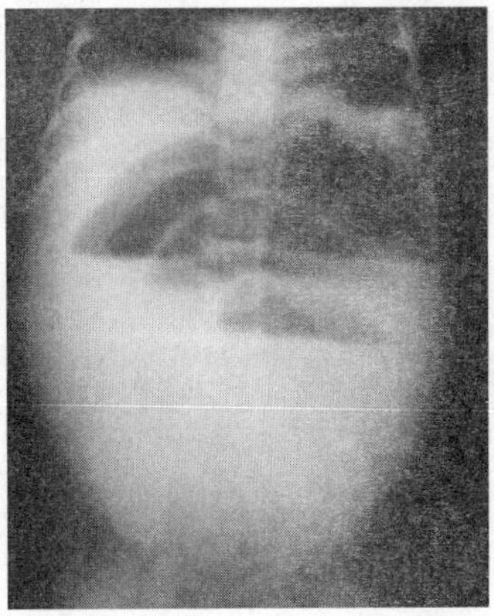

(a) Intussusception (b) Anal atresia
(c) Chron's disease
(d) Intestinal perforation with multiple air fluid levels

187. What is X-ray diagnosis?

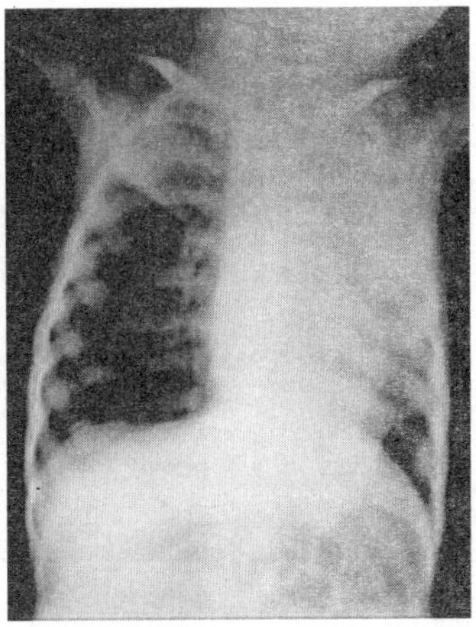

(a) Lobar pneumonia (lt) (b) Left pleural effusion
(c) Left pneumothorax (d) None

188. What is X-ray diagnosis?

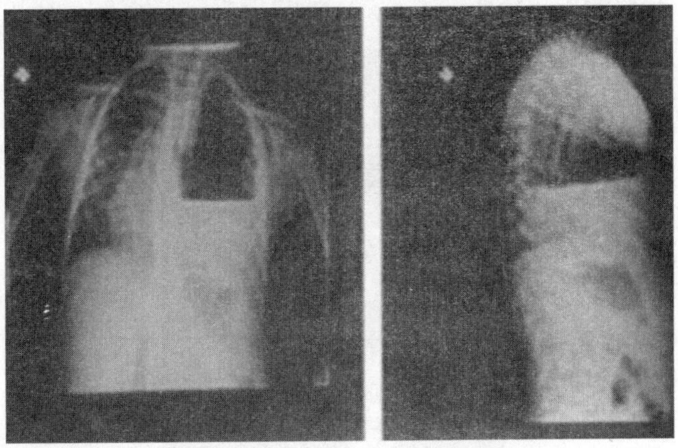

(a) Pleural effusion (b) Pneumonia
(c) TB (d) Hydropneumothorax

189. What is X-ray diagnosis?

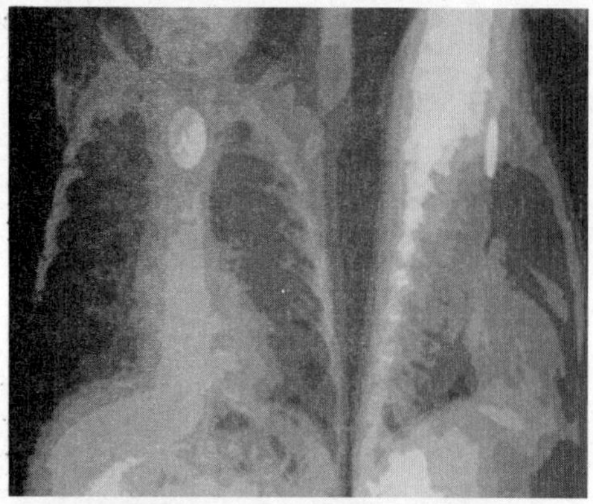

(a) Foreign body in oesophagus
(b) Foreign body in trachea
(c) Spinal calcification
(d) Ghons foci

190. What is X-ray diagnosis?

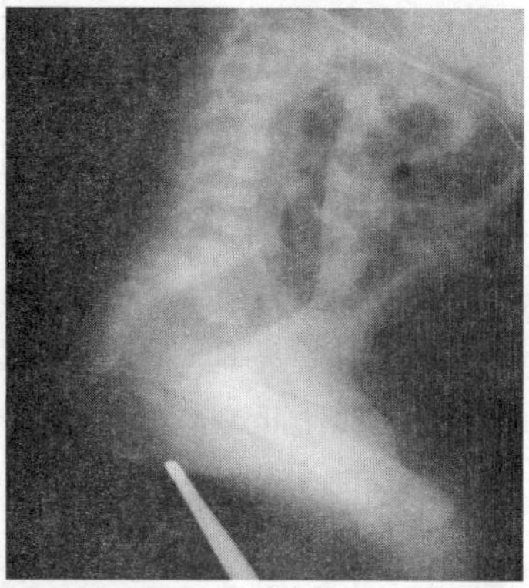

(a) Coanal atresia
(b) Imperforated anus–invertogram
(c) NEC
(d) Deuodenal atresia

191. What is X-ray diagnosis?

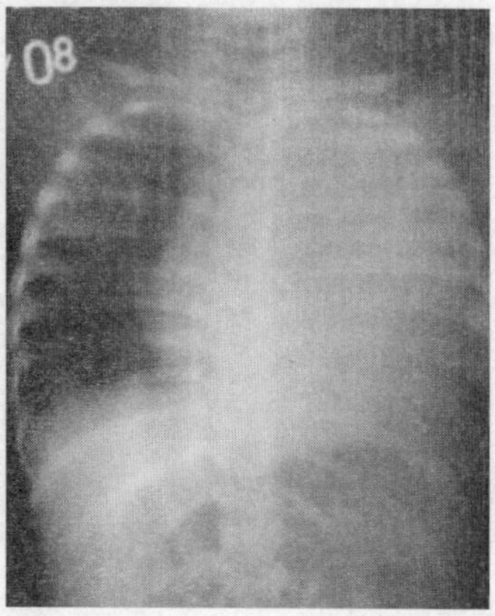

(a) Cardiac temponade
(b) Consolidation
(c) Pleural effusion
(d) Lobar pneumonia

192. What is X-ray diagnosis?

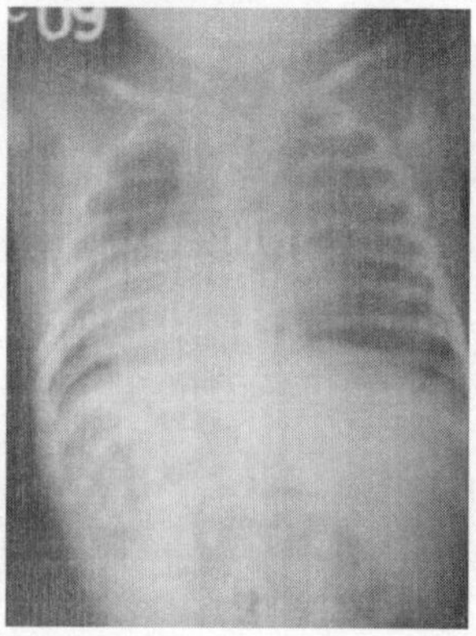

(a) Diaphragmatic hernia
(b) Fallot's tetralogy
(c) Situs inversus
(d) Both (a) and (b)

193. What is X-ray diagnosis?

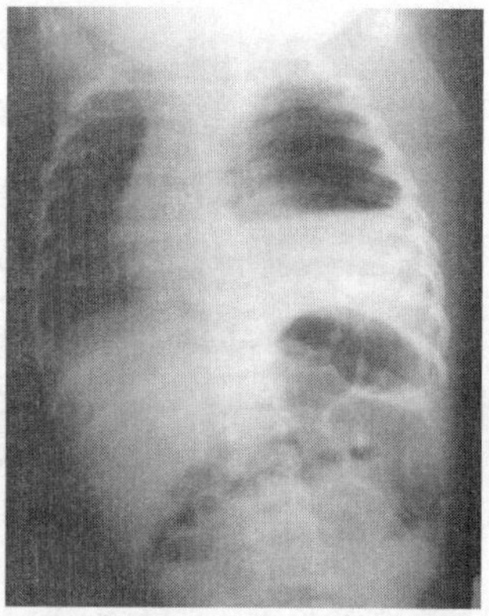

(a) Left pleural effusion
(b) Left middle consolidation
(c) TAPVC
(d) Left hydropneumothorax

194. What is X-ray diagnosis?

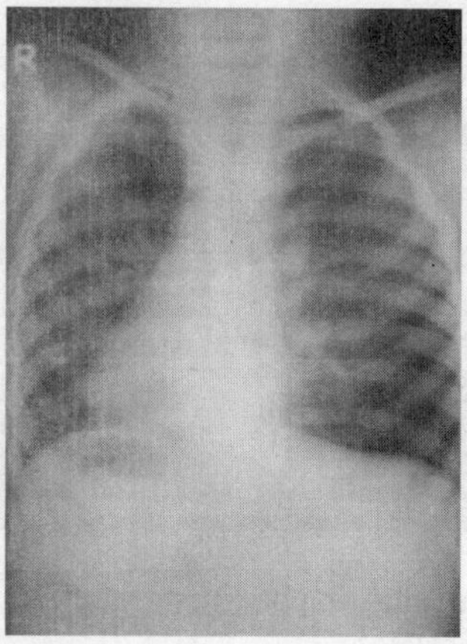

(a) Dextocardia
(b) Left effusion
(c) Right consolidation
(d) Butterfly ribs

195. What is X-ray suggestive of?

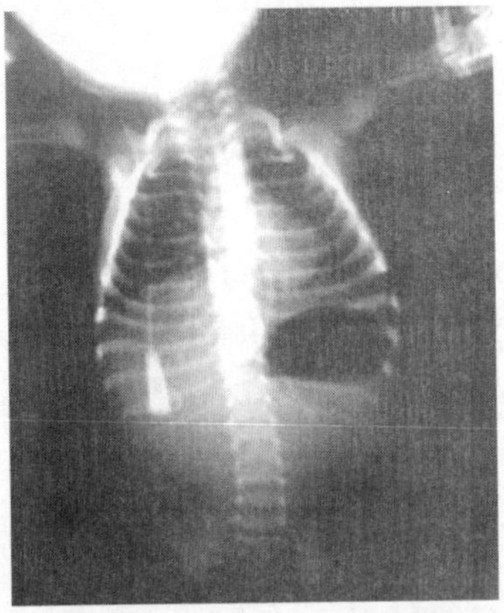

(a) Diaphragmatic hernia (b) Intussusception
(c) Dextrocardia (d) Fundaic gas shadow

196. What is X-ray diagnosis?

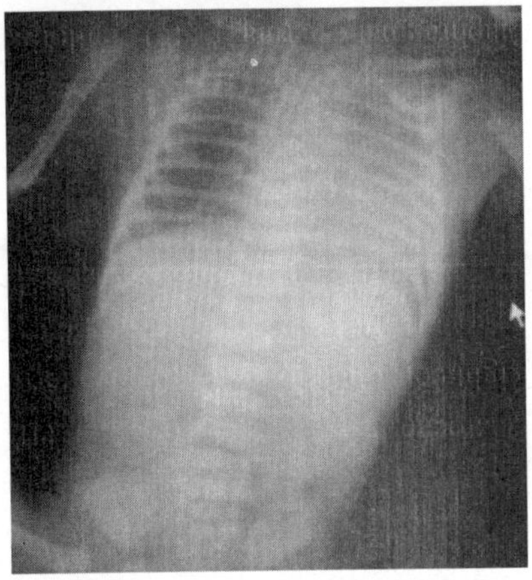

(a) Pneumothorax
(b) Pyopneumothorax
(c) Diaphragmatic hernia
(d) Congenital left sided pneumonia

197. What is X-ray diagnosis?

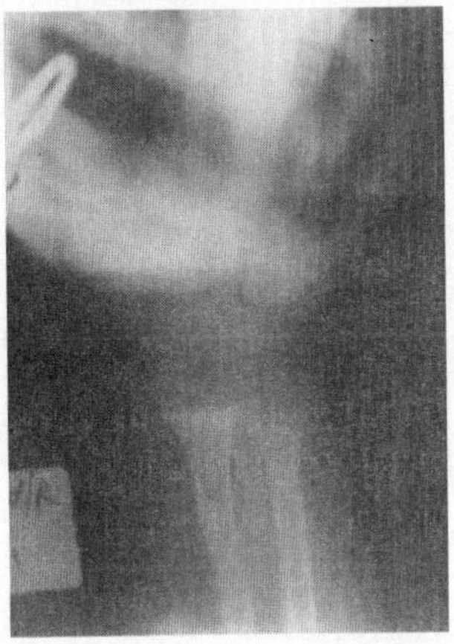

(a) Osteoporosis (b) Osteopetrosis
(c) Rickets (d) Hypothyroidism

198. What is X-ray diagnosis?

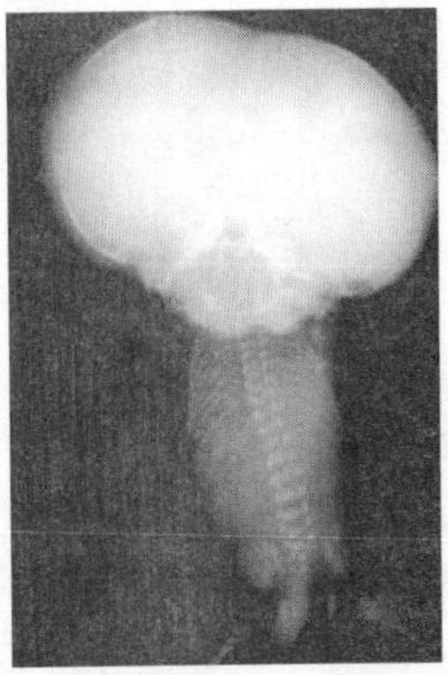

(a) Craniophagus (b) Hydrocephalus
(c) Thalassemia (d) Spina bifida

199. What is X-ray diagnosis?

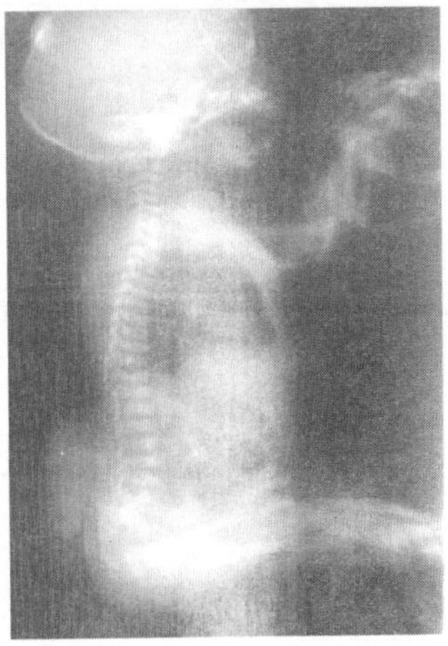

(a) Wilm's tumor (b) Spina bifida
(c) Thalassemia (d) Hydrocephalus

200. What is X-ray diagnosis?

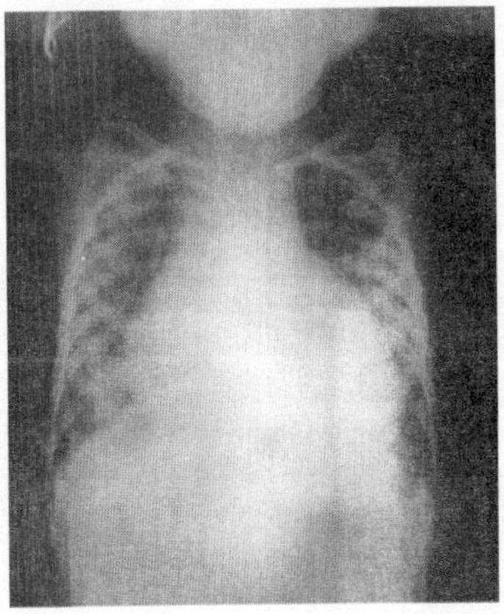

(a) Fallot's tetralogy (b) Cardiomegaly–CCF
(c) Pleural effusion (d) None

201. What is X-ray diagnosis?

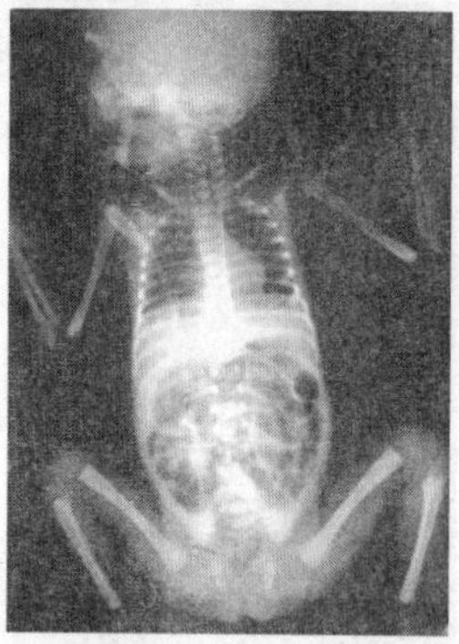

(a) Necrotizing enterocolitis
(b) Diaphragmatic hernia
(c) Rickets
(d) Hirschprung's disease

202. Contraindication for use of Diazepam:

(a) Respiratory depression
(b) Myasthenia gravis
(c) Acute narrow angle glaucoma
(d) All of the above

Answers

1. **(a)** 90°
2. **(a)** 45°
3. **(a)** 25°
4. **(a)** 10-15°
5. **(d)** All of the above
6. **(a)** L3-4 interspaces
7. **(c)** 70 – 180
8. **(d)** All of the above
9. **(b)** Paul Ehrlich
10. **(c)** Louis K. Diamond
11. **(d)** All of the above
12. **(c)** 1
13. **(a)** Diaphragmatic hernia
14. **(a)** Meconium aspiration
15. **(c)** 4.0 mm
16. **(d)** All of the above
17. **(d)** All of the above
18. **(c)** 10
19. **(b)** 100-150 mg/kg/day
20. **(b)** Neonatal hyperbilirubinemia
21. **(c)** Chloramphenicol
22. **(b)** 5 to 7.5 mg/kg/day
23. **(b)** 15 to 25 mg/kg/day
24. **(d)** All of the above
25. **(b)** 10 mg/kg/day
26. **(b)** 10 mg/kg/day
27. **(a)** Pyrazinamide
28. **(a)** Retrobulbar neuritis
29. **(a)** Myasthenia gravis
30. **(a)** Two years
31. **(c)** Albendazole
32. **(d)** All of the above
33. **(c)** Staining of teeth
34. **(a)** 15 mg/kg/dose
35. **(d)** 115 kcal
36. **(d)** All of the above
37. **(a)** Distal water
38. **(d)** All of the above
39. **(d)** All of the above
40. **(d)** Aminophylline
41. **(d)** All of the above
42. **(d)** All of the above
43. **(c)** Phenobarbitone sodium
44. **(d)** 5-8 mg/kg/day
45. **(d)** 10-15 mg/kg/day
46. **(a)** Triclofos
47. **(b)** Metoclopramide
48. **(c)** Ondansatron
49. **(a)** Cloxacillin
50. **(b)** 25,000 units/kg/day
51. **(a)** Procaine penicillin
52. **(a)** Intradermal
53. **(a)** 6
54. **(b)** Ringer lactate
55. **(a)** 5
56. **(c)** Pulmonary edema
57. **(c)** Edward Anthony Jenner
58. **(b)** 1974
59. **(a)** 1985
60. **(d)** All of the above
61. **(a)** Freezing compartment
62. **(d)** All of the above
63. **(d)** All of the above
64. **(a)** Albert Calmette
65. **(d)** TB meningitis
66. **(b)** 50%
67. **(d)** Intradermal
68. **(b)** 6-12 weeks
69. **(c)** 0.05 ml
70. **(a)** Left deltoid
71. **(d)** Albert Bruce Sabin
72. **(b)** 2 years

73. **(c)** Two drops
74. **(d)** All of the above
75. **(d)** Jonas Edward Salk
76. **(a)** 0.5 ml
77. **(a)** Aluminum hydroxide/phosphate
78. **(a)** 6 weeks
79. **(b)** 0.5 ml
80. **(d)** Progressive neurological disease
81. **(d)** All of the above
82. **(a)** Subcutaneously
83. **(b)** Staphylococcal toxic shock syndrome
84. **(d)** All of the above
85. **(c)** 0.5 ml
86. **(b)** Ty 21a
87. **(b)** 6 weeks
88. **(c)** Oka strain
89. **(a)** H M 175
90. **(d)** All of the above
91. **(a)** Oral
92. **(b)** 0.5 ml
93. **(a)** 240 ml
94. **(a)** 200 ml
95. **(d)** 5 ml
96. **(c)** 15 ml
97. **(b)** 96
98. **(c)** 96
99. **(b)** 66
100. **(b)** 596
101. **(b)** 299
102. **(d)** 43.2 grams
103. **(d)** 22.9 grams
104. **(d)** 11.6 grams
105. **(d)** 7.5 grams
106. **(a)** Laryngoscope
107. **(d)** All of the above
108. **(d)** All of the above
109. **(d)** 40%
110. **(a)** Bag valve mask
111. **(d)** All of the above
112. **(c)** Infant feeding tube
113. **(b)** Oxygen hood
114. **(d)** Metered dose inhaler
115. **(d)** Rotahaler
116. **(a)** Endotracheal tube
117. **(a)** 16
118. **(a)** 60
119. **(a)** 10
120. **(d)** Right side
121. **(a)** Right ventricle
122. **(b)** Right ventricle
123. **(c)** Right
124. **(d)** All of the above
125. **(b)** 80
126. **(d)** 30 ms
127. **(a)** Right ventricular hypertrophy
128. **(c)** 8 years
129. **(d)** Right ventricular hypertrophy
130. **(d)** All of the above
131. **(d)** All of the above
132. **(d)** All of the above
133. **(d)** All of the above
134. **(d)** All of the above
135. **(d)** All of the above
136. **(d)** All of the above
137. **(d)** All of the above
138. **(d)** All of the above
139. **(d)** All of the above
140. **(d)** All of the above
141. **(d)** All of the above
142. **(d)** All of the above
143. **(c)** Polydactyle
144. **(a)** Bilateral inguinal hernia
145. **(a)** Preauricular skin tag
146. **(c)** Cleft palate
147. **(b)** Micrognathia
148. **(b)** Cavernous hemangioma
149. **(a)** Congenital hypothyroidism
150. **(d)** Thalidomide
151. **(a)** Syndactyle
152. **(c)** Genu valgum

153. **(b)** Neural tube defect

154. **(d)** Tongue tie

155. **(c)** Orchidometer

156. **(c)** Orchidometer

157. **(a)** CML smudge cell

158. **(b)** Reticulocytosis-hemolytic anemia

159. **(b)** Eliptocytes

160. **(a)** Acute myeloid leukemia

161. **(a)** Malarial parasite ring form

162. **(d)** Hypersegmented neutrophil–megaloblastic anemia

163. **(d)** Macrocytes–macrocytic anemia

164. **(d)** Microcyte–microcytic hypochromic anemia

165. **(a)** Hydrocephalus

166. **(a)** Sunset sign

167. **(d)** Kyphoscoliosis

168. **(b)** Marasmus

169. **(a)** Single umbilical artery

170. **(b)** Paraphimosis

171. **(d)** Bilateral CTEV

172. **(a)** Simian crease

173. **(a)** Steroid therapy

174. **(d)** Right sided undescended testis

175. **(a)** Hydrocephalous

176. **(a)** Hydrocephalous

177. **(c)** Fallot's tetralogy

178. **(a)** Miliary tuberculosis

179. **(a)** Right side pyopneumothorax

180. **(a)** Hyaline membrane disease

181. **(d)** Hydrocephalous

182. **(a)** Thalassemia

183. **(d)** Congenital syphilis

184. **(c)** Esophageal atresia

185. **(a)** Congenital diaphragmatic hernia

186. **(d)** Intestinal perforation with multiple air fluid levels

187. **(a)** Lobar pneumonia (lt)

188. **(d)** Hydropneumothorax

189. **(b)** Foreign body in trachea

190. **(b)** Imperforated anus–invertogram

191. **(d)** Lobar pneumonia

192. **(c)** Situs inversus

193. **(d)** Left hydropnumothorax

194. **(a)** Dextocardia

195. **(d)** Fundaic gas shadow

196. **(d)** Congenital left sided pneumonia

197. **(c)** Rickets

198. **(a)** Craniophagus

199. **(b)** Spina bifida

200. **(b)** Cardiomegaly—CCF

201. **(a)** Necrotizing enterocolitis

202. **(d)** All of the above